HEALTH TECHNOLOGY

SOURCEBOOK

THIRD EDITION

Health Reference Series

HEALTH TECHNOLOGY
SOURCEBOOK

THIRD EDITION

Provides Consumer Health Information about Digital Health, Telehealth, Artificial Intelligence, Health Information Technology, Digital Innovations in Preventive Medicine, Screening and Detection Technologies, Diagnostic Technology, Nanotechnology, Robots in Health Care, and Rehabilitative and Assistive Devices

Along with Information about the Future of Heath Technology, Laws and Regulations Governing Health Technology, Tips for Cybersafety, a Glossary of Terms Related to Health Technology, and a List of Resources for Additional Help and Information

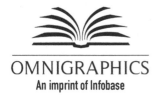

OMNIGRAPHICS
An imprint of Infobase

Bibliographic Note

Because this page cannot legibly accommodate all the copyright notices, the Bibliographic Note portion of the Preface constitutes an extension of the copyright notice.

* * *

OMNIGRAPHICS
An imprint of Infobase
132 W. 31st St.
New York, NY 10001
www.infobase.com
James Chambers, *Editorial Director*

* * *

Copyright © 2023 Infobase
ISBN 978-0-7808-2016-6
E-ISBN 978-0-7808-2017-3

Library of Congress Cataloging-in-Publication Data

Names: Chambers, James (Editor), editor.

Title: Health technology sourcebook / edited by James Chambers.

Description: Third edition. | New York, NY: Omnigraphics, an imprint of Infobase, [2023] | Series: Health reference series | Includes index. | Summary: "Provides basic consumer health information about the application of science to develop solutions to health problems or issues such as the prevention or delay of onset of diseases or the promotion and monitoring of good health. Includes index, glossary of related terms, and other resources"-- Provided by publisher.

Identifiers: LCCN 2022045210 (print) | LCCN 2022045211 (ebook) | ISBN 9780780820166 (library binding) | ISBN 9780780820173 (ebook)

Subjects: LCSH: Medical technology. | Medical care--Data processing.

Classification: LCC R855.3 .H437 2023 (print) | LCC R855.3 (ebook) | DDC 610.285--dc23/eng/20221128

LC record available at https://lccn.loc.gov/2022045210
LC ebook record available at https://lccn.loc.gov/2022045211

Electronic or mechanical reproduction, including photography, recording, or any other information storage and retrieval system for the purpose of resale is strictly prohibited without permission in writing from the publisher.

The information in this publication was compiled from the sources cited and from other sources considered reliable. While every possible effort has been made to ensure reliability, the publisher will not assume liability for damages caused by inaccuracies in the data, and makes no warranty, express or implied, on the accuracy of the information contained herein.

This book is printed on acid-free paper meeting the ANSI Z39.48 Standard. The infinity symbol that appears above indicates that the paper in this book meets that standard.

Printed in the United States

Table of Contents

Preface xiii

Part 1. Introduction to Health Technology

Chapter 1 — Understanding Medical Technology
and Digital Health 3

    Section 1.1 — Overview of Medical
Technology 5

    Section 1.2 — What Is Digital Health? 7

Chapter 2 — Artificial Intelligence in Health Care 11

    Section 2.1 — Role of Artificial
Intelligence and
Machine Learning 13

    Section 2.2 — Machine Learning in
Drug Development 19

    Section 2.3 — Artificial Intelligence
for Global Health 24

Chapter 3 — Medical Chatbots 31

Chapter 4 — Health Technology Assessment 35

Part 2. Understanding Telehealth

Chapter 5 — Telehealth 43

    Section 5.1 — Telehealth: An
Overview 45

    Section 5.2 — Benefits of Telehealth 47

    Section 5.3 — Implementation and
Future of Telehealth 51

v

Section 5.4—Medicare Benefits and
Telehealth........................ 53
Section 5.5—Health Equity in
Telehealth........................ 60
Chapter 6—Preparing for Telehealth Visits.....................................67
Chapter 7—Remote Patient Monitoring.....................................75
Chapter 8—Getting Help with Accessing Telehealth
Services...81
Chapter 9—Virtual Health-Care Services.....................................85
Section 9.1—Telehealth and
Cancer Care...................... 87
Section 9.2—Telerehabilitation for
Advanced Cancer............. 90
Section 9.3—Telehealth for Chronic
Conditions...................... 94
Section 9.4—Telehealth for
COVID-19...................... 102
Section 9.5—Telehealth for
HIV Care 106
Section 9.6—Telehealth for Maternal
Health Services.............. 111
Section 9.7—Telehealth for Children
with Special
Health-Care Needs........ 118
Section 9.8—School-Based
Telehealth Services 122
Section 9.9—Use of Telehealth in
Emergency
Departments................... 125

Part 3. Health Information Technology
Chapter 10—Understanding Health Information
Technology..133
Section 10.1—Information and
Communication
Technology 135

Section 10.2—Benefits of Health
Information
Technology 138
Chapter 11—Integrating Technology and Health Care................141
Section 11.1—Implementation and
Integration of Health
Information
Technology 143
Section 11.2—Basics of Health
Information Exchange
Technology 145
Section 11.3—E-prescription 148
Chapter 12—Digital Health Records 151
Section 12.1—Electronic Health
Records and Electronic
Medical Records............. 153
Section 12.2—Blue Button 157
Section 12.3—Medical Scribes
and Patient Safety 160

Part 4. Technology and Preventive Health Care

Chapter 13—Digital Innovations in Preventive Medicine.............169
Section 13.1—Sensors 171
Section 13.2—Body Area Networks 173
Section 13.3—Wearable Devices........... 176
Section 13.4—Wireless Medical
Devices 180
Section 13.5—Mobile Medical
Applications.................... 186
Section 13.6—Continuous Glucose
Monitoring..................... 198
Section 13.7—Wireless Patient
Monitoring..................... 206
Chapter 14—Predictive Analytics in Health Care 209
Section 14.1—Big Data and Its
Applications in
Health Care..................... 211

vii

Section 14.2—Big Data in the Age
of Genomics 214
Section 14.3—Big Data for Infectious
Disease Surveillance 217
Chapter 15—Screening and Detection Technologies 223
Section 15.1—Advanced Molecular
Detection 225
Section 15.2—GI Genius in Detection
of Colon Cancer 231
Section 15.3—OsteoDetect in Wrist
Fracture Analysis 233
Section 15.4—Prediction of Abdominal
Aneurysm Using
Machine Learning 234
Chapter 16—Genetics 237
Section 16.1—Genomics 239
Section 16.2—Genetic Testing 245
Section 16.3—DNA Microarray
Technology 249
Section 16.4—Genome Editing
and CRISPR 251
Section 16.5—Messenger RNA 258
Section 16.6—Cloning 264
Chapter 17—Neurotechnology 273
Chapter 18—Clinical Decision Support 277

Part 5. Diagnostic Technology

Chapter 19—Advances in Imaging 283
Section 19.1—Detection of Diabetic
Retinopathy 285
Section 19.2—Artificial Intelligence
in Diagnostic Imaging ... 286
Section 19.3—Neuroimaging
Technique to Predict
Autism among
High-Risk Infants 290

Section 19.4—Artificial-Intelligence-
Based Analysis of
Cardiovascular Disease
Risk 291
Section 19.5—Virtual Colonoscopy 293
Section 19.6—Liver Elastography 297
Chapter 20—Advanced Imaging in Laboratory
Technology 303
Section 20.1—Live Cell Imaging 305
Section 20.2—Nonlinear Optical
Imaging 306
Section 20.3—Surface Plasmon
Resonance Imaging 309
Chapter 21—Point-of-Care Diagnostic Testing 311

Part 6. Role of Technology in Treatment

Chapter 22—Artificial Intelligence Tools to Augment
Patient Care 319
Chapter 23—Technology and the Future of Mental Health
Treatment 327
Chapter 24—Artificial Pancreas Device System 335
Chapter 25—Technology in Cancer Treatment 341
Section 25.1—Enabling New Cancer
Technologies 343
Section 25.2—Proton Beams for
Cancer Therapy 347
Section 25.3—Nanotechnology
for Cancer 350
Section 25.4—Biomarker Testing for
Cancer Treatment 370
Chapter 26—What Is Precision Medicine? 377
Chapter 27—Human Genome Project 381
Chapter 28—Robots and Their Use in Health Care 387
Section 28.1—Image-Guided Robotic
Interventions 389

Section 28.2—Robot-Assisted
Surgery 392
Section 28.3—Fiber-Optic-Enabled
Sensitive Surgery
Tools 395
Chapter 29—Advanced Therapies...401
Section 29.1—Tissue Engineering
and Regenerative
Medicine 403
Section 29.2—NIST and the National
Biotechnology and
Biomanufacturing
Initiative 410
Section 29.3—Cartilage Engineering ... 412
Section 29.4—Light Therapy and
Brain Function 413
Section 29.5—Radiofrequency Thermal
Ablation as Tumor
Therapy........................... 416

Part 7. Rehabilitation and Assistive Technologies

Chapter 30—Rehabilitation Engineering...427
Chapter 31—Vision and Hearing Loss...433
Section 31.1—Low Vision and
Blindness
Rehabilitation 435
Section 31.2—Artificial Retina.............. 446
Section 31.3—Cochlear Implants:
Different Kinds
of Hearing....................... 449
Chapter 32—Prosthetic Engineering..459
Chapter 33—Brain–Computer Interface...465
Chapter 34—Assistive Devices 469
Section 34.1—Rehabilitative and
Assistive Technology:
An Overview 471

Section 34.2—Assistive Devices for
Communication............ 476
Section 34.3—Hearing Aids 482
Section 34.4—Mobility Aids................. 483
Section 34.5—GPS and Wayfinding
Apps for People with
Visual Impairment......... 489

Part 8. Future of Health Technology

Chapter 35—Internet of Things in Health Care.............................499
Chapter 36—Use of Blockchain Technology
in Health-Care Industry...503
Chapter 37—Nanotechnology...507
Section 37.1—What Is
Nanotechnology?........... 509
Section 37.2—Nanomedicine................ 510
Chapter 38—Stem Cells and Artificial Intelligence:
Better Together...515
Chapter 39—Deep Learning for Better Medical Images.................519
Chapter 40—Emerging Artificial Intelligence
Applications in Oncology 523
Chapter 41—Drug Delivery Systems...527
Chapter 42—Smart Operating Rooms of the Future....................533
Chapter 43—Telecritical Care...537

Part 9. Health Technology: Legal and Ethical Concerns

Chapter 44—Health Information Privacy Law and Policy............541
Chapter 45—Health Information Technology Legislation
and Regulations...543
Chapter 46—HIPAA Privacy Rule's Right of Access
and Health Information Technology.......................547
Chapter 47—Telehealth Privacy and Legal Considerations 553
Chapter 48—Security and Privacy Risks of
Wearable Devices...557
Chapter 49—Tips for Cybersecurity in Health Care 563

Part 10. Additional Help and Information

Chapter 50—Glossary of Terms Related to
Health Technology...579
Chapter 51—Directory of Agencies That Provide
Information about Health Technology.....................591

Index..**601**

Preface

ABOUT THIS BOOK

Technology has revolutionized the way health care is delivered today, from preventive medicine to rehabilitation. The digitization of health records allows health-care professionals to provide better patient care with enhanced precision. It has increased the quality of life for patients suffering from terminal illnesses. The use of technology-enabled devices helps people track their health status on a day-to-day basis and allows health-care professionals to monitor patient health efficiently. It enables patients to make informed health choices and improves overall well-being.

Health Technology Sourcebook, Third Edition provides information on digital health, telehealth, artificial intelligence and its application in health care, health information technology, innovations in preventive medicine, big data in predictive analysis, screening and detection technologies, and wireless patient monitoring services. It further discusses various treatment technologies in cancer, precision medicine, robotics, and various rehabilitation and assistive devices in health care. In addition, it provides insight into the future of health technology and its ethical and legal limitations. The book concludes with a glossary of related terms and a directory of resources for additional information.

HOW TO USE THIS BOOK

This book is divided into parts and chapters. Parts focus on broad areas of interest. Chapters are devoted to single topics within a part.

Part 1: Introduction to Health Technology gives an overview of the technologies used to drive the health-care industry and provides information on the impact of technology on health expenditures.

Part 2: Understanding Telehealth addresses the basics of telehealth, its benefits, implementation, and scope. It also provides information on remote patient monitoring (RPM) and health-care services delivered through tele-health for various medical conditions.

Part 3: Health Information Technology deals with the basics, benefits, and applications of health information technology. Facts about information and communication technologies (ICTs) and digital health records are also discussed.

Part 4: Technology and Preventive Health Care offers detailed information about various digital health innovations, such as sensors, body area networks (BANs), wearable devices, and so on. It discusses the use of big data and artificial intelligence in preventive health care. Recent advancements in medicine, such as genome editing and the development of mRNA vaccines, are also discussed. The part concludes with information on how clinical decision support (CDS) systems help improve health-care decision-making.

Part 5: Diagnostic Technology discusses advanced imaging technologies, such as virtual colonoscopy, liver elastography, surface plasmon resonance imaging, point-of-care testing, artificial-intelligence-based diagnostic imaging, and wireless patient monitoring services.

Part 6: Role of Technology in Treatment provides information on various technologies used in cancer treatment, nanotechnology, precision medicine, and the use of robots in health care. It also details regenerative medicine; advanced therapies, such as tissue and cartilage engineering; and light therapy.

Part 7: Rehabilitation and Assistive Technologies discusses various rehabilitative technologies for low vision and blindness, prosthetic engineering, and brain–computer interface (BCI). Assistive technologies for communication, vision, hearing, and mobility are also discussed.

Part 8: Future of Health Technology provides insight into the various advancements in health technology, such as the use of blockchain technology and the Internet of Things (IoT) in health care; nanotechnology; and emerging applications in the field of oncology using artificial intelligence. The part concludes with information on drug delivery systems, smart operating rooms, and TeleCritical Care.

Part 9: Health Technology: Legal and Ethical Concerns discusses the privacy and security issues in using various digital technologies and provides tips to protect your digital privacy.

Part 10: Additional Help and Information provides a glossary of terms related to health technology and a directory of agencies that provide information about health technology.

BIBLIOGRAPHIC NOTE

This volume contains documents and excerpts from publications issued by the following U.S. government agencies: ADA.gov; Agency for Healthcare Research and Quality (AHRQ); Argonne National Laboratory (ANL); Center for Limb Loss and Mobility (CLiMB); Centers for Disease Control and Prevention (CDC); Centers for Medicare & Medicaid Services (CMS); Clinical Center (CC); *Eunice Kennedy Shriver* National Institute of Child Health and Human Development (NICHD); Fogarty International Center (FIC); HealthIT.gov; International Trade Administration (ITA); MedlinePlus; National Aeronautics and Space Administration (NASA); National Cancer Institute (NCI); National Eye Institute (NEI); National Human Genome Research Institute (NHGRI); National Institute of Biomedical Imaging and Bioengineering (NIBIB); National Institute of Dental and Craniofacial Research (NIDCR); National Institute of Diabetes and Digestive and Kidney Diseases (NIDDK); National Institute of Mental Health (NIMH); National Institute of Standards and Technology (NIST); National Institute on Aging (NIA); National Institutes of Health (NIH); National Nanotechnology Initiative (NNI); National Science Foundation (NSF); Office of Disease Prevention and Health Promotion (ODPHP); Office of Technology Transfer (OTT); Substance Abuse and Mental Health Services Administration (SAMHSA); U.S. Agency for International Development (USAID); U.S. Consumer Product Safety Commission (CPSC); U.S. Department of Energy (DOE); U.S. Department of Health and Human Services (HHS); U.S. Department of Homeland Security (DHS); U.S. Department of Veterans Affairs (VA); U.S. Food and Drug Administration (FDA); U.S. Government Accountability Office (GAO); U.S. Library of Congress (LOC); and U.S. National Library of Medicine (NLM).

It also contains original material produced by Infobase and reviewed by medical consultants.

ABOUT THE *HEALTH REFERENCE SERIES*

The *Health Reference Series* is designed to provide basic medical information for patients, families, caregivers, and the general public. Each volume provides comprehensive coverage on a particular topic. This is especially important for people who may be dealing with a newly diagnosed disease or a chronic disorder in themselves or in a family member. People looking for preventive guidance, information about disease warning signs, medical statistics, and risk factors for health problems will also find answers to their questions in the *Health Reference Series*. The *Series*, however, is not intended to serve as a tool for diagnosing illness, in prescribing treatments, or as a substitute for the physician–patient relationship. All people concerned about medical symptoms or the possibility of disease are encouraged to seek professional care from an appropriate health-care provider.

A NOTE ABOUT SPELLING AND STYLE

Health Reference Series editors use *Stedman's Medical Dictionary* as an authority for questions related to the spelling of medical terms and *The Chicago Manual of Style* for questions related to grammatical structures, punctuation, and other editorial concerns. Consistent adherence is not always possible, however, because the individual volumes within the *Series* include many documents from a wide variety of different producers, and the editor's primary goal is to present material from each source as accurately as is possible. This sometimes means that information in different chapters or sections may follow other guidelines and alternate spelling authorities. For example, occasionally a copyright holder may require that eponymous terms be shown in possessive forms (Crohn's disease vs. Crohn disease) or that British spelling norms be retained (leukaemia vs. leukemia).

MEDICAL REVIEW

Infobase contracts with a team of qualified, senior medical professionals who serve as medical consultants for the *Health Reference Series*. As necessary, medical consultants review reprinted and originally written material for currency and accuracy. Citations including the phrase "Reviewed (month, year)" indicate material reviewed by this team. Medical consultation services are provided to the *Health Reference Series* editors by:

Dr. Vijayalakshmi, MBBS, DGO, MD
Dr. Senthil Selvan, MBBS, DCH, MD
Dr. K. Sivanandham, MBBS, DCH, MS (Research), PhD

HEALTH REFERENCE SERIES UPDATE POLICY

The inaugural book in the *Health Reference Series* was the first edition of *Cancer Sourcebook* published in 1989. Since then, the *Series* has been enthusiastically received by librarians and in the medical community. In order to maintain the standard of providing high-quality health information for the layperson, the editorial staff felt it was necessary to implement a policy of updating volumes when warranted.

Medical researchers have been making tremendous strides, and it is the purpose of the *Health Reference Series* to stay current with the most recent advances. Each decision to update a volume is made on an individual basis. Some of the considerations include how much new information is available and the feedback we receive from people who use the books. If there is a topic you would like to see added to the update list, or an area of medical concern you feel has not been adequately addressed, please write to: custserv@infobaselearning.com.

Part 1 | Introduction to Health Technology

Chapter 1 | Understanding Medical Technology and Digital Health

Chapter Contents

Section 1.1—Overview of Medical Technology 5
Section 1.2—What Is Digital Health? 7

Section 1.1 | **Overview of Medical Technology**

This section contains text excerpted from the following sources: Text in this section begins with excerpts from "Medical Technologies," International Trade Administration (ITA), U.S. Department of Commerce (DOC), September 24, 2020. Text under the heading "Contributions to Medical Technology" is excerpted from "Medical Imaging, Diagnostics, and Treatment," U.S. Department of Energy (DOE), May 6, 2022.

Medical technology companies research, develop, and manufacture devices used in the prevention, diagnosis, or treatment of illness or disease or for detecting, measuring, restoring, correcting, or modifying the structure or function of the body for some health purpose. Typically, this purpose is not achieved by pharmacological, immunological, or metabolic means. The industry has several distinct subsectors:

- Electro-medical or electrotherapeutic equipment, including pacemakers, hearing aids, electrocardiographs, magnetic resonance imaging (MRI), and medical ultrasound devices
- Irradiation apparatus for medical diagnostic, medical therapeutic, industrial, research, and scientific evaluation, including x-ray devices and computed tomography equipment
- Surgical and medical instruments, covering anesthesia apparatus, orthopedic instruments, blood transfusion devices, syringes, hypodermic needles, and catheters
- Surgical appliances and supplies, including artificial joints and limbs, stents, orthopedic surgical dressings, disposable surgical drapes, hydrotherapy appliances, surgical kits, rubber medical and surgical gloves, and wheelchairs
- Dental equipment and supplies consisting of equipment, instruments, and supplies used by dentists, dental hygienists, and laboratories
- In vitro (i.e., not taken internally) diagnostic systems, including chemical, biological, and radiological substances used for diagnostic tests, machines, and other test devices
- Ophthalmic goods comprising eyeglass frames, lenses, and related optical products

The U.S. exports of medical devices exceeded $45 billion in 2019. The R&D spending continues to represent a high percentage of medical device industry expenditures, averaging seven percent of revenue.

Innovative ways to treat and diagnose medical conditions, coupled with increasing patient life expectancy and aging populations globally, bode well for future medical technology sector growth. The industry also directly and indirectly supports two million jobs across the United States, and more than 80 percent of medical device manufacturers are considered small and medium-sized enterprises (SMEs).

CONTRIBUTIONS TO MEDICAL TECHNOLOGY

Exciting new medical tools and treatments offer great promise to millions of Americans who now face a variety of serious diseases or conditions. A surprising number of today's medical breakthroughs evolved from basic and applied research that was conducted at the National Laboratories of the U.S. Department of Energy (DOE) to advance national economic, energy, and security interests. Many products and therapies later became even more effective, affordable, and user-friendly through the efforts of academia and industry.

Roots in Basic and Applied Research

The DOE's National Laboratory System pursues basic research to push the limits of science and help meet future challenges. Scientists engaged in basic research often cannot anticipate how their findings will be used. Medical isotopes were an unexpected benefit of early basic DOE research.

The National Laboratories also conduct applied research, often with government, industry, and university partners, tapping into their unique facilities and expertise to solve pressing national problems. Many solutions developed by the National Laboratories have directly and indirectly improved medical technology in the following four areas:

- **Isotopes or radioisotopes** are essential to modern imaging technologies and treatments. The DOE's

Understanding Medical Technology and Digital Health

National Laboratories played a key role in their discovery and continue to support their safe production, effectively helping shape the field of nuclear medicine as we know it today.

- **Diagnostics advances** originating from the National Laboratories include mainstays, such as positron emission tomography–computed tomography (PET–CT) and MRI, as well as highly specialized instrumentation for identifying genetic conditions, health risks, and infectious diseases.
- **Treatment of disease** has improved with the development of better drugs, therapies, and management techniques. The National Laboratories have worked with industrial partners to develop options for successfully treating critical health risks, such as cancer and heart disease.
- **Precision medicine** is based on recent advancements in the understanding of human deoxyribonucleic acid (DNA) and proteins—enabling individualized patient treatment and management. This field was made possible by the completion of the Human Genome Project, which received significant support from the National Laboratories.

Section 1.2 | What Is Digital Health?

This section includes text excerpted from "What Is Digital Health?" U.S. Food and Drug Administration (FDA), September 22, 2020.

The broad scope of digital health includes categories such as mobile health (mHealth), health information technology (health IT), wearable devices, telehealth and telemedicine, and personalized medicine.

From mobile medical apps and software that support the clinical decisions doctors make every day to artificial intelligence (AI) and

Health Technology Sourcebook, Third Edition

machine learning, digital technology has been driving a revolution in health care. Digital health tools have the vast potential to improve our ability to accurately diagnose and treat disease and to enhance the delivery of health care for the individual.

Digital health technologies use computing platforms, connectivity, software, and sensors for health care and related uses. These technologies span a wide range of uses, from applications in general wellness to applications as medical devices. They include technologies intended for use as a medical product, in a medical product, as companion diagnostics, or as an adjunct to other medical products (devices, drugs, and biologics). They may also be used to develop or study medical products.

WHAT ARE THE BENEFITS OF DIGITAL HEALTH TECHNOLOGIES?

Digital tools are giving providers a more holistic view of patient health through access to data and giving patients more control over their health. Digital health offers real opportunities to improve medical outcomes and enhance efficiency.

These technologies can empower consumers to make better-informed decisions about their own health and provide new options for facilitating prevention, early diagnosis of life-threatening diseases, and management of chronic conditions outside of traditional health-care settings. Providers and other stakeholders are using digital health technologies in their efforts to:

- Reduce inefficiencies.
- Improve access.
- Reduce costs.
- Increase quality.
- Make medicine more personalized for patients.

Patients and consumers can use digital health technologies to better manage and track their health- and wellness-related activities.

The use of technologies, such as smartphones, social networks, and Internet applications, is not only changing the way we communicate but also providing innovative ways for us to monitor our health and well-being and giving us greater access to information.

Understanding Medical Technology and Digital Health

Together, these advancements are leading to a convergence of people, information, technology, and connectivity to improve health care and health outcomes.

THE U.S. FOOD AND DRUG ADMINISTRATION'S FOCUS IN DIGITAL HEALTH

Many medical devices now have the ability to connect to and communicate with other devices or systems. Devices that are already approved, authorized, or cleared by the U.S. Food and Drug Administration (FDA) are being updated to add digital features. New types of devices that already have these capabilities are being explored.

Many stakeholders are involved in digital health activities, including patients, health-care practitioners, researchers, traditional medical device industry firms, and firms new to the FDA regulatory requirements, such as mobile application developers.

The FDA's Center for Devices and Radiological Health (CDRH) is excited about these advances and the convergence of medical devices with connectivity and consumer technology. The following are topics in the digital health field on which the FDA has been working to provide clarity using practical approaches that balance benefits and risks:
- Software as a medical device (SaMD)
- Artificial intelligence and machine learning (AI/ML) in SaMD
- Cybersecurity
- Device software functions, including mobile medical applications
- Health IT
- Medical device data systems
- Medical device interoperability
- Telemedicine
- Wireless medical devices

As another important step in promoting the advancement of digital health technology, the CDRH has established the Digital Health Center of Excellence, which seeks to empower digital health stakeholders to advance health care.

Chapter 2 | **Artificial Intelligence in Health Care**

Chapter Contents
Section 2.1—Role of Artificial Intelligence and
Machine Learning 13
Section 2.2—Machine Learning in Drug Development.............. 19
Section 2.3—Artificial Intelligence for Global Health................. 24

Section 2.1 | Role of Artificial Intelligence and Machine Learning

This section contains text excerpted from the following sources: Text beginning with the heading "What Is Artificial Intelligence and Machine Learning?" is excerpted from "Artificial Intelligence and Machine Learning in Software as a Medical Device," U.S. Food and Drug Administration (FDA), September 22, 2021; Text beginning with the heading "How Is AI Being Used to Improve Medical Care and Biomedical Research?" is excerpted from "Artificial Intelligence (AI)," National Institute of Biomedical Imaging and Bioengineering (NIBIB), January 9, 2020; Text under the heading "Machine Learning in AI Innovation" is excerpted from "Artificial Intelligence in Health Care," U.S. Government Accountability Office (GAO), December 2019.

WHAT ARE ARTIFICIAL INTELLIGENCE AND MACHINE LEARNING?

Artificial intelligence (AI) has been broadly defined as the science and engineering of making intelligent machines, especially intelligent computer programs. AI can use different techniques, including models based on a statistical analysis of data, expert systems that primarily rely on if-then statements, and machine learning.

Machine learning (ML) is an AI technique that can be used to design and train software algorithms to learn from and act on data. Software developers can use ML to create an algorithm that is "locked" so that its function does not change or "adaptive" so its behavior can change over time based on new data.

Some real-world examples of AI and ML technologies include:

- An imaging system that uses algorithms to give diagnostic information for skin cancer in patients
- A smart sensor device that estimates the probability of a heart attack

HOW ARE ARTIFICIAL INTELLIGENCE AND MACHINE LEARNING TRANSFORMING MEDICAL DEVICES?

AI and ML technologies have the potential to transform health care by deriving new and important insights from the vast amount of data generated during the delivery of health care every day. Medical device manufacturers are using these technologies to innovate their products to better assist health-care providers and improve patient care. One of the greatest benefits of AI/ML in software resides in its ability to learn from real-world use and experience and its capability to improve its performance.

HOW IS THE FDA CONSIDERING REGULATION OF ARTIFICIAL INTELLIGENCE AND MACHINE LEARNING MEDICAL DEVICES?

Traditionally, the U.S. Food and Drug Administration (FDA) reviews medical devices through an appropriate premarket pathway, such as premarket clearance (510(k)), De Novo classification, or premarket approval. The FDA may also review and clear modifications to medical devices, including software as a medical device (SaMD), depending on the significance or risk posed to patients by that modification.

The FDA's traditional paradigm of medical device regulation was not designed for adaptive AI and ML technologies. Under the FDA's current approach to software modifications, the FDA anticipates that many of these AI- and ML-driven software changes to a device may need a premarket review.

On April 2, 2019, the FDA published a discussion paper, "Proposed Regulatory Framework for Modifications to Artificial Intelligence/Machine Learning (AI/ML)-Based Software as a Medical Device (SaMD): Discussion Paper and Request for Feedback" (www.fda.gov/media/122535/download) that describes the FDA's foundation for a potential approach to premarket review for AI- and ML-driven software modifications.

The ideas described in the discussion paper leverage practices from the FDA's current premarket programs and rely on IMDRF's risk categorization principles, the benefit–risk framework, risk management principles described in the software modifications guidance, and the organization-based total product lifecycle approach (also envisioned in the Digital Health Software Precertification (Pre-Cert) Program).

In the framework described in the discussion paper, the FDA envisions a "predetermined change control plan" in premarket submissions. This plan would include the types of anticipated modifications—referred to as the "Software as a Medical Device Pre-Specifications"—and the associated methodology being used to implement those changes in a controlled manner that manages risks to patients—referred to as the "Algorithm Change Protocol."

In this potential approach, the FDA would expect a commitment from manufacturers on transparency and real-world performance monitoring for AI- and ML-based SaMD, as well as

Artificial Intelligence in Health Care

periodic updates to the FDA on what changes were implemented as part of the approved prespecifications and the algorithm change protocol.

Such a regulatory framework could enable the FDA and manufacturers to evaluate and monitor a software product from its premarket development to postmarket performance. This approach could allow for the FDA's regulatory oversight to embrace the iterative improvement power of AI- and ML-based SaMD while assuring patient safety.

As part of the AI/ML Action Plan, the FDA highlights its intention to develop an update to the proposed regulatory framework presented in the AI-/ML-based SaMD discussion paper, including through the issuance of draft guidance on the predetermined change control plan.

HOW IS ARTIFICIAL INTELLIGENCE BEING USED TO IMPROVE MEDICAL CARE AND BIOMEDICAL RESEARCH?

- **Radiology.** The ability of AI to interpret imaging results may aid in detecting a minute change in an image that a clinician might accidentally miss.
- **Imaging.** One example is the use of AI to evaluate how an individual will look after facial and cleft palate surgery.
- **Telehealth.** Wearable devices allow for constant monitoring of a patient and the detection of physiological changes that may provide early warning signs of an event, such as an asthma attack.
- **Clinical care.** A large focus of AI in the health-care sector is on clinical decision support (CDS) systems, which use health observations and case knowledge to assist with treatment decisions.

HOW ARE NIBIB-FUNDED RESEARCHERS USING ARTIFICIAL INTELLIGENCE IN THEIR BIOMEDICAL RESEARCH?
Early Diagnosis of Alzheimer Disease Using Analysis of Brain Networks

Neurological degeneration related to Alzheimer disease (AD) begins long before the appearance of clinical symptoms.

Information provided by functional magnetic resonance imaging (fMRI) neuroimaging data, which can detect changes in brain tissue during the early phases of AD, holds potential for early detection and treatment. The researchers are combining the ability of fMRI to detect subtle brain changes with the ability of machine learning to analyze multiple brain changes over time. This approach aims to improve the early detection of AD, as well as other neurological disorders, including schizophrenia, autism, and multiple sclerosis (MS).

Prediction of Blood Glucose Levels Using Wearable Sensors

The researchers funded by the National Institute of Biomedical Imaging and Bioengineering (NIBIB) are building ML models to better manage blood glucose levels by using data obtained from wearable sensors. New portable sensing technologies provide continuous measurements that include heart rate, skin conductance, temperature, and body movements. The data will be used to train an AI network to help predict changes in blood glucose levels before they occur. Anticipating and preventing blood glucose control problems will enhance patient safety and reduce costly complications.

Enhanced Image Analysis for Improved Colorectal Cancer Screening

This project aims to develop an advanced image scanning system with high detection sensitivity and specificity for colon cancers. The researchers will develop deep neural networks that can analyze a wider field of the radiographic images obtained during surgery. The wider scans will include the suspected lesion areas and more surrounding tissue. The neural networks will compare patient images with images of past diagnosed cases. The system is expected to outperform current computer-aided systems in the diagnosis of colorectal lesions. Broad adoption could advance the prevention and early diagnosis of cancer.

Artificial Intelligence in Health Care

Smart Clothing to Reduce Low-Back Pain
Smart, cyber-physically assistive clothing (CPAC) is being developed in an effort to reduce the high prevalence of low-back pain. Forces on back muscles and discs that occur during daily tasks are major risk factors for back pain and injury. The researchers are gathering a public data set of more than 500 movements measured from each subject to inform an ML algorithm. The information will be used to develop assistive clothing that can detect unsafe conditions and intervene to protect low-back health. The long-term vision is to create smart clothing that can monitor lumbar loading, train safe movement patterns, directly assist wearers in reducing the incidence of low-back pain, and reduce costs related to health-care expenses and missed work.

MACHINE LEARNING IN ARTIFICIAL INTELLIGENCE INNOVATION
Machine learning systems are a central focus of the current AI innovation in drug development. AI has been conceptualized as having three waves of development:
- **Wave 1**. Expert or rules-based systems.
- **Wave 2**. Statistical learning and perceiving and prediction systems.
- **Wave 3**. Abstracting and reasoning capability, including explainability.

ML, the basis for second-wave AI technology, begins with data—generally in vast amounts—and infers rules or decision procedures that accurately predict specified outcomes on the basis of the data provided. In other words, ML systems can learn from data, known as the "training set," in order to perform a task. Increased availability of large data sets and computing power has enabled recent machine learning advances such as voice recognition by personal assistants on smartphones, an example of natural language processing, and image recognition, an example of computer vision.

Health Technology Sourcebook, Third Edition

Researchers use several methods to train machine learning algorithms, including:

- **Supervised machine learning**. The data scientist presents an algorithm with labeled data or input; the algorithm identifies logical patterns in the data and uses those patterns to predict a specified answer to a problem. For example, an algorithm trained on many labeled images of cats and dogs could then classify new, unlabeled images as containing either a cat or a dog.
- **Unsupervised machine learning**. The data scientist presents an algorithm with unlabeled data and allows the algorithm to identify structure in the inputs, for example, by clustering similar data, without a preconceived idea of what to expect. In this technique, for example, an algorithm could cluster images into groups based on similar features, such as a group of cat images and a group of dog images, without being told that the images in the training set are those of cats or dogs.
- **Semisupervised learning**. The data scientist provides an algorithm with a training set that is partially labeled. The algorithm uses the labeled data to determine the pattern and apply labels to the remaining data.
- **Reinforcement learning**. An algorithm performs actions and receives rewards or penalties in return. It learns by developing a strategy to maximize rewards.

While classical ML algorithms have been used in drug development for years, recent interest in this area stems from advances in deep learning. An artificial neural network is a ML algorithm that, inspired by the brain, contains an input layer that receives data, hidden layers that process data, and an output layer. Deep learning uses deep neural networks, which contain a large number of hidden layers. By contrast, classical artificial neural networks were technologically limited to one or two hidden layers. The types of deep neural networks that are seeing success in

Artificial Intelligence in Health Care

other applications are also finding uses in drug development. For example:

- Techniques that are widely used in computer vision can also be used to process biological images, such as images of cells from microscopes.
- Techniques often used with sequential data—for example, natural language processing of a text document—can be used to mine scientific literature or process molecular data such as the chemical code in a molecule of DNA.
- Unsupervised learning techniques can be used to generate new chemical structures with desirable therapeutic properties.

Deep learning algorithms, as well as many classical machine learning algorithms, are considered black box systems, meaning users are unable to understand why the system makes a specific decision or recommendation, why a decision may be in error, or how an error can be corrected. Researchers are actively investigating ways to increase the interpretability or explainability of these algorithms.

Section 2.2 | Machine Learning in Drug Development

This section includes text excerpted from "Benefits and Challenges of Machine Learning in Drug Development," U.S. Government Accountability Office (GAO), January 21, 2020.

Drug companies spend 10–15 years bringing a drug to market, often at a high cost. Machine learning could reduce time and cost by finding new insights in large biomedical or health-related data sets.

Machine learning is already used throughout drug development, from discovery to clinical trials. Experts say further advances could be transformative. But a lack of high-quality data hinders its use, as do research gaps, obstacles to data access and sharing, human capital challenges, and regulatory uncertainty.

Health Technology Sourcebook, Third Edition

WHAT THE U.S. GOVERNMENT ACCOUNTABILITY OFFICE FOUND

Machine learning—a field of artificial intelligence (AI) in which software learns from data to perform a task—is already used in drug development and holds the potential to transform the field, according to stakeholders, such as agency officials, industry representatives, and academic researchers. Machine learning is used throughout the drug development process and could increase its efficiency and effectiveness, decreasing the time and cost required to bring new drugs to market. These improvements could save lives and reduce suffering by getting drugs to patients in need more quickly and could allow researchers to invest more resources in areas such as rare or orphan diseases.

This set of technologies could screen more chemical compounds and zero in on promising drug candidates in less time than the current process.

Examples of machine learning in the early steps of drug development are as follows:

- **Drug discovery**. Researchers are identifying new drug targets, screening known compounds for new therapeutic applications, and designing new drug candidates, among other applications.
- **Preclinical research**. Researchers are augmenting preclinical testing and predicting toxicity before testing potential drugs in humans.
- **Clinical trials**. Researchers are beginning to improve clinical trial design, a point where many drug candidates fail. Their efforts include applying machine learning to patient selection, recruitment, and stratification.

The U.S. Government Accountability Office (GAO) identified several challenges that hinder the adoption and impact of machine learning in drug development. Gaps in research in biology, chemistry, and machine learning limit the understanding of and impact in this area. A shortage of high-quality data, which are required for machine learning to be effective, is another challenge. Accessing and sharing these data is also difficult due to costs, legal issues, and a lack of incentives for sharing. Furthermore, a low supply of

Artificial Intelligence in Health Care

skilled and interdisciplinary workers creates hiring and retention challenges for drug companies. Lastly, uncertainty about the potential regulation of machine learning used in drug development may limit investment in this field.

The GAO developed six policy options in response to these challenges. Five policy options are centered around research, data access, standardization, human capital, and regulatory certainty. The last is the status quo, whereby policymakers—federal agencies, state and local governments, academic and research institutions, and industry, among others—would not intervene with current efforts. The policy options and the relevant opportunities are discussed in Table 2.1.

Table 2.1. Policy Options to Address Challenges to the Use of Machine Learning in Drug Development

	Opportunities	**Considerations**
Research Policymakers could promote basic research to generate more and better data and improve understanding of machine learning in drug development.	• Could result in increased scientific and technological output by solving previously challenging problems. • Could result in the generation of additional high-quality, machine-readable data.	• Basic research is generally considered a long-term investment, and its potential benefits are uncertain. • Would likely require an assessment of available resources and may require the reallocation of resources from other priorities.
Data Access Policymakers could create mechanisms or incentives for increased sharing of high-quality data held by public or private actors while also ensuring the protection of patient data.	• Could shorten the length of the drug development process and reduce costs. • Could help companies identify unsuccessful drug candidates sooner, conserving resources.	• Would likely require coordination between various stakeholders and incur setup and maintenance costs. • Improper data sharing or use could have legal consequences. • Cybersecurity risks could increase, and those threats would likely take additional time and resources to mitigate. • Organizations with proprietary data could be reluctant to participate.

Health Technology Sourcebook, Third Edition

Table 2.1. Continued

	Opportunities	Considerations
Standardization Policymakers could collaborate with relevant stakeholders to establish uniform standards for data and algorithms.	• Could improve interoperability by more easily allowing researchers to combine different data sets. • Could help efforts to ensure algorithms remain explainable and transparent, as well as aid data scientists with benchmarking.	• Could be time- and labor-intensive because standards development typically requires consensus from a multitude of public and private sector stakeholders. This process can result in standards development taking anywhere from 18 months to a decade to complete and require multiple iterations.
Human Capital Policymakers could create opportunities for more public and private sector workers to develop appropriate skills.	• Could provide a larger pool of skilled workers for agencies, companies, and other research organizations, allowing them to better leverage advances in the use of machine learning in drug development. • Interdisciplinary teamwork could improve as workers with different backgrounds learn to communicate better with one another.	• Data-science-trained workers could exit the drug development field in search of higher-paying opportunities. • Would likely require an investment of time and resources. Companies and agencies will need to decide if the opportunities and challenges justify the investment or shifting of existing resources and how best to provide such training.
Regulatory Certainty Policymakers could collaborate with relevant stakeholders to develop a clear and consistent message regarding the regulation of machine learning in drug development.	• Could help increase the level of public discourse surrounding the technology and allow regulators and the public to better understand its use. • Drug companies could better leverage the technology if they have increased certainty surrounding how, if at all, regulators will review or approve the machine learning algorithms used in drug development.	• Would likely require coordination within and among agencies and other stakeholders, which can be challenging and require additional time and costs. • If new regulations are promulgated, compliance costs and review times could be increased.

Artificial Intelligence in Health Care

Table 2.1. Continued

	Opportunities	Considerations
Status Quo Policymakers could maintain the status quo (i.e., allow current efforts to proceed without intervention).	• Challenges may be resolved through current efforts. • Companies are already using machine learning and may not need action from policymakers to continue expanding its use.	• The challenges described in this report may remain unresolved or be exacerbated.

WHY DID THE U.S. GOVERNMENT ACCOUNTABILITY OFFICE DO THIS STUDY?

Developing and bringing a new drug to market is lengthy and expensive. Drug developers study the benefits and risks of new compounds before seeking the approval of the U.S. Food and Drug Administration (FDA). Only about one out of 10,000 chemical compounds initially tested for drug potential makes it through the research and development pipeline and is then determined by the FDA to be safe and effective and approved for marketing in the United States. Machine learning is enabling new insights in the field.

The GAO was asked to conduct a technology assessment on the use of AI technologies in drug development with an emphasis on foresight and policy implications. The assessment report discusses (1) current and emerging AI technologies available for drug development and their potential benefits, (2) challenges to the development and adoption of these technologies, and (3) policy options to address challenges to the use of machine learning in drug development.

The GAO assessed AI technologies used in the first three steps of the drug development process: drug discovery, preclinical research, and clinical trials; interviewed a range of stakeholder groups, including government, industry, academia, and nongovernmental organizations; convened a meeting of experts in conjunction with the National Academies; and reviewed key reports and scientific literature.

Health Technology Sourcebook, Third Edition

Section 2.3 | Artificial Intelligence for Global Health

This section includes text excerpted from "Artificial Intelligence in Global Health," U.S. Agency for International Development (USAID), August 10, 2022.

Artificial intelligence (AI) has begun to create change in health care across developed markets and has the potential to drive game-changing improvements for underserved communities in global health. From enabling community-health workers to better serve patients in remote areas to helping governments in low- and middle-income countries (LMICs) prevent deadly disease outbreaks before they occur, there is growing recognition of the tremendous potential of AI tools to break fundamental trade-offs in health access, quality, and cost. Health systems in LMICs face obstacles, including daunting shortages of workers, medical equipment, and other resources that require strategic and innovative approaches to overcome. AI tools have the exciting potential not only to optimize existing resources and help overcome these workforce resource shortages but also to greatly improve health-care delivery and outcomes in low-income settings in ways never previously imagined.

ARTIFICIAL INTELLIGENCE USE CASES WITH HIGH POTENTIAL FOR IMPACT ON GLOBAL HEALTH
Groupings of Artificial Intelligence Use Cases and Opportunity Areas

The researchers of the United States Agency for International Development (USAID) began with a broad scan of instances where AI is being used, tested, or considered in health care, resulting in a catalog of over 240 examples. As they looked across these examples, they determined that they were stratified across four broad functional areas depending on the role they play in the health-care value chain. These functions include population health, individual care (including care routing and care services), health systems, and pharma and MedTech, as shown in Figure 2.1.

Artificial Intelligence in Health Care

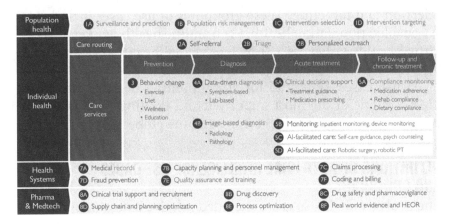

Figure 2.1. Framework of All AI Use Cases in Health Care

The researchers of the USAID then distilled this broad catalog of examples down to a framework of 27 use cases for AI in global health, with use cases aligned to the four functional areas described above. Then they conducted a rapid assessment of impact and feasibility to prioritize a subset of these use cases. Within impact, they considered the extent to which each use case might increase healthcare access, quality, and efficiency. For feasibility, they considered the current activity and maturity of the technology, the extent to which it is already being tested in an LMIC context, and the eventual suitability for LMICs. These relative rankings allowed them to look across the long list of use cases and deprioritize those which were likely to have lower impact and feasibility. For example, use cases around billing improvements were deprioritized as they are less likely to improve patient outcomes and are less well suited to low-income contexts.

Through this prioritization exercise, they found that the remaining use cases fall somewhat naturally into groupings of use cases. These groupings are largely defined by the primary user and include use cases that are often combined to create maximum impact. For example, population health use cases around surveillance and prediction unlock even more potential when linked to intervention

Health Technology Sourcebook, Third Edition

selection and targeting. These groupings of use cases include (1) AI-enabled population health, (2) frontline health worker (FHW) virtual health assistants, (3) patient virtual health assistants, and (4) physician clinical decision support.

AI use cases' potential for strengthening health systems in LMICs is one of the most important and exciting ways in which AI could transform health care around the globe.

DEFINITIONS OF ARTIFICIAL INTELLIGENCE USE CASES AND GROUPINGS

The analysis of AI use cases included relative assessments of the potential impact and feasibility for scale in LMICs—including the relative level of maturity of technologies and current level of penetration in LMICs for each AI case. The relative impact assessment considered the extent to which each use case might increase healthcare access, quality, and efficiency. The feasibility study helped the researchers to better understand which use cases have already been executed in both high- and low-income contexts, which may already be common in developing world contexts but have yet to be tailored to low-resource settings, and which are still nascent and in need of further development in order to scale.

The analysis yielded the following insights across the four groupings of AI use cases:

- **The AI-enabled precision public health use cases** were identified as technologies that are relatively nascent and less widely used (in both high- and low-income contexts) than many other AI technologies— but that are well suited for global health and LMIC contexts in the future.
- **The patient and frontline health worker** (FHW) **groupings** of AI use cases were identified as relatively more advanced technologies that are increasingly common in developed markets but that need to be tailored and scaled in LMICs.
- **Clinical decision support (CDS) AI tools** are relatively mature technologies that have greater levels of penetration in high-income markets than other AI

26

Artificial Intelligence in Health Care

technologies in question but that need greater scaling and adaptation in LMIC contexts. In addition, some of these CDS use cases are relatively less suitable for low-resource settings at present due to broader resource gaps in these markets (i.e., image diagnostics tools that rely on expensive radiology equipment that is rare in LMICs).

Artificial-Intelligence-Enabled Population Health

TOOLS FOR INGESTING, ANALYZING, AND PROVIDING RECOMMENDATIONS ON POPULATION HEALTH DATA

This grouping involves tools that leverage AI to monitor and assess population health and select and target public health interventions based on AI-enabled predictive analytics. It includes AI-driven data processing methods that map the spread and burden of disease, while AI predictive analytics are then used to project future disease spread of existing and possible outbreaks. It also includes risk management tools that use AI to better understand risk across different groups of a given population and stratify these groups according to risk levels. One example of the potential of tools in this opportunity area is Artificial Intelligence in Medical Epidemiology (AIME), an AI-enabled platform that helps a country's Ministry of Health predict future outbreaks of diseases, such as Zika and dengue in a specific geography months before their possible occurrence, and helps the Ministry of Health select the most appropriate vector control method to prevent the outbreak. While AIME is a very early-stage venture and its technologies and tools have not been validated at scale, its work reflects the potential of AI predictive analytics tools in global health.

These AI-enabled population health tools can provide value to populations, governments, and health systems across LMIC contexts. These tools help governments better understand health burdens and potential disease outbreaks across their geographies and thus enable them to allocate their resources more effectively to prevent and manage outbreaks. These AI-enabled tools can also help diverse stakeholders (beyond a country's Ministry of Health) determine which communities are most in need of care and public health interventions and optimize their resources accordingly.

27

Frontline Health Worker Virtual Health Assistant
TOOLS AUGMENTING FHW EXPERTISE TO DIRECT PATIENT CARE, SUCH AS TRIAGE AND SYMPTOM-BASED DIAGNOSTICS AND CARE RECOMMENDATIONS

This grouping of use cases involves placing AI in the hands of frontline health workers (FHWs), enabling them to better serve—and bring top-notch medical technology and advice to—their patients. FHWs in LMICs use AI-enabled tools to triage and diagnose patients (often outside of health facilities), assist with clinical decision support, and monitor the compliance of their patients. Rapid and accurate triage and diagnosis functions are enabled when AI is applied to real-time patient data collected by FHWs. FHWs are then able to provide targeted health recommendations for patients on whether, where, and how to seek care.

Overall, the AI uses cases in this opportunity area to provide value by strengthening FHWs' abilities to serve their patients by providing health information and advice (and eventually even possibly diagnoses) without them having to visit a facility. This, in turn, reduces the patient burden on already overburdened facilities and enables FHWs to focus on their most at-risk patients, helping them optimize their time and effort.

This grouping of tools illustrates how AI technologies can overcome prior constraints of access, cost, and quality. Patients without easy access to health facilities and with little ability to pay may be able to better access quality health advice and avoid unnecessary trips to health facilities.

Patient Virtual Health Assistant
TOOLS HELPING PATIENTS DIRECT THEIR OWN CARE AND WELLNESS, INCLUDING DATA-DRIVEN DIAGNOSTICS AND RECOMMENDATIONS

The use cases in this opportunity area put AI in patients' hands for self-referral, behavioral change, data-driven self-diagnosis, personalized outreach, medical record collection, and AI-facilitated self-care functions. Through the collection of real-time data at the

Artificial Intelligence in Health Care

patient level, these AI-enabled tools can help identify the type and severity of a patient's condition and provide health recommendations directly to the patient. Recommendations may include how and where to seek care if it is needed or guidelines for self-care and behavioral changes to address health issues outside of the health system. It is important to note that these AI tools are not intended to replace humans in the provision of diagnosis and care. Rather, these tools can provide helpful recommendations on if, how, and where someone should seek formal care from a health-care professional—and what they can do in the meantime to best manage the situation. This can be critical for patients who may have to wait days to see a doctor or reach quality care.

These AI use cases provide tremendous value to patients by enabling them to access medical information, behavioral and lifestyle recommendations, care routing advice, and even potential diagnoses without having to go to a health facility, which can be time-consuming and expensive in LMIC health systems. They can also provide value and efficiency gains to the broader health system by ensuring that only patients who truly need to go to health facilities do so, freeing up health providers' time for acute patients, and by remotely collecting ongoing patient data, which can be linked to a patient's broader medical record.

An example of a patient-facing AI tool reshaping health care in LMIC contexts is Babyl, a subsidiary of Babylon, operating in certain LMIC geographies, such as Rwanda. Developed in the U.K., Babylon provides an integrated AI platform for patients, including an AI triage symptom checker, health assessment, and virtual consultations with a physician when a referral is needed. In Rwanda, Babyl aims to build toward the AI-powered services available in the U.K. but has started with virtual consultations, prescriptions, and lab tests through mobile phones, including special phone options to reach underserved populations. The Babyl experience in Rwanda also provides broader value to the global health field by studying how AI-enabled technologies can be ported from developed country markets to LMIC markets.

Physician Clinical Decision Support
A TOOL PROVIDING SPECIALIZED EXPERTISE TO PHYSICIANS, FOR EXAMPLE, BY ENABLING A GENERAL PRACTITIONER TO READ DIAGNOSTIC IMAGES

This grouping includes AI use cases that support and improve the decisions of clinical physicians. Examples of AI tools in this grouping are image-based diagnosis support for radiologists and pathologists, decision support tools for clinicians, and quality assurance and training to provide insights for clinicians on past performance and indicate where errors may have been made.

Just as with the patient virtual health assistant use case, it is important to note that AI tools in this use case are not intended to replace the physician. Overall, the AI use cases in this clinical decision support (CDS) grouping provide value by augmenting physicians' roles and their capacity to serve their patients, helping them provide faster and more accurate diagnoses to patients, and widening a significant bottleneck in the provision of care in LMIC contexts, enabling them to focus on their patients most in need of care. Given the often extreme scarcity of health-care providers in LMIC contexts and how overburdened providers in these contexts are, this function of helping doctors optimize their time and focus on those most at risk can save patients' lives and provide catalytic impact across health systems.

AI tools like this "give superpowers" to health-care providers and can greatly improve the quality of care they provide to their patients.

Chapter 3 | Medical Chatbots

WHAT ARE MEDICAL CHATBOTS?

Medical chatbots are interactive communicative platforms that use conversational artificial intelligence (AI), algorithms, and natural language processing (NLP) to produce human-like responses to users' queries. Medical or health-care chatbots function as the communicative medium between patients and health-care providers. They are often the first point of contact for incoming patients and are designed to ask patients basic questions about their medical histories, such as details about previous occurrences, symptoms, and chronic conditions. Based on the answers provided and the set of solutions programmed into the system, the AI-powered chatbot will provide remedies on the same interactive platform, automatically schedule an appointment with a health-care provider, or give details on emergency care services in critical cases.

TYPES OF MEDICAL CHATBOTS

The kind of services a health-care provider wants to offer determines the degree of communication required with patients and the style of conversation. Health-care chatbots are usually categorized into three types:

- **Informative chatbots** provide customer support and helpful information to patients, such as regular notifications and pop-up alerts on the user's screen. They allow businesses to interact with customers

"Medical Chatbots," © 2023 Infobase. Reviewed November 2022.

Health Technology Sourcebook, Third Edition

without the use of human representatives. They are programmed to perform automated tasks, such as answering questions by delivering a selection from a preprogrammed set of answers.

- **Prescriptive chatbots** are based on NLP. These chatbots have a self-learning software wireframe that alters their conditional algorithms after deriving information from the latest learning experience. These chatbots can access a patient's medical history and provide more sophisticated health-care information.
- **Conversational chatbots** simulate human conversations based on text and voice responses provided by the user. This type of chatbot is programmed to respond to the user's specific intention or query. Conversational chatbots utilize concepts of NLP, contextual awareness, episodic memory, and natural language understanding (NLU) to recall previous conversations and use them to tailor responses.

BENEFITS OF MEDICAL CHATBOTS

Medical chatbots have revolutionized the health-care industry. Using a medical chatbot as the first point of contact for patients significantly reduces waiting time and overcrowding in health-care spaces. Chatbots help reduce overhead costs and hiring costs by taking on work otherwise done by humans. Medical chatbots enable patients to get answers immediately for minor concerns and keep them connected to the health-care provider around the clock. Waiting time for critical problems is also significantly reduced. Some chatbots can instantly access a patient's medical information and refer to their medical history to make an accurate recommendation.

In contrast, other chatbots can give doctors access to a patient's medical records in emergencies where the patient cannot describe their condition or circumstances. Chatbots are designed to provide anonymity and maximum security against the theft of medical records and other personal details of patients. Given the AI-powered efficiency of chatbots, they can handle many patient

Medical Chatbots

cases simultaneously without compromising case integrity and accuracy. Chatbots can efficiently send reminders to patients, suggest treatments, or provide resources to monitor their health.

MEDICAL CHATBOTS IN THE FIGHT AGAINST COVID-19

Health-care chatbots were of immense use during the global COVID-19 pandemic. Chatbots helped keep patients at home and clear of health-care spaces to reduce the spread of the virus. During the pandemic, as hospitals filled up with symptomatic and asymptomatic patients, chatbots became a valuable tool for segregating critical patients from those exhibiting mild and nonsevere flu cases. Chatbots helped provide initial symptom assessment tools and speed up the screening process for health-care professionals. They helped provide necessary care for patients at immediate risk for COVID-19 and timely reminders and follow-up alerts for those under quarantine or monitoring their health from their homes.

Chatbots were also used extensively by most health-care organizations, such as the World Health Organization (WHO), to propagate accurate information about the virus, its symptoms, and when to contact a local health-care provider. Medical chatbots provide on-demand services for people affected by COVID-19 by bringing medicine delivery and home testing services to their doorstep to minimize interpersonal contact and curtail the spread of the virus. Such uses of chatbots help reduce demands on health-care systems and improve patients' access to information and care.

FUTURE OF MEDICAL CHATBOTS

Chatbots offer many advantages, such as cost savings and improved returns on investments for health-care providers. They are predicted to be the future of remote health care. Chatbots will potentially make health care more accessible, accurate, relevant, and affordable. Tech experts project that medical chatbots in the form of therapy chatbots will, in the future, help mental health patients manage symptoms and mood disorders, provide healthy lifestyle management tips, and provide real-time alerts and updates to patients and doctors, respectively. Some chatbots may also be capable of integrating telemedicine strategies into their functions, such as scheduling video consultations with doctors. Medical chatbots of the future might also function like a nurse, taking a patient's vital signs and monitoring their condition. They will likely also help health-care organizations automate specific business tasks and improve administrative accuracy.

As health care progresses and integrates technological advancements, medical chatbots will be a valuable tool in making health care more efficient and accurate.

References

"Healthcare Chatbot: The Future of the Health Industry through AI," Xenioo, August 2, 2021.

"How Are Intelligent Healthcare Chatbots Being Used? [New Uses for 2022]," Engati, June 27, 2022.

"Overview: What Is the Role of Chatbots in the Healthcare Industry?" Folio3 Digital Health, February 8, 2022.

Teo Peiru. "AI Chatbots in Healthcare," Key Reply, February 22, 2022.

Chapter 4 | **Health Technology Assessment**

Technological innovation has yielded remarkable health-care advances during the past five decades. In recent years, breakthroughs in a variety of areas have helped improve health-care delivery and patient outcomes, including antivirals, anticlotting drugs, antidiabetic drugs, antihypertensive drugs, antirheumatic drugs, vaccines, pharmacogenomics and targeted cancer therapies, cardiac rhythm management, diagnostic imaging, minimally invasive surgery, joint replacement, pain management, infection control, and health information technology (health IT).

The proliferation of health-care technology and its expanding uses have contributed to burgeoning health-care costs, and the former has been cited as the "culprit" for the latter. However, this relationship is variable, complex, and evolving. The U.S. Congressional Budget Office (CBO) concluded that "roughly half of the increase in health-care spending during the past several decades was associated with the expanded capabilities of medicine brought about by technological advances."

Few patients or clinicians are willing to forego access to state-of-the-art health-care technology. In wealthier countries and those with growing economies, the adoption and use of technology have been stimulated by patient and physician incentives to seek any potential health benefit with limited regard to cost and by third-party payment, provider competition, effective marketing of technologies, and consumer awareness.

This chapter includes text excerpted from "HTA 101: Introduction to Health Technology Assessment," U.S. National Library of Medicine (NLM), July 22, 2019.

Health Technology Sourcebook, Third Edition

In this era of increasing cost pressures, restructuring of health-care delivery and payment, and heightened consumer demand—yet continued inadequate access to care for many millions of people—technology remains the substance of health care. The culprit or not, technology can be managed in ways that improve patient access and health outcomes while continuing to encourage useful innovation. The development, adoption, and diffusion of technology are increasingly influenced by a widening group of policymakers in the health-care sector. Health product makers, regulators, clinicians, patients, hospital managers, payers, government leaders, and others increasingly demand well-founded information to support decisions about whether or how to develop technology, allow it on the market, acquire it, use it, pay for its use, ensure its appropriate use, and more. The growth and development of health technology assessment (HTA) in government and the private sector reflect this demand.

HTA methods are evolving, and their applications are increasingly diverse. This chapter introduces fundamental aspects and issues of a dynamic field of inquiry. Broader participation of people with multiple disciplines and different health-care roles enriches the field. The heightened demand for HTA, particularly from the for-profit and not-for-profit private sectors and government agencies, is pushing the field to evolve more systematic and transparent assessment processes and reporting to diverse users. The body of knowledge about HTA cannot be found in one place and is not static. Practitioners and users of HTA should not only monitor changes in the field but also have considerable opportunities to contribute to its development.

ORIGINS OF TECHNOLOGY ASSESSMENT

Technology assessment (TA) arose in the mid-1960s from an appreciation of the critical role of technology in modern society and its potential for unintended, and sometimes harmful, consequences. Experience with the side effects of many chemical, industrial and agricultural processes, and services, such as transportation, health, and resource management, contributed to this understanding. Early assessments concerned topics such as offshore oil drilling,

Health Technology Assessment

pesticides, automobile pollution, nuclear power plants, supersonic airplanes, weather modification, and the artificial heart. TA was conceived as a way to identify the desirable first-order, intended effects of technologies and the higher-order, unintended social, economic, and environmental effects.

The term "technology assessment" was introduced in 1965 during deliberations of the Committee on Science and Astronautics of the U.S. House of Representatives. Congressman Emilio Daddario emphasized that the purpose of TA was to serve policy making: "technical information needed by policymakers is frequently not available, or not in the right form. A policymaker cannot judge the merits or consequences of a technological program within a strictly technical context. He has to consider social, economic, and legal implications of any course of action."

Congress commissioned independent studies by the National Academy of Sciences, the National Academy of Engineering (NAE), and the Legislative Reference Service of the Library of Congress that significantly influenced the development and application of TA. These studies and further congressional hearings led the National Science Foundation (NSF) to establish a TA program and, in 1972, Congress to authorize the congressional Office of Technology Assessment (OTA), which was founded in 1973, became operational in 1974, and established its health program in 1975.

Many observers were concerned that TA would be a means by which government would impede the development and use of technology. However, this was not Congress's intent or the agencies that conducted the original TAs. In 1969, an NAE report to Congress emphasized that TA would aid Congress in becoming more effective in assuring that broad public and private interests are fully considered while enabling technology to make the maximum contribution to our society's welfare.

With somewhat different aims, the private industry used TA to aid in competing in the marketplace, understanding the future business environment, and producing options for decision makers.

Technology assessment methodology drew upon various analytical, evaluative, and planning techniques. Among these were

Health Technology Sourcebook, Third Edition

systems analysis, cost-benefit analysis, consensus development methods (e.g., Delphi method), engineering feasibility studies, clinical trials, market research, technological forecasting, and others. TA practitioners and policymakers recognize that TA is evolving and flexible and should be tailored to the task.

EARLY HEALTH TECHNOLOGY ASSESSMENT

Health technologies had been studied for safety, effectiveness, cost, and other concerns long before the advent of HTA. The development of TA as a systematic inquiry in the 1960s and 1970s coincided with the introduction of some health technologies that prompted widespread public interest in matters that transcended their immediate health effects. Health-care technologies were among the topics of early TAs. Multiphasic health screening was one of three topics of "experimental" TAs conducted by the NAE at the request of Congress. In response to a request by the NSF to further develop the TA concept in the area of biomedical technologies, the National Research Council (NRC) conducted TAs on in vitro fertilization, predetermination of the sex of children, retardation of aging, and modifying human behavior by neurosurgical, electrical, or pharmaceutical means. The OTA issued a report on drug bioequivalence in 1974, and the OTA Health Program issued its first formal report in 1976.

Since its early years, HTA has been fueled partly by the emergence and diffusion of technologies that have evoked social, ethical, legal, and political concerns. Among these technologies are contraceptives, organ transplantation, artificial organs, life-sustaining technologies for critically or terminally ill patients, and, more recently, genetic testing, genetic therapy, ultrasonography for fetal sex selection, and stem cell research. These technologies have challenged certain societal institutions, codes, and other norms regarding fundamental aspects of human life, such as parenthood, heredity, birth, bodily sovereignty, freedom and control of human behavior, and death.

Despite the comprehensive approach originally intended for TA, its practitioners recognized early on that "partial TAs" may be preferable in circumstances where selected impacts are of particular

Health Technology Assessment

interest or were necessitated by resource constraints. In practice, relatively few TAs have encompassed the full range of possible technological impacts; most focus on certain sets of impacts or concerns.

FACTORS THAT REINFORCE THE MARKET FOR HEALTH TECHNOLOGY

- Advances in science and engineering
- Intellectual property, especially patent protection
- Aging populations
- Increasing prevalence of chronic diseases
- Emerging pathogens and other disease threats
- Third-party payment, especially fee-for-service payment
- Financial incentives for technology companies, clinicians, hospitals, and others
- Public demand driven by direct-to-consumer advertising, mass media reports, social media, and consumer awareness and advocacy
- Off-label use of drugs, biologics, and devices
- "Cascade" effects of unnecessary tests, unexpected results, or patient or physician anxiety
- Clinician specialty training at academic medical centers
- Provider competition to offer state-of-the-art technology
- Malpractice avoidance
- Strong or growing economies

Part 2 | **Understanding Telehealth**

Chapter 5 | Telehealth

Chapter Contents
Section 5.1—Telehealth: An Overview... 45
Section 5.2—Benefits of Telehealth... 47
Section 5.3—Implementation and Future of Telehealth 51
Section 5.4—Medicare Benefits and Telehealth 53
Section 5.5—Health Equity in Telehealth 60

Section 5.1 | Telehealth: An Overview

This section includes text excerpted from "What Is Telehealth?" U.S. Department of Health and Human Services (HHS), September 14, 2022.

Hearing a lot about telehealth and telemedicine lately? Connecting with your health-care provider online is a great way to get the health care you need from the comfort and safety of your own home.

WHAT DOES TELEHEALTH MEAN?

Telehealth—sometimes called "telemedicine"—lets your health-care provider provide care for you without an in-person office visit. Telehealth is done primarily online with Internet access on your computer, tablet, or smartphone.

There are several options for telehealth care:
- Talk to your health-care provider live over the phone or through video chat.
- Send and receive messages from your health-care provider using secure messaging, e-mail, and secure file exchange.
- Use remote monitoring so your health-care provider can check on you at home. For example, you might use a device to gather vital signs or other vitals to help your health-care provider stay informed on your progress.

WHAT TYPES OF CARE CAN YOU GET USING TELEHEALTH?

You can get a variety of specialized care through telehealth. Telehealth is especially helpful in monitoring and improving ongoing health issues, such as medication changes or chronic health conditions.

Telehealth care can be obtained for the following:
- Lab test or x-ray results
- Mental health treatment, including online therapy, counseling, and medication management

Health Technology Sourcebook, Third Edition

- Recurring conditions such as migraines or urinary tract infections
- Skin conditions
- Prescription management
- Urgent care issues such as colds, coughs, and stomach aches
- Postsurgical follow-up
- Treatment and follow-up appointments for attention deficit disorder (ADD) and attention deficit hyperactivity disorder (ADHD)
- Physical therapy and occupational therapy
- Remote monitoring services that help you track your health goals and manage chronic conditions such as diabetes, high blood pressure (HBP), and high cholesterol

Your health-care provider will decide whether telehealth is right for your health needs. Ask your health-care provider's office what your telehealth options are, especially if you are concerned about the health risk of COVID-19.

Your health-care provider may also ask you to send information that will help improve your health, for example:
- Your weight, blood pressure, blood sugar, or vital information
- Images of a wound or eye or skin condition
- A diary or document of your symptoms
- Medical records that may be filed with another health-care provider, such as x-rays

Health-care providers can send you the following information to manage your health at home:
- Notifications or reminders to do rehabilitation exercises or take medication
- New suggestions for improving diet, mobility, or stress management
- Detailed instructions on how to continue your care at home
- Encouragement to stick with your treatment plan

Telehealth

Section 5.2 | **Benefits of Telehealth**

This section includes text excerpted from "Telehealth for the Treatment of Serious Mental Illness and Substance Use Disorders," Substance Abuse and Mental Health Services Administration (SAMHSA), June 2, 2021.

Telehealth supports team-based care and its interrelated care objectives. The Quadruple Aim is a conceptual framework to understand, measure, and optimize health system performance. The Quadruple Aim organizes the benefits of telehealth into the following four categories:

- **Health-care provider experience**. Health-care providers may improve the quality of care they provide and experience the following benefits from implementing telehealth methods:
  - **Provision of timely client care**. Health-care providers may have increased flexibility in appointment scheduling by using telehealth. They can extend care beyond a clinic's normal operating hours and its four walls and leverage "virtual walk-in visits." Increased flexibility can help clinics more effectively manage client "no-shows" and cancellations.
  - **Effective and efficient coordination of care**. An estimated 40–60 percent of civilian clients (not inclusive of military populations) with mental and substance use disorders are treated in primary care offices rather than specialty care settings. Health-care providers can use telehealth methods for tele-consultation, tele-supervision, and tele-education to coordinate, integrate, and improve care (e.g., through the "hub-and-spoke" model).
  - **Reduction in workforce shortages**. This is especially true for underserved and rural areas.
  - **Ability to assess the client's home environment**. Rather than relying on a client's report of their home and living conditions, telehealth makes it possible for health-care providers to see, with appropriate

47

Health Technology Sourcebook, Third Edition

permission, inside a client's home; meet family support systems; and determine if an in-person visit at a person's home is needed.

- **Ability to share information for psychoeducation and assessment.** Psychoeducation, or the didactic communication of information to the client about therapeutic intervention or diagnosis, can be done through screen-sharing, thus allowing the clinician to seamlessly display videos, slideshows, and other visuals to the client. Mental health and substance use assessments can also be done this way, allowing the clinician to track the client's responses in real time.
- **Efficient connections to crisis services.** In emergencies, telehealth providers can instruct clients to call emergency response systems (e.g., 911, 988) while the health-care providers remain connected via telephone or video. Enhanced 911 (E911) automatically provides emergency dispatchers with the location of the client rather than the client needing to provide their address to the dispatcher.
- **Reductions in provider burnout.** This is a pervasive issue in the health-care field and is exacerbated by numerous factors, including time pressures, fast-paced environments, family responsibilities, and time-consuming documentation. Telehealth may lead to reductions in provider stress and burnout by promoting more manageable schedules, greater flexibility, and reductions in commute time.
- **Client experience.** Clients may experience many benefits from receiving mental health and substance use treatment through telehealth.
  - **Increased access to experienced providers and high-quality care.** Through telehealth, clients can access experienced providers that may be geographically distant from their homes. Through telehealth modalities, clients can access providers with expertise in their particular conditions and

Telehealth

treatment plans that can provide care appropriate for their culture, race, gender, sexual orientation, and living experience.

- **Improved access to and continuity of care.** Telehealth provides a mechanism to increase access to quality care and reduce travel costs for clients, increasing the likelihood that clients will see their health-care provider regularly and attend scheduled appointments.
- **Increased convenience that removes traditional barriers to care.**
  - **Geographic barriers** (e.g., transportation and distance to health-care providers). Telehealth increases the opportunity for individuals in remote locations to access the care they need.
  - **Psychological barriers.** Clients who experience anxiety about leaving their homes to access treatment (e.g., clients experiencing panic disorder or agoraphobia) are able to receive care in a safe environment.
  - **Accessibility.** Individuals with physical, visual, or hearing impairments and clients who are isolated (e.g., older adults) or incarcerated are able to access needed health care through the use of telehealth.
  - **Employment.** The use of telehealth allows clients to receive care while not requiring them to take significant leave from employment or other essential activities.
  - **Childcare and caregiver responsibilities.** Receiving home-based telehealth can help reduce the burden of finding childcare. For family caregivers, telehealth technologies, such as remote monitoring, can relieve some caregiver responsibilities, thereby decreasing stress and improving quality of life.
  - **Team-based services and group-based interventions.** Team-based and coordinated care is

critical to high-quality client treatment. However, geographic distances between health-care providers and clients can limit communication. Telehealth enhances team-based care across geographic barriers by remotely connecting multiple providers with a client, promoting health-care provider collaboration and the exchange of health information. Similarly, telehealth improves access to group-based interventions, which demonstrate similar treatment outcomes as in-person groups.

- **Reduction in stigma associated with experiencing and accessing treatment.** Through telehealth, clients can disclose their health information from the privacy of their own home. In rural communities with fewer behavioral health providers, telehealth can connect clients with providers in other geographic locations, which can increase their privacy and protect their anonymity when accessing care.
- **Satisfaction with care consistent with in-person treatment**. Despite some initial client hesitancy toward using telehealth, clients often report comparable satisfaction between telehealth and in-person care.

- **Population health**. Treatments delivered through telehealth have been shown to improve health outcomes, including improved quality of life and access to health care. For people experiencing severe mental illness (SMI), telehealth has the potential to improve quality of life and general mental health, reduce depressive symptoms, build more confidence in managing depression, and increase satisfaction with mental health and coping skills (when compared to treatment offered in-person only). For people experiencing substance use disorders (SUD), treatments delivered through telehealth have resulted in reductions in alcohol consumption, increased tobacco cessation, and increased engagement and retention in opioid use disorder treatment.

Telehealth

- **Costs.** In rural communities, in particular, implementing telehealth services reduces organizational costs by replacing the budget for a full-time, onsite behavioral health provider with as-needed hourly fees.

Section 5.3 | Implementation and Future of Telehealth

This section includes text excerpted from "Telehealth for the Treatment of Serious Mental Illness and Substance Use Disorders," Substance Abuse and Mental Health Services Administration (SAMHSA), June 2, 2021.

While the use of telehealth as a mode of service delivery is increasing, health-care providers, clients, and health-care settings continue to experience challenges related to adoption and implementation. For example, the uptake of telehealth can be hindered by disparities in access to appropriate and needed technology.

Recent advances in technology and access to personal computing devices and mobile phones have led to a rapid increase in the application of telehealth across the continuum of care (i.e., assessment, treatment, medication management/monitoring, recovery supports). Both health-care providers and clients need access to appropriate technology to benefit from synchronous or asynchronous telehealth. Practitioners can provide synchronous treatment through relatively low-tech options, including telephones, smartphones, tablets, and laptops.

The age, usability, and functionality of clients' devices may inhibit their use (e.g., ability to utilize various mobile health applications, appropriate data plans). Additionally, clients may be sharing devices with family members or others in a household, limiting the types of data a client would want to store or share through a device. For health-care providers, some clinics struggle to have enough laptops to support staff working from home or outside of typical shared office space and may not have updated devices or software systems to utilize available telehealth applications.

Table 5.1 discusses the various barriers associated with access to technology that are compounded by challenges experienced on multiple interrelated levels.

Table 5.1. Barriers Associated with Access to Technology

Individual client and provider	• Increasing access to and comfort using telehealth
Interpersonal client–provider relationships	• Preparing clients to use telehealth • Building a therapeutic relationship
Organizational	• Assessing organizational needs • Increasing organizational readiness and workforce capacity to participate in telehealth • Ensuring security and confidentiality
Regulatory and reimbursement environments	• Complying with federal, state, and local regulations

FUTURE OF TELEHEALTH

The use of telehealth has increased substantially in recent years and has accelerated rapidly with the COVID-19 pandemic. While the landscape of telehealth is continually evolving and health-care provider, client, population, and cost benefits are emerging, the practices and programs have demonstrated efficacy in improving client mental health outcomes in multiple settings and contexts.

Telehealth

Section 5.4 | **Medicare Benefits and Telehealth**

This section contains text excerpted from the following sources: Text in this section begins with excerpts from "CMS Next Generation ACO Beneficiary Telehealth Expansion Waiver Frequently Asked Questions," Centers for Medicare & Medicaid Services (CMS), January 26, 2018. Reviewed November 2022; Text under the heading "Expansion of Telehealth Benefits for Rural Population" is excerpted from "Trump Administration Proposes to Expand Telehealth Benefits Permanently for Medicare Beneficiaries Beyond the COVID-19 Public Health Emergency and Advances Access to Care in Rural Areas," Centers for Medicare & Medicaid Services (CMS), August 3, 2020.

Medicare only covers certain telehealth services under certain situations (e.g., with some health-care providers or in some areas). This typically involves visits and consultations that are provided using an interactive two-way telecommunications system (with real-time audio and video) by a doctor or certain other health-care provider who is not at your location. Advancing telehealth capabilities and the increased opportunities for communications that it affords allow health-care professionals to assess patients' status and change and reiterate parts of their care plan routines as frequently as needed. Medicare's Next Generation Accountable Care Organization (ACO) Model has an expanded benefit allowing beneficiaries who are associated with a Next Generation ACO to receive telehealth services from their doctor from their homes, regardless of geographic location, using a two-way telecommunications system. In addition, these beneficiaries are allowed to receive certain dermatology and ophthalmology services using asynchronous (i.e., store and forward) telehealth technology.

TELEHEALTH EXPANSION BENEFIT
How Do You Know If You Are a Beneficiary Associated with a Next Generation ACO and If You Can Receive This Benefit?

Medicare beneficiaries are those who receive care from a doctor participating in a Next Generation ACO and should receive a letter from the ACO notifying them that they are associated with the ACO. If the beneficiary's doctor (or a number of her or his doctors) participates in the Next Generation ACO, then the beneficiary may be associated with the ACO and may be eligible for expanded telehealth services under this benefit. You can also call

Health Technology Sourcebook, Third Edition

800-MEDICARE (800-633-4227) to ask whether you are associated with a Next Generation ACO.

What Types of Telehealth Services Are Covered by This Benefit?

The telehealth expansion benefit allows for two things. First, a beneficiary is allowed to receive some services via telecommunication devices that allow for interactive or "real-time" communication. For example, a home care worker can remotely check in on a beneficiary using a smartphone, tablet, smart TV, or other technology devices that the beneficiary also has in their home to assess a beneficiary's health status, monitor their medication routines, or instruct a relative or caregiver on how to administer the beneficiary's medication. Overall, technology gives those who are less mobile the ability to connect with a doctor, a nurse, a psychologist, or other health-care professionals via technology devices. Second, a beneficiary is allowed to receive some dermatology or ophthalmology services using asynchronous (i.e., store and forward) telehealth technology. Asynchronous telehealth includes the transmission of recorded health history (e.g., retinal scanning and digital images) through a secure electronic communications system to a doctor, usually a specialist, who uses the information to evaluate the beneficiary's case or provide a service outside of real-time interaction.

How Do You Know If a Health-Care Provider or Facility Is Participating with a Next Generation ACO in This Telehealth Expansion Benefit?

Your Next Generation ACO is required to maintain on its website a current list of health-care providers and facilities participating in the ACO's care network. You can also ask your doctor if she or he is participating in the Next Generation ACO and whether she or he is participating in this benefit with the ACO.

Can You Still Go to Your Doctor for an Office Visit, or Do You Have to Use Technology Instead?

You can still visit your doctor in their office. A health-care provider should not restrict you from coming into the office under normal

54

Telehealth

operations if that is your preference. If you suspect that your doctor is restricting you from visiting them in their office, please contact 800-MEDICARE (800-633-4227).

Medicare Telehealth Service Sounds Great; How Much Does It Cost?

Medicare telehealth service costs (e.g., coinsurance) remain the same with or without the waiver.

You Are Covered under Medicare: Does This Limit Your Choice of Doctors and Hospitals?

You still have your choice of doctors and hospitals, but this waiver applies only to beneficiaries who receive their care from a health-care provider or facility partner of a Next Generation ACO. If you choose a health-care provider or other facilities in which your ACO does not have a partnership, the normal Medicare telehealth rules apply.

How Is This Benefit Different from Regular, Existing Medicare Telehealth-Care Benefits?

The use of telehealth care in Medicare is often limited to rural areas (also known as "Health Professional Shortage Areas" (HSPA)) that are designated by the Health Resources and Services Administration (HRSA) as having shortages of primary care, dental care, or mental illness providers and may be geographic (a county or service area), population (e.g., low income or Medicaid eligible), or facilities (e.g., federally qualified health centers or state or federal prisons). The regular telehealth benefit is also limited to the following sites (i.e., where the service is received by the patient): the offices of physicians or practitioners, hospitals, critical access hospitals (CAHs), rural health clinics, federally qualified health centers, hospital- or CAH-based renal dialysis centers (including satellites), skilled nursing facilities (SNFs), community mental health centers (CMHCs), renal dialysis facilities, homes of beneficiaries with end-stage renal disease (ESRD) getting home dialysis, and mobile stroke units.

Health Technology Sourcebook, Third Edition

The use of telehealth care in Medicare is also regularly limited to an interactive two-way telecommunications system (with real-time audio and video) except in federal demonstration programs in Alaska and Hawaii, where asynchronous (i.e., store and forward) telehealth technology is permitted. The telehealth expansion benefit in the Next Generation ACO Model removes the rural area location requirements and allows eligible Medicare beneficiaries to receive telehealth care in their home and to receive certain dermatology and ophthalmology services using asynchronous (i.e., store and forward) technology.

EXPANSION OF TELEHEALTH BENEFITS FOR RURAL POPULATION

The Centers for Medicare & Medicaid Services (CMS) has proposed changes to expand telehealth permanently, consistent with the Executive Order on Improving Rural and Telehealth Access that President Trump signed. The Executive Order and proposed rule advance efforts to improve access and convenience of care for Medicare beneficiaries, particularly for those living in rural areas. Additionally, the proposed rule implements a multiyear effort to reduce clinician burden under the Patients over Paperwork initiative and to ensure appropriate reimbursement for time spent with patients. This proposed rule also takes steps to implement President Trump's Executive Order on Protecting and Improving Medicare for Our Nation's Seniors and continues the commitment to ensure that the Medicare program is sustainable for future generations.

Expanding Beneficiary Access to Care through Telehealth

Over the past three years, as part of the Fostering Innovation and Rethinking Rural Health strategic initiatives, the CMS has been working to modernize Medicare by unleashing private sector innovations and improving beneficiary access to services furnished via telecommunications technology. Starting in 2019, Medicare began paying for virtual check-ins, meaning patients across the country can briefly connect with doctors by phone or video chat to see whether they need to come in for a visit. In response to the COVID-19 pandemic, the CMS moved swiftly to significantly

Telehealth

expand payment for telehealth services and implement other flexibilities so that Medicare beneficiaries living in all areas of the United States can get convenient and high-quality care from the comfort of their home while avoiding unnecessary exposure to the virus. Before the public health emergency (PHE), only 14,000 beneficiaries received a Medicare telehealth service in a week, while over 10.1 million beneficiaries received a Medicare telehealth service during the public health emergency from mid-March through early July.

As directed by President Trump's Executive Order on Improving Rural and Telehealth Access, the CMS has taken steps to extend the availability of certain telemedicine services after the PHE ends, giving Medicare beneficiaries more convenient ways to access health care, particularly in rural areas where access to health-care providers may otherwise be limited.

"Telemedicine can never fully replace in-person care, but it can complement and enhance in-person care by furnishing one more powerful clinical tool to increase access and choices for America's seniors," said CMS Administrator Seema Verma. "The Trump Administration's unprecedented expansion of telemedicine during the pandemic represents a revolution in health-care delivery, one to which the health-care system has adapted quickly and effectively. Never one merely to tinker around the edges when it comes to patient-centered care, President Trump will not let this opportunity slip through our fingers."

During the PHE, the CMS added 135 services, such as emergency department visits, initial inpatient and nursing facility visits, and discharge day management services, that could be paid for when delivered by telehealth. The CMS is proposing to permanently allow some of those services to be done by telehealth, including home visits for the evaluation and management (E/M) of a patient (in the case where the law allows telehealth services in the patient's home) and certain types of visits for patients with cognitive impairments. The CMS is seeking public input on other services to add permanently to the telehealth list beyond the PHE in order to give clinicians and patients time as they get ready to provide in-person care again. The CMS is also proposing to temporarily extend payment for other telehealth services, such as emergency department visits, for a specific time period, through the calendar year in which the PHE ends. This will also give the community time to consider whether these services should be delivered permanently through telehealth outside of the PHE.

Prioritizing Investment in Preventive Care and Chronic Disease Management

Under the Patients over Paperwork initiative, the Trump Administration has taken steps to eliminate burdensome billing and coding requirements for E/M (or office/outpatient visits) that make up 20 percent of the spending under the Physician Fee Schedule. These billing and documentation requirements for E/M codes were established 20 years ago and have been subject to long-standing criticism from clinicians that they do not reflect current care practices and needs. After extensive stakeholder collaboration with the American Medical Association (AMA) and others, simplified coding and billing requirements for E/M visits have gone into effect since January 1, 2021, saving clinicians 2.3 million hours per year in burden reduction. As a result of this change, clinicians will be able to make better use of their time and restore the doctor–patient relationship by spending less time documenting visits and more time treating their patients.

Additionally, the Trump Administration finalized historic changes to increase payment rates for office/outpatient E/M visits beginning in 2021. The higher payment for E/M visits takes into account the changes in the practice of medicine, recognizing that additional resources are required of clinicians to take care of Medicare patients, of which two-thirds have multiple chronic conditions. The prevalence of certain chronic conditions in the Medicare population is growing. For example, as of 2018, 68.9 percent of beneficiaries have two or more chronic conditions. In addition, between 2014 and 2018, the percentage of beneficiaries with six or more chronic conditions grew from 14.3 to 17.7 percent.

In this rule, the CMS proposed to similarly increase the value of many services that are comparable to or include office/outpatient E/M visits, such as maternity care bundles, emergency department

Telehealth

visits, end-stage renal disease (ESRD) capitated payment bundles, physical and occupational therapy evaluation services, and others. The proposed adjustments, which implemented recommendations from the AMA, helped ensure that the CMS appropriately recognizes the kind of care where clinicians need to spend more face-to-face time with patients, such as primary care and complex or chronic disease management.

Bolstering the Health-Care Workforce/Patients over Paperwork

The CMS is also taking steps to ensure that health-care professionals can practice at the top of their professional training. During the COVID-19 public health emergency, the CMS announced several temporary changes to expand workforce capacity and reduce clinician burden so that staffing levels remain high in response to the pandemic. As part of its Patients over Paperwork initiative to reduce the regulatory burden for health-care providers, the CMS is proposing to make some of these temporary changes permanent following the PHE. Such proposed changes include nurse practitioners, clinical nurse specialists, physician assistants, and certified nurse-midwives (instead of only physicians) to supervise others performing diagnostic tests consistent with state law and licensure, providing that they maintain the required relationships with supervising/collaborating physicians as required by state law, clarifying that pharmacists can provide services as part of the professional services of a practitioner who bills Medicare, allowing physical and occupational therapy assistants (instead of only physical and occupational therapists) to provide maintenance therapy in outpatient settings, and allowing physical or occupational therapists, speech-language pathologists, and other clinicians who directly bill Medicare to review and verify (sign and date), rather than redocument, information already entered by other members of the clinical team into a patient's medical record.

Health Technology Sourcebook, Third Edition

Section 5.5 | **Health Equity in Telehealth**

This section includes text excerpted from documents published by two public domain sources. Text under the headings marked 1 are excerpted from "Health Equity in Telehealth," U.S. Department of Health and Human Services (HHS), June 3, 2022. Text under the heading marked 2 is excerpted from "Telehealth for the Treatment of Serious Mental Illness and Substance Use Disorders," Substance Abuse and Mental Health Services Administration (SAMHSA), June 2, 2021.

WHAT IS HEALTH EQUITY?[1]

Health equity in telehealth is the opportunity for everyone to receive the health care they need and deserve, regardless of social or economic status. Providing health equity in telehealth means making changes in digital literacy, technology, and analytics. This will help telehealth providers reach the underserved communities that need it the most.

Underserved communities often include:
- Low-income Americans
- Rural Americans
- People of color
- Immigrants
- People who identify as LGBTQ
- People with disabilities
- Older patients
- People with limited knowledge of the English language
- People with limited digital literacy
- People who are underinsured or uninsured

Underserved communities often lack equal access to health care, leading to consequences such as:
- Higher mortality rates
- Higher rates of disease
- More disease and illness severity
- Higher medical costs
- Lack of access to treatment
- Lack of access to health insurance

Barriers to telehealth access may include:
- Lack of video sharing technology, such as a smartphone, tablet, or computer

Telehealth

- Spotty or no Internet access
- Lack of housing or private space to participate in virtual visits
- Few local health-care providers who offer telehealth practices
- Language barriers, including oral, written, and sign language
- Lack of adaptive equipment for people with disabilities

HEALTH EQUITY AND TELEHEALTH[2]

While telehealth has many benefits, concerns around access to telehealth and telemedicine services, especially for those with low technology literacy or disabilities, remain.

- Americans aged 65 and older (18% of the population) are most likely to have a chronic disease, but almost half (40–45%) do not own a smartphone or have broadband Internet access.
- People experiencing poverty report lower rates of smartphone ownership (71%), broadband Internet access (59%), and digital literacy (53%) compared to the general population.
- People who are Black or Hispanic report having lower computer ownership (Black: 58% and Hispanic: 57%) or home broadband Internet access (Black: 66% and Hispanic: 61%) than White respondents (82 and 79%, respectively) although smartphone access is nearly equal (Black: 80%, Hispanic: 79%, and White: 82%).

Due to these limitations, some clients may not benefit from telehealth.

EQUAL ACCESS IN TELEHEALTH[1]

There are many ways health-care providers can use to improve access to telehealth. This will help new patients feel welcome and comfortable.

- Make materials accessible in different formats and multiple languages.

Health Technology Sourcebook, Third Edition

- Use images and words in your online communications for patients with low literacy.
- Measure patient satisfaction with postvisit surveys to improve service. Knowing what your patients need will help them feel more comfortable with virtual visits.
- Use inclusive patient intake forms that ask about access to technology and patient preferences. This could include language and pronoun preferences.
- Ask if your patients need assistive devices to participate in virtual visits.
- Encourage staff to learn how to broaden telehealth access. Consider sending internal news and progress related to accessibility.
- Include accessibility options within your telehealth programs. This could include screen readers or closed captioning options.
- Allow extra time in virtual visit appointments for patients that may need support in getting online.
- Use technology designed with equity in mind when it comes to speech recognition and health prediction algorithms.
- Encourage all patients to get involved in planning and implementing health equity. This could include:
  - Sitting on a board or committee.
  - Providing input on materials or procedures.
  - Conducting sensitivity training.
- Look for skills and experiences within your team, including:
  - Cultural competency
  - Connections with the local community
  - Experience working with underserved patient groups
  - Fluency in languages other than English

STAFF AND HEALTH-CARE PROVIDER HEALTH EQUITY EDUCATION[1]

A successful telehealth practice includes health-care providers and staff who know how to meet their patients' needs. Health-care

Telehealth

providers can support their staff in understanding accessibility challenges and how to overcome them.

Here are a few ways to promote health equity:

- **Create a flexible telehealth workflow that allows for quick changes and improvements.** This will help health-care providers meet the needs of their local community with little disruption.
- **Plan time for staff and health-care provider training.** This includes training in areas such as cultural sensitivity and accessibility requirements. Allow additional time to implement this training.
- **Consider a dedicated telehealth support team or staff member.** This might mean shifting staff roles or hiring additional employees. Having telehealth support will help more patients successfully participate in virtual visits.

HEALTH EQUITY FOR SPECIAL POPULATIONS[1]

There are numerous ways telehealth can support and improve health care for underserved patients.

Telehealth and LGBTQ+ Patients

Telehealth appointments are a safe, convenient way for LGBTQ+ patients to access health care. Telehealth can also be a necessary lifeline for some patients who do not have LGBTQ+-affirming health care available nearby.

The following are a few of the several ways to offer LGBTQ+-specific telehealth care.

PRESCRIPTIONS

This could include depression and anxiety medication or pre-exposure prophylaxis (PrEP). Health-care providers can also pre-scribe gender-affirming hormones for patients whose gender does not align with their sex assigned at birth, such as transgender and gender nonbinary people.

COUNSELING AND THERAPY

LGBTQ+ Americans, especially LGBTQ+ youth, have markedly higher rates of suicide than their heterosexual, cisgender counterparts. But there are not always LGBTQ+-focused health-care providers in less populated areas. Inclusive behavioral telehealth care can change lives and save lives.

HIV/AIDS MANAGEMENT AND TREATMENT

There are fewer numbers of HIV specialists in rural areas. Telehealth can offer patients a variety of HIV/AIDs prevention, treatment, and management options:

- Prescriptions for PrEP and post-exposure prophylaxis (PEP)
- Lab orders for testing
- HIV case management
- Prevention counseling
- HIV/AIDs counseling and therapy

Telehealth and Older Adults

There are more than 54 million Americans aged 65 or older. They account for about 16 percent of the population. This figure is expected to rise to more than 21 percent by 2040.

Telehealth is one way to meet the substantial health-care needs of this growing population. It is safe, convenient, and more cost-effective for your patients who may have mobility and transportation concerns that make getting to the office difficult.

BEST PRACTICES FOR TREATING OLDER AMERICANS THROUGH TELEHEALTH

It is important that older patients do not get left behind as the prominence of telehealth grows. Here are a few tips for making sure they get the attention and care they need through telehealth:

- Be understanding that your patients might not be digitally literate or have a basic understanding of how video calls work.

Telehealth

- Be flexible and consider other nonvideo telehealth options, such as phone calls or answering follow-up questions via e-mail.
- Allow extra time during the first few telehealth appointments with older patients. They may need more time to figure out how to get online and log into the video chat.
- Use remote monitoring devices to cut down on the amount of times you need to see your patient in person. These devices could measure blood pressure, breathing, and cardiac activity.

Chapter 6 | **Preparing for Telehealth Visits**

Most telehealth visits will include video. All you will need for this is a smartphone or a device, such as a tablet or a computer with an Internet connection and audio/video capabilities.

GETTING COMFORTABLE WITH TELEHEALTH

It might be hard to imagine what a virtual visit or e-visit will be like, especially if you have never had a health-care visit that was not in person.

A video visit is the closest telehealth option to an in-person visit. There are many reasons why telehealth may be a great option:

- You may live far away from health-care providers.
- You may have difficulty traveling for an in-person appointment.
- You may be responsible for children or elderly family members.
- You may feel too sick to leave home.
- You may need to stay a safe distance away from others.

There are many types of health care that can be offered through telehealth, including:

- Primary care
- Urgent care
- Diabetes care and management
- Prenatal care

This chapter includes text excerpted from "Preparing for a Virtual Visit," U.S. Department of Health and Human Services (HHS), June 29, 2022.

Health Technology Sourcebook, Third Edition

- Mental health care
- Cardiology
- Neurology
- Genetic counseling

Whatever your reason for choosing telehealth, the goal is to make your virtual visit feel like an in-person visit as much as possible.

PREPARING FOR YOUR VIRTUAL VISIT

Use these tips to help your virtual health visit run smoothly, especially if you are using video to talk with a health-care provider.

- **Write it down**. Just like an in-person visit, you will want to write down important information to make the best use of your time with the provider:
  - Make a list of your current medications (or gather the actual bottles).
  - Write down any symptoms, questions, or concerns you want to discuss during the appointment so you do not forget them.
  - If your health-care provider has requested information, such as your temperature or weight, have this information ready.
  - Keep paper nearby to take notes about what your health-care provider says during the e-visit.
- **Request any assistive technology or programs you may need to participate with**. Needing assistance, whether it is a screen reader, closed captioning, or another method, will allow you to communicate confidently.
  - If English is not your first language, you can also request a native speaker of your language if there is someone available. Or you can let your health-care provider's office know that a trusted family member or friend will be translating for you.
- **Be truthful on your medical forms and answering questions**. Your health-care provider needs to know the truth to be able to treat you properly. If you are

Preparing for Telehealth Visits

concerned about your privacy, let your health-care provider know ahead of time or even at the beginning of the appointment. It includes topics such as:

- Drinking
- Smoking
- Drug use
- Domestic violence
- Past surgeries
- Hospitalization
- Hormone use
- Medications and supplements
- **Check your e-mail for instructions**. Be sure to review any e-mails, texts, or other communication from your health-care provider's office. The office may send you details about your upcoming appointment and how to log on or use their technology.
- **Reduce background noise**. This can be tricky when there are a lot of people in the house. Try to find a quiet activity for the kids in a separate room and ask other adults to speak quietly if you can.
- **Close other applications**. Some applications on your phone, tablet, or computer will slow down your Internet connection. Closing them will also cut down on distractions.

Getting Ready for Your Video Appointment

- **Choose a spot with plenty of light**. If you are using the camera on your phone, you can try using the flash for extra light. If you are near a window, make sure the light is not coming in from behind you so your health-care provider can see your face clearly.
- **Make sure the camera is steady**. Set your computer or laptop on a flat service or prop up your phone or tablet on a desk or table.
- **Get comfortable**. Wear something that is easy to move in case your health-care provider asks you to show part of your skin or another area of your body.

Health Technology Sourcebook, Third Edition

- **Stay focused on your appointment**. Make your virtual visit a priority. Try to avoid eating or drinking during your appointment and avoid distractions, such as driving or riding in a car or running errands.
- **Choose a spot with plenty of privacy**. You want to be able to discuss your health-care issue in private.
- **Be patient while waiting for your health-care provider to appear for your visit**. Just like a regular in-person office visit, health-care providers sometimes run behind schedule.

FEELING EMPOWERED WITH TELEHEALTH

Feeling empowered means that you have the confidence, the ability, and the opportunity to advocate for your health during appointments, either in-person or over telehealth.

Talking to a health-care provider about your medical concerns, your history, and your symptoms may feel overwhelming. Some people may feel embarrassed. Others may be unsure what questions to ask. The first step to feeling empowered is to remember the following:

- The right health-care provider for you will take your concerns seriously.
- The right health-care provider for you has your best interests in mind.
- You have the right to absolute privacy in what you choose to discuss with your health-care provider during a telehealth or in-person appointment.

Telehealth has many benefits that can help you feel more confident and in control, including:

- Logging on to the appointment from the comfort of your own home or even your office or car
- Decreased stress from less travel or less need for childcare
- More control over your environment, such as a comfortable temperature and not having to change into medical gowns

Preparing for Telehealth Visits

- The ability to select a health-care provider who makes you feel comfortable, even if they are not in your local area

Empowerment and Health Equity

Empowerment in telehealth and health equity are important ideals in getting you the quality health care you deserve. Health equity in telehealth is the opportunity for everyone to receive the health care they need and deserve, regardless of social or economic status.

Feeling empowered when it comes to your health care will help you achieve health equity for yourself, your family, and others in your community.

Here are a few ways you can be empowered while using telehealth and working toward health equity:

- **Choose a telehealth provider that best fits your needs**. This could be a provider who is welcoming and affirming of LGBTQ+ patients. They could be a provider of color who understands the needs of the Black and Latinx community. You could also choose a provider who speaks your native language or ask for an interpreter if you think speaking English could be a barrier to care.
- **Be honest with your health-care provider if you are uninsured or underinsured**. Your health-care provider will likely know of programs or clinics where you can get low-cost or free services. This could include mobile vaccination clinics or free wellness checks.
- **Give feedback to help your health-care provider work toward more health equity in telehealth**. This could be through virtual discussions about community-specific topics or suggestions for online training.

Feel Empowered during Your Appointment

This is your time with your health-care provider. You should not be made to feel rushed or unheard. Here are a few ways you can feel empowered during the appointment:

- **Ask all the questions you need**. And make sure you feel comfortable with the answers you get. If the

Health Technology Sourcebook, Third Edition

health-care provider tells you something you do not fully understand, ask them to explain further.

- **Get information about how telehealth works if you need it.** Whether it is your first telehealth appointment or you are seeing a new health-care provider, feel free to ask what to expect.
- **Tell them you are uncomfortable talking about a specific topic.** It can help the provider take the lead and also reassure you that they are there to help.
- **Tell them your pronouns and the name you prefer they use.** It is your right to be recognized and treated well by your providers.

After Your Appointment

Your telehealth care does not stop when you log off from your appointment. Continue participating with the following tips:

- **Call the office or e-mail your health-care provider through a patient portal.** Do not worry if you forgot to ask a question, think of something later, or need help understanding your care. Your health-care provider will be happy to get you the information you need.
- **Make sure your health-care provider's office follows up as promised.** Your health-care provider may want to refer you to another physician, send you for lab work or imaging, or call in prescriptions to the pharmacy. If you have not heard back, call your health-care provider or e-mail through a patient portal to check in.
- **Give feedback and suggestions.** If there was something you liked about your appointment, your health-care provider's care, or their telehealth program, make sure to let them know. Conversely, feel confident in making suggestions if you feel certain parts of your telehealth experience could be improved. Feedback is the best way for providers to know how they can best serve their patients.

Preparing for Telehealth Visits

PAYING FOR YOUR TELEHEALTH VISIT

Paying for your telehealth appointment varies depending on your insurance status and insurance coverage. Telehealth insurance varies from state to state and continues to expand across the country. Medicare covers the cost of virtual visits for appointments related to COVID-19. Many private insurance companies cover telehealth appointments with the same benefits as in-person visits.

Check with your insurance company to find out whether you are covered for a virtual visit and how much it will cost. Even if a virtual visit costs you a bit more, it could still save you money if you consider travel costs, lost wages, and childcare costs for in-person visits.

TROUBLESHOOTING TELEHEALTH TECHNOLOGY

Here are common troubleshooting tips you can use if you are having trouble logging in to your telehealth appointment or if you have technology issues during the appointment itself:

- Restart your computer or device.
- Make sure the device is plugged in and charged.
- Check if the Internet connection is working and is strong enough to work with the telehealth platform.
- Close all other applications.
- Update your Internet browser (if the telehealth platform is web-based).
- Try connecting with a different device.
- Check your e-mail or call your health-care provider's office to reach someone who can provide help.

Chapter 7 | **Remote Patient Monitoring**

The ability to monitor certain aspects of a patient's health from their own home has become an increasingly popular telehealth option. Remote patient monitoring (RPM) lets health-care providers manage acute and chronic conditions, and it cuts down on patients' travel costs and infection risk.

HOW TO USE REMOTE PATIENT MONITORING WITH TELEHEALTH

Remote patient monitoring pairs well with telehealth when patients need to be monitored for certain health conditions. It can also prevent health complications in patients who are not able to travel easily.

There are many symptoms and conditions that can be tracked through remote patient monitoring, including:

- High blood pressure (HBP)
- Diabetes
- Weight loss or gain
- Heart conditions
- Chronic obstructive pulmonary disease (COPD)
- Sleep apnea (SA)
- Asthma

This chapter contains text excerpted from the following sources: Text in this chapter begins with excerpts from "Telehealth and Remote Patient Monitoring," U.S. Department of Health and Human Services (HHS), August 26, 2022; Text under the heading "Physical Therapy and Remote Patient Monitoring" is excerpted from "Physical Therapy and Remote Patient Monitoring," U.S. Department of Health and Human Services (HHS), August 26, 2022.

Health Technology Sourcebook, Third Edition

Many of the devices that patients will use may be familiar to them, including:

- Weight scales
- Pulse oximeters
- Blood glucose meters
- Blood pressure monitors

Other conditions require more complicated devices that will require patient training, including:

- Apnea monitors
- Heart monitors
- Specialized monitors for dementia and Parkinson disease (PD)
- Breathing apparatuses
- Fetal monitors

As the popularity and convenience of telehealth grow, so does remote patient monitoring. More providers are implementing remote patient monitoring for several reasons, including:

- Advanced medical technology
- A growing awareness of telehealth for health-care providers and patients
- More insurance coverage during the COVID-19 public health emergency
- The ability to monitor and prevent serious complications in remote locations

HOW TO HELP PATIENTS USE AT-HOME HEALTH MONITORS

Remote monitoring may be new for your patients and for you also. The best way to help your patients is to be informed about the devices you will be using. This includes how they work and how you will receive the data from the device.

Make Sure the Patient Understands Why You Are Prescribing At-Home Health Monitors

The following are a few among a number of ways to share information with your patients:

- A telehealth appointment before they begin using the device

Remote Patient Monitoring

- A follow-up telehealth appointment after they have been using the device for several days
- An e-mail or downloadable PDF explaining remote patient monitoring for their condition or symptoms

Help Your Patient Understand How to Use Their Device

Some products, such as a weight scale, may not need a lot of explanation. But other devices may be more high tech or confusing for patients. Here are a few tips:

- Walk your patient through operating the device in a telehealth appointment.
- Refer your patient to an at-home medical equipment provider in their area who can set them up with the device and provide support.
- Tell your patient what types of readings you will get from their device and how you will receive that information.
- Make sure your patient has written instructions they can refer to, including paper copies, e-mail, or downloadable PDFs.
- Encourage your patient to write down their questions and either call your office, e-mail you the questions through a patient portal, or request a follow-up telehealth appointment.
- Have a member of your staff let your patient know when you are receiving their information correctly from the device.

Talk to Your Patients about the Benefits of Remote Patient Monitoring

Some patients will need in-person testing, diagnostics, or monitoring. This depends on their condition, Internet capabilities, or personal preferences and abilities. But there are many ways that remote patient monitoring can help with chronic conditions, pregnancy complications, and short-term illnesses.

Health Technology Sourcebook, Third Edition

These benefits include:
- Reduced hospitalizations
- Shorter hospital stays if the patient can be discharged with a remote monitoring device to use at home
- Fewer visits to the emergency room
- Better health outcomes for patients in rural areas
- Better preventative management for chronic conditions
- Reduced risk of COVID-19 exposure, along with other illnesses, for patients and health-care workers

Tip: Medicare uses the term "remote physiologic monitoring" in its coding and billing language. Remote physiologic monitoring (RPM) is a set of codes that describes non-face-to-face monitoring and analysis of physiologic factors used to understand a patient's health status. For example, the RPM codes allow remote monitoring of oxygen saturation levels in patients with COVID-19.

BILLING AND PAYMENT FOR REMOTE PHYSIOLOGIC MONITORING
Billing for Medicare
While private insurance companies set their own terms, Medicare has its own payment policies. They include:
- An established patient–physician relationship is required. But there does not have to be an established relationship between the patient and physician for the duration of the public health emergency.
- Consent to receive RPM services at the time services are furnished is allowed.
- Physicians and nonphysicians practitioners who are eligible to furnish evaluation and management (E/M) services may bill for RPM services.

Guidelines for Remote Physiologic Monitoring Services
- Physiologic data must be electronically collected and automatically uploaded to a secure location where the data can be available for analysis and interpretation by the billing practitioner.

Remote Patient Monitoring

- The device used to collect and transmit the data must meet the definition of a medical device as defined by the U.S. Food and Drug Administration (FDA).
- RPM data must be collected for at least 16 days out of 30 days. During a public health emergency for COVID-19, if a patient is suspected or diagnosed with COVID-19, the data can be collected over as few as two days.
- RPM services must monitor acute care or chronic condition.
- The services may be provided by auxiliary personnel under the general supervision of the billing practitioner.

PHYSICAL THERAPY AND REMOTE PATIENT MONITORING

Remote patient monitoring technology can help you gather and analyze health information without a face-to-face appointment or in-person testing.

Practical Applications

With RPM, an individual's health and medical data can be collected and transmitted in real time to a health-care provider.

The latest RPM technology for physical therapy often comes in the form of mobile applications. These apps guide patients through exercises and monitor their movements to ensure they are doing them correctly. The data are transmitted directly to your EHR system, and the patient receives real-time feedback and tips as they perform the exercises.

Bluetooth-enabled "smart scales" are also popular with patients because they can connect to wearable fitness tracking devices, among other reasons.

Remote Patient Monitoring versus Remote Therapeutic Monitoring

As telehealth becomes an essential component of the health-care system in the United States, the classification of certain services continues to evolve to best fit the needs of patients and providers. For physical therapists and their staff, remote therapeutic monitoring (RTM) is one of those new classifications.

Health Technology Sourcebook, Third Edition

According to the Centers for Medicare & Medicaid Services (CMS), "new RTM coding was created to allow practitioners who cannot bill [remote patient monitoring] (RPM) codes to furnish and bill for services that look similar to those of RPM."

The main difference between RPM and RTM is the type and amount of data collected. Unlike RPM codes, which only cover physiologic data (e.g., heart rate, blood pressure, body temperature), RTM codes monitor and collect nonphysiological data, such as pain tolerance and medication adherence.

Chapter 8 | **Getting Help with Accessing Telehealth Services**

Even if you might like to try telehealth, you may have trouble accessing online services.

IF YOU DO NOT HAVE INTERNET ACCESS

Patients can maximize cost savings on Internet bills. The Affordable Connectivity Program (ACP; www.affordableconnectivity.gov) and Lifeline (www.lifelinesupport.org) are federal government programs that help eligible households pay for Internet services and Internet-connected devices. Eligible families who pair their benefits with one of the partnered Internet providers can receive high-speed Internet at no cost.

Who Is Eligible for Internet Services?

Eligibility for ACP and Lifeline programs is based on income or meeting other criteria. Individuals and families are automatically eligible if they belong to programs such as:

- Supplemental Nutrition Assistance Program (SNAP)
- Medicaid
- Federal public housing assistance
- Supplemental Security Income (SSI)
- Veterans pension or survivor benefits

This chapter includes text excerpted from "Getting Help with Access," U.S. Department of Health and Human Services (HHS), August 10, 2022.

Health Technology Sourcebook, Third Edition

- Tribal-specific assistance programs
- Other

How to Apply for Internet Services

For the Affordable Connectivity Program, eligible households can enroll through a participating broadband provider or using an online or mail-in application. To apply for Lifeline (nv.fcc.gov/lifeline), households can apply online, by mail, or through a phone or Internet company.

If your health-care provider uses a secure, password-protected portal, you may also be able to access telehealth services at libraries, community centers, or other places offering Internet access to the public. Video or phone discussions may not be advisable in a public environment.

IF YOU DO NOT HAVE HEALTH INSURANCE

Since the COVID-19 pandemic, more people have qualified for financial help and lower premiums on health insurance plans. Most customers can qualify for a plan that includes health-care provider visits, prescription medications, and preventive services for $10 per month or less.

- Visit HealthCare.gov (www.healthcare.gov/get-coverage).
- Check your state's website to see if it has its own insurance marketplace.
- See if you qualify for Medicaid or the Children's Health Insurance Program (CHIP).
- Find a health center near you.

IF YOU ARE NOT CONFIDENT USING TECHNOLOGY FOR TELEHEALTH

Meeting your health-care provider online may feel a bit uncomfortable at first. With practice, telehealth appointments can be as easy as making a phone call.

Getting Help with Accessing Telehealth Services

Video Meetings

Your health-care provider will likely ask you to confirm your telehealth visit in the days before your appointment. Confirmation is typically done by text message, phone call, or messages in a patient portal.

Before you log on to your appointment, you may receive instructions on how to sign onto the video chat with your health-care provider. Give yourself plenty of time to get set up for your appointment. If you are having trouble getting online, you can message your provider or call them for help.

There are a lot of telehealth video platforms out there. Each one will look a bit different than the others, but all of them have a few common features. Once you are logged in, here are a few things to look for:

- **Camera icon**. This button controls your camera. When you see a slash through it, it means your health-care provider cannot see you.
- **Microphone icon**. This button controls your microphone. When you see a slash through it, it means your health-care provider cannot hear you.
- **Messaging icon**. When you click this button, a chat box will open up. The chat box lets you type and send messages to your health-care provider.
- **Hang-up icon**. This button is usually red. Clicking on it will end your telehealth video meeting.

Accessing Documents for Telehealth

Your health-care provider may ask you to fill out forms before or after your telehealth appointment. Some health-care providers allow you to provide information directly on their website or through their patient portal, but some may ask you to download documents.

The most common kind of document you will receive is a portable document format (PDF) file. If you see ".pdf" at the end of a file name, it means that it is a PDF file. You will need a document reader to view, print, and fill out PDFs.

Health Technology Sourcebook, Third Edition

What to Do When You Are Having Trouble

Technical issues happen to everyone, and a lot of the time, the issues are not your fault. If you are having technical problems during your telehealth appointment, here are a few things you can do to fix them:

- **Close your web browser, then open it again**. Your health-care provider's telehealth website may need a quick reset.
- **Turn off your Internet connection, then turn it on again**. There might be a temporary issue with your network.
- **Call your health-care provider's office on the phone**. Someone should be available to walk you through your technical issues or help you reschedule your telehealth appointment.

Improving Digital Literacy

Digital literacy means safely sharing information online. Telehealth involves sharing personal medical information online. So feeling certain that your details are private is important.

Below are some online resources that help you learn digital literacy skills:

- Internet Skills (allofus.nnlm.gov/learn-internet-skills)—from the National Institutes of Health (NIH)
- Digital Health Literacy Curriculum (allofus.nnlm.gov/digital-health-literacy)—from the NIH

The following are the places to look for improving digital literacy skills:

- Public libraries
- Local government community and human services departments
- Nonprofit groups that provide English as a second language (ESL) classes
- Job training programs
- Public schools that provide support services for parents and guardians
- Community colleges and adult education centers

Chapter 9 | Virtual Health-Care Services

Chapter Contents

Section 9.1—Telehealth and Cancer Care..................................87
Section 9.2—Telerehabilitation for Advanced Cancer 90
Section 9.3—Telehealth for Chronic Conditions.......................94
Section 9.4—Telehealth for COVID-19 102
Section 9.5—Telehealth for HIV Care......................................106
Section 9.6—Telehealth for Maternal Health Services.............111
Section 9.7—Telehealth for Children with Special
          Health-Care Needs...118
Section 9.8—School-Based Telehealth Services.......................122
Section 9.9—Use of Telehealth in Emergency
          Departments 125

Chapter 4 | Virtual
Health-Care Services

Section 9.1 | **Telehealth and Cancer Care**

This section includes text excerpted from "Introduction to Telehealth and Cancer Care," U.S. Department of Health and Human Services (HHS), August 26, 2022.

Every year, nearly two million people in the United States are diagnosed with cancer. As telehealth technology grows and evolves, more health-care providers are integrating telehealth as part of their cancer care programs, also known as "tele-oncology." Tele-oncology may offer patients, their family members, and their caregivers convenience (i.e., time and travel), lower costs, and flexible scheduling. Telehealth also reduces germ exposure for immunocompromised individuals.

TELEHEALTH AND CANCER TREATMENT

Many cancer care services can be performed without an in-person visit.

Distress Screening via Telehealth

The standard of care for all cancer programs includes a method to screen all newly diagnosed patients for their level of distress and, based on the results, offer appropriate levels of psychosocial care. Like many other forms of behavioral health care, these distress screenings and follow-ups can be conducted through telehealth. Follow these steps to ensure that your cancer patients are receiving the mental health support that they need.

SELECT A DISTRESS SCREENING TEAM LEAD

This person or these persons can be an oncology social worker, clinical psychologist, or other licensed mental health professional trained in the psychosocial aspects of cancer care.

If your practice cannot accommodate this type of staffing, work with community organizations and other specialty providers to develop a virtual distress screening care network.

CREATE A STANDARDIZED PROTOCOL

Having a protocol ensures that screenings are completed and distress can be addressed in a timely and organized fashion. Protocol considerations include the telehealth platform where screenings will be conducted, how to determine the need for a follow-up clinical assessment, and developing a referral plan.

CHOOSE A SCREENING TOOL

Three distress screening measurement tools are commonly used in the United States. Each has unique metrics, and the tool that you select should be based on individual patient needs.
- The Psychosocial Screen for Cancer (PSCAN) measures general distress.
- Patient Health Questionnaire-4 (PHQ-4) measures anxiety and depression.
- The Edmonton Symptom Assessment System (ESAS-r) assesses nine common symptoms in cancer patients, such as anxiety, depression, nausea, and fatigue.

Chemotherapy and Telehealth

Intravenous chemotherapy requires an in-person visit and healthcare provider supervision. Telehealth visits can be used to assess treatment requirements and potential side effects of chemotherapy before each cycle of treatment. You can also use telehealth to review patient progress and determine if dosing adjustments are needed.

As oral chemotherapy becomes more widely adopted, your telehealth cancer practice may consider including it as part of a patient's care plan when appropriate.

Both oral and intravenous chemotherapy require strong health IT and remote patient monitoring (RPM) infrastructure to track patient progress and side effects as well as keep them connected with their care team. RPM allows you to respond to a patient's symptoms in a timely manner with evidence-based care recommendations.

Ongoing monitoring and clinical response to patient feedback can be assessed during scheduled telehealth follow-ups, which can ensure the appropriate use of the monitoring tools.

Virtual Health-Care Services

Palliative Care with Telehealth

Tele-palliative care, or palliative care conducted primarily through telehealth, has the potential to provide a variety of benefits to palliative and hospice care patients, especially those who are susceptible to infection and/or rely upon interdisciplinary care. These patients can receive care with minimal disruption to their daily lives from the comfort of their homes—which is particularly valuable to those living in remote or rural areas.

Cancer patients in palliative care benefit from continuous monitoring and symptom management, both of which can be completed through either videoconferencing or audio-only telehealth services.

Periodic virtual visits can help providers address additional care needs and assess symptoms that may require hospitalization. RPM can be used to manage and treat symptoms such as pain and respiratory distress. Outpatient services or hospitalizations can be coordinated earlier to address symptoms, such as pain control or fluid needs to prevent emergency visits.

IMPLEMENTATION CONSIDERATIONS FOR TELE-PALLIATIVE CARE

Tele-palliative care requires careful planning for successful implementation. As you consider integrating tele-palliative care into your practice, be sure to keep the following in mind.

Scheduling Flexibility

Take advantage of the relationship consistency telehealth can provide. Tele-palliative visits can be scheduled around chemotherapy infusions to promote better continuity of care.

Communication Barriers

Designate one or more members of your staff to review virtual login instructions with patients ahead of a scheduled call to prevent delays that can impact your care schedule. To address potential audio delays that can happen with video visits, allow for deliberate pauses in speech.

Health Technology Sourcebook, Third Edition

Access Disparities

Keep in mind that video-based tele-palliative care may not be an option for many patients due to a lack of technological access. In these cases, work closely with patients to determine alternative approaches, such as in-person visits and audio-only care.

TELE-PALLIATIVE CARE IN PRACTICE

When symptom reports reach predetermined thresholds, notify the patient's palliative care team for further treatment and symptom management. In response to these notifications, the patient could participate in videoconferences with their nurse as an alternative to an in-person office visit when medically appropriate to do so.

Section 9.2 | Telerehabilitation for Advanced Cancer

This section includes text excerpted from "Telerehabilitation for Advanced Cancer," National Cancer Institute (NCI), April 29, 2019.

TELEPHONE-BASED REHAB PROGRAM HELPS PEOPLE WITH ADVANCED CANCER MAINTAIN INDEPENDENCE

As cancer progresses, it often leads to physical disability and pain that can threaten a person's independence and devastate their quality of life (QOL).

Yet most people with advanced cancer do not receive physical therapy or engage in exercise that can help maintain function, said Dr. Andrea Cheville, M.D., a rehabilitation physician at the Mayo Clinic in Rochester, MN. For these patients, she said, small changes in physical fitness can mean the difference between being able to live independently and losing one's independence and may also affect their ability to receive certain treatments.

An NCI-funded clinical trial led by Dr. Cheville found that a six-month physical rehabilitation program delivered by telephone modestly improved function and reduced pain for people with advanced cancer. The telerehabilitation program also reduced the

Virtual Health-Care Services

time patients spent in hospitals and long-term care facilities such as nursing homes.

"Overall, the study findings add to the growing evidence that low-tech interventions can effectively improve the delivery of supportive cancer care services," wrote Dr. Manali Patel, M.D., M.P.H., of the Stanford University School of Medicine, in a commentary on the study. Embracing these low-tech approaches "may be a smart move ... to improve patient-reported outcomes and keep patients at home," she concluded.

The findings, published April 4 in *JAMA Oncology*, also "reiterate the importance of supportive care for patients, and particularly for patients with advanced cancer," said Dr. Karen Mustian, Ph.D., M.P.H., of the University of Rochester's Wilmot Cancer Institute, who was not involved with the study.

"We need to think of new and creative ways to be able to support patients, their care providers, and their family members [in] the process of managing cancer," Dr. Mustian said.

PHYSICAL THERAPY FOR PATIENTS WITH ADVANCED CANCER

Various factors explain why many people with advanced stages of cancer do not receive physical therapy or other rehabilitation services.

It is often hard to find physical therapists or other professionals with the specialized training needed to work with people with advanced cancer. Also, these patients may have difficulty traveling to a specialty center for care, Dr. Cheville said.

Furthermore, she said that patients may feel too overwhelmed by the disease and its treatments to seek such care.

And Dr. Patel said, "Oncologists and other health-care providers may also be reluctant to refer patients with cancer, especially those with advanced cancer, to physical therapy" due to concerns that the patient may be too debilitated to benefit from such a program or could even be harmed by it.

Dr. Patel, an oncologist who mainly sees patients with advanced stages of cancer, said the new findings would change her practice. It includes being more likely to refer eligible patients for physical therapy and to consider physical therapy as "a way to also provide

Health Technology Sourcebook, Third Edition

symptom relief from pain without having to rely on pain medications alone," including opioids, she said.

REMOTELY-DELIVERED CARE

For the trial, dubbed Cognitive and Physical Exercise (COPE), Dr. Cheville and her colleagues enrolled 516 adults (257 women and 259 men) with advanced-stage cancer and moderate functional impairment. People with moderate impairment can independently get around their home and, to a more limited extent, their communities and manage activities of daily living such as grocery shopping, but they do so with some difficulty. The average age of study participants was approximately 66 years.

To assess the value of a telerehabilitation program that addressed function and pain, patients eligible for the trial—all of whom had been seen at one of the three Mayo Clinic medical centers (in Minnesota, Arizona, or Florida)—were randomly assigned to one of three groups.

Those in the control group (group 1) continued their usual care and activities. Those in group 2 received an individualized telerehabilitation program delivered by a physical therapist with extensive experience in cancer rehabilitation—referred to as a fitness care manager. They also received targeted rehabilitation to manage pain. Those in group 3 received the individualized telerehabilitation program plus medication-based pain management coordinated by a nurse.

At the time of enrollment, fitness care managers phoned group 2 and group 3 participants to discuss symptoms, identify goals, and discuss any physical impairments and barriers to staying active.

With supervision from a rehabilitation physician (Dr. Cheville), fitness care managers instructed patients in a simple set of strength training exercises using resistance bands and a walking program that used a pedometer to track steps. The fitness care managers monitored patients' progress and coordinated with their primary clinical team.

When needed, patients were referred to a local physical therapist to fine-tune their exercise programs or address physical impairments in consultation with the fitness care manager.

Virtual Health-Care Services

All participants were monitored for function, pain, and QOL using short questionnaires that they could opt to answer either online or by telephone.

MODEST BUT MEANINGFUL IMPROVEMENTS WITH TELEREHABILITATION

Over the six-month study period, group 2 participants (the telerehabilitation-only group) reported improvements in function, pain, and QOL compared with patients in the control group.

The researchers expected that group 3 participants, who received telerehabilitation plus medication-based pain management, would see the greatest improvement in pain. But, to their surprise, pain control was similar in groups 2 and 3. Also, unexpectedly, telerehabilitation alone was most effective in improving function, and QOL was not markedly better in group 3 than in the control group.

Telerehabilitation was associated with fewer and shorter hospitalizations, and hospitalized telerehabilitation participants were more likely than those in the control group to be discharged from the hospital to home rather than to a long-term care facility.

Although the changes in function seen with telerehabilitation alone were modest, they were clinically meaningful, Dr. Cheville said.

"Even a [small] change can correlate with the ability to get in and out of a chair independently, go up stairs on your own, or get in and out of a car without help. These changes can make the difference between going home from the hospital rather than going to a nursing home," she said.

Dr. Cheville's team has some ideas as to why patients in group 2 fared better overall than those in group 3 and plans to explore this question in future studies.

CANCER THERAPIES ALONE ARE NOT ENOUGH

"One of the key lessons we learned from our study is the importance of helping patients to understand that cancer care isn't only about treating the cancer. We need to strategically care for the person as well" to assure their well-being, Dr. Cheville said. "Convincing

Health Technology Sourcebook, Third Edition

patients that they need to take ownership for maintaining muscle strength and protecting their ability to function is very important."

"We shouldn't underestimate the power of implementing telephone-based supportive care services, as was done in this study," Dr. Mustian emphasized. "We have not really adopted those models in cancer care much."

One question that remains is whether health insurance would cover such services and, if not, whether the telerehabilitation approach is cost-effective for health-care providers, Dr. Patel noted in her commentary. Indeed, Dr. Cheville said that she and her colleagues are preparing to submit a paper that analyzes the program's cost-effectiveness.

Even without that information, the improvements in outcomes shown by the study "may be enough [for cancer care providers] to consider the integration of collaborative telerehabilitation into routine cancer care," Dr. Patel wrote.

Another key limitation of the study is that most of the participants were non-Hispanic Whites who had in-home caregivers. So it is unclear whether the telerehabilitation approach can be generalized to other patient populations.

"Our next steps will involve taking what we have learned and engaging representatives from other communities to find out how we can make [this approach] better and tailor it so that it is embraced by other patient populations," Dr. Cheville said. "We see that as a critical need."

Section 9.3 | Telehealth for Chronic Conditions

This section includes text excerpted from "Introduction to Telehealth for Chronic Conditions," U.S. Department of Health and Human Services (HHS), March 25, 2022.

CHRONIC HEALTH CONDITIONS AND TELEHEALTH

More than half of Americans have been diagnosed with at least one chronic health condition, according to the Centers for Disease Control and Prevention (CDC). Chronic diseases are the leading

Virtual Health-Care Services

cause of death and disability and are also responsible for driving the cost of health care.

The severity and even the occurrence of chronic health conditions can often be mitigated by telehealth-care services.

There are many common chronic conditions that can be treated and managed, in part, through telehealth.

Asthma

Getting a patient's asthma under control is a top priority, but it can often require multiple appointments to check symptoms, tweak medications, and test breathing levels. This can be difficult for patients to manage if they live a long distance from a doctor's office or clinic. Some patients also cannot afford to travel, take time off work, or find childcare. Telehealth can help.

There are several ways telehealth providers can help a patient control their asthma to avoid hospitalizations or life-threatening events.

- Remote patient monitoring (RPM) with devices, such as a pulse oximeter and a peak flow meter
- Follow-up appointments to discuss medication, review asthma diaries, or order new medication
- Messaging through a secure patient portal for topics, such as nebulizer use questions, identifying triggers, or questions about dosages

Diabetes

More than 37 million Americans have diabetes, according to the Centers for Disease Control and Prevention (CDC), and most of them have type 2 diabetes.

Prevention is key to treating patients, as well as the promotion of a healthy lifestyle, both of which can be done via telehealth appointments. For patients with type 1 or type 2 diabetes, doctors can also use telehealth to monitor blood sugar and insulin levels. Here are a few ways to manage diabetes via telehealth:

- Diet and nutrition counseling
- Weight loss and exercise counseling

Health Technology Sourcebook, Third Edition

- Remote patient monitoring with blood glucose devices
- Secure patient messaging to check in on progress
- Remote orders and evaluation of diagnostic testing and blood work

Long-Haul COVID-19

Researchers are still studying the cause, effects, risk factors, and treatment of long-haul COVID-19, known officially as "post-acute sequelae of SARS-CoV-2" (PASC). Post-COVID-19 symptoms typically appear 3–4 weeks following COVID-19 infection. Long-haul COVID-19 can affect anyone who was infected, even those who had mild symptoms or no symptoms at all.

Telehealth providers can be on the lookout for these symptoms of long-haul COVID-19:

- Difficulty breathing or shortness of breath
- Fatigue or lightheadedness
- Symptoms that get worse after physical or mental activities
- Difficulty thinking or concentrating (sometimes referred to as "brain fog")
- Cough
- Pain in the stomach, chest, joints, or muscles
- Heart palpitations
- Headache
- Pins-and-needles feeling
- Diarrhea
- Sleep problems
- Fever
- Rash
- Mood changes
- Change in smell or taste
- Changes in menstrual cycles

Telehealth providers may choose to follow up with long-haul COVID-19 patients more frequently. Telehealth treatment options may also include:

- Referral to a specialist
- Prescription medication for certain symptoms, such as cough, headache, stomachache, or trouble sleeping

Virtual Health-Care Services

- Orders for diagnostic testing or evaluation for chest pain, heart palpitations, difficulty breathing, and dizziness

Obesity

More than 42 million Americans are considered obese, according to the CDC, and are at increased risk for heart disease, type 2 diabetes, certain cancers, and premature death. Talking to patients about their weight can be a sensitive but necessary conversation.

Using telehealth to manage and treat obesity can help patients feel more comfortable tackling their health challenges from the comfort of their own homes. Telehealth treatment options may include:

- RPM using a digital scale that sends automated results
- Counseling with a registered dietician
- At-home exercise plans
- Mental health counseling and/or online support groups
- Secure messaging to share food or exercise diaries and progress updates

Other Conditions

There are many other chronic medical conditions that can be at least partially treated or managed with telehealth, including:

- High blood pressure (HBP)
- Certain cardiovascular diseases (CVDs)
- Respiratory conditions
- Human immunodeficiency virus (HIV)
- End-stage renal disease (ESRD)
- Dermatological conditions
- Rheumatological conditions
- Mental health conditions
- Parkinson disease (PD)
- Certain cancers
- Migraine
- Oral health

Benefits of Managing Chronic Conditions with Telehealth

Telehealth is not a substitute for in-person care of chronic health conditions, but it is an important tool in providing consistent, convenient care for patients who need ongoing medical attention.

There are several telehealth benefits for patients, including:

- Access to more preventative care for rural or low-economic patients
- More access to specialists and subspecialists
- Increased comfort and convenience for patients who have mobility or pain issues
- Increased confidence for patients who may feel embarrassed to be often seen in person for their chronic conditions

Cost Savings with Telehealth Programs

Telehealth for chronic conditions saves money for patients and health-care providers. It also reduces strain on the overall health-care industry.

Cost savings for patients include:

- Lower costs in travel, childcare, and time off work for routine follow-up appointments
- Fewer hospitalizations and emergency room (ER) visits
- The potential for less medication if their chronic disease is more under control or even eliminated through routine telehealth care and monitoring

Cost savings for health-care providers include:

- Fewer in-person appointments, which means fewer in-house resources and expenses
- Fewer missed appointments because patients cannot travel or find childcare
- The ability to see more patients because there is not as much turnaround time in exam rooms
- Less need for late office hours to accommodate patients who work during normal business hours

Virtual Health-Care Services

MANAGING CHRONIC CONDITIONS THROUGH TELEHEALTH

Telehealth treatment options are vast, but they vary depending on the condition and the patient's needs and abilities.

There are some instances where patients will need in-person office appointments. Examples include:

- Examination of surgical incisions or permanent ports
- Certain diagnostic or imaging tests, such as biopsies or cardiac imaging
- Suspected infection
- Acute illness or the inability to control the chronic condition through telehealth

Improvements to technology mean there are a lot more options for telehealth care that will benefit both patients and their providers. Patients are more likely to follow their treatment and management plan with routine telehealth follow-ups, which gives providers a better look at the patient's health and well-being.

More frequent check-ins through telehealth, and the possibility of remote patient monitoring, can also help providers catch any complications faster. It could lead to fewer hospitalizations and ER visits.

Make an Emergency Plan

Creating a plan for emergency care is necessary when treating chronically ill patients with telehealth. You may notice that your patient's remote monitoring devices are picking up alarming data or that the symptoms they are describing sound like a life-threatening event.

Keep an emergency plan in the patient's file that includes the following information:

- The patient's phone number and street address for emergency officials
- The names and numbers of family or close friends of the patient
- The closest hospital or medical facility and the number of air transport helicopters
- An up-to-date list of the patient's medications and allergies

Telehealth Video Appointments to Manage Chronic Conditions

Video appointments between providers and patients are the most common type of telehealth. This digital type of "face-to-face" lets providers see any outwardly physical symptoms. And patients can be comforted by seeing their provider and being able to ask questions.

There are several ways telehealth video appointments can be used to treat and manage chronic conditions, including:

- Follow-up appointments to see how a patient is doing on a new diet, medications, or other modification
- Telebehavioral care and therapy
- Routine check-ins for patients with certain cancers, rheumatological diseases, diabetes, and migraines
- Explanation of test or imaging results
- Explanation of how patients use remote monitoring devices
- Nutrition and fitness counseling

Provider-to-Provider Telehealth

Providers can also use telehealth to collaborate with other providers involved in the patient's care. This could be done via video chat, phone conversations, or asynchronous communication. Providers can also use telehealth with other providers for tele-mentoring new, updated, or complex topics.

The benefits include:

- Collaboration between a patient's local primary care doctor and a specialist that could be in another city, state, or region
- Reduced strain on local providers, especially if they are located in a rural area or a busy urban area with too few providers for their patient load
- The ability for consultations on patient imaging, diagnostic tests, or lab work
- Collaboration between small, local health centers and larger hospitals and universities

Virtual Health-Care Services

Asynchronous Telehealth Care to Reduce Patient Visits

Patients and providers can share important information without having to set up an appointment. This could include a patient filling out a form to gauge their symptom progression or improvement. It could be messaging updates through a secure portal. The ability to communicate asynchronously with a patient saves time and resources for your practice with fewer phone calls, less paper filing, and fewer appointments to schedule.

Examples of asynchronous telehealth care for chronic conditions include:

- Respiratory-compromised patients sending regular peak flow meter results
- Patients with neurological or rheumatological conditions sending back forms that keep track of symptoms and their severity
- Text messaging with chronically ill patients who do not have access to broadband Internet
- Sending x-ray images or lab results through a secure messaging portal
- Patients uploading their food logs if on a specific dietary plan

Remote Patient Monitoring to Keep Track of Symptoms and Vital Signs

Advancements in technology allow providers and patients the flexibility to monitor their chronic conditions without routine trips to the office. Certain remote patient monitoring is also now covered by Medicare, Medicaid, and many private insurers.

There are guidelines, however, for Medicare coverage. Devices must be FDA-approved, and they must be able to automatically transmit data and information to the provider without patient interference.

Many serious chronic illnesses require frequent testing and monitoring to keep the patient stable and feeling well. RPM options for chronically ill patients include:

- Blood sugar levels for diabetes management
- Blood pressure for cardiac patients

Health Technology Sourcebook, Third Edition

- Pulse oximeter readings for patients with respiratory illnesses
- Weight scales for patients being treated for obesity

Specialist Telehealth Appointments to Improve and Manage Chronic Conditions

Patients living with chronic conditions often benefit from evaluations, treatment, and care from providers who specialize in that area of medicine. But there may be several barriers to access for millions of Americans.

Rural or underserved areas may not have the medical facilities or teaching hospitals that attract certain specialists or subspecialists. Some patients may not be able to afford the time off work, gas, or childcare needed to travel to see a specialist. Specialists may also not be covered by the patient's insurance plan.

Telehealth can help remove some or all of those barriers.

- Patients can find a specialist who will work with the underinsured or uninsured.
- Specialists who use telehealth can see patients who may live more than an hour away.
- Specialists can see patients over telehealth and then work with the patient's local doctor to manage care and treatment of the condition.
- Specialists can order remote patient monitoring and make recommendations to local physicians based on their findings.

Section 9.4 | Telehealth for COVID-19

This section includes text excerpted from "Telehealth and COVID-19," U.S. Department of Health and Human Services (HHS), July 27, 2022.

It is important to protect yourself and your health-care provider during the COVID-19 public health emergency. Telehealth can help you get access to your provider without spreading or getting COVID-19.

Virtual Health-Care Services

IF YOU ARE INTERESTED IN THE COVID-19 VACCINE

The COVID-19 vaccine is the best way to protect yourself and others from getting the virus. Use these resources if you have questions about the COVID-19 vaccine, where to get one, or how to make an appointment.

- Talk to your health-care provider.
- Have you already received a COVID-19 vaccine? If it has been at least six months since you received your final dose that means you are eligible for a vaccine booster, which can give you additional protection.

Tip: The COVID-19 vaccine is free of charge to everyone regardless of income, immigration, or health insurance status. Health-care providers' office visit fees may still apply.

IF YOU ARE WORRIED THAT YOU HAVE COVID-19

It is extremely important that you self-isolate if you think you may have COVID-19 or have been exposed. Self-isolation means staying home from work or school and distancing yourself from friends and family, even the people who live in your home.

Follow the steps provided below to get the care you need.

Start by Using a COVID-19 Self-Assessment Tool

Use an online COVID-19 self-assessment tool before you contact your health-care provider. This protects everyone's health and safety and reduces the burden on the health-care system.

This self-assessment tool was developed based on information from the Centers for Disease Control and Prevention (CDC).

A self-assessment tool will ask you a few questions about the following:

- Symptoms you have
- Whether you have been in close physical contact with someone who has been diagnosed with COVID-19
- Whether you live in a community where many people have been diagnosed with COVID-19
- Any medical conditions that put you at high risk for complications if you get COVID-19

Know Your Telehealth Options

Many health-care providers now provide telemedicine services. Contact your provider or health insurance company to ask about your options.

There are also health centers and on-demand telehealth services available to everyone, including people who do not have health insurance.

Before You Meet with Your Health-Care Provider Online

Your health-care provider will need several important pieces of information when you schedule a telemedicine visit to discuss COVID-19. Consider writing down this information before your virtual visit:

- **Your symptoms.** What they are and when they started.
- **Your health.** Any other health conditions you have and how you have been managing them during the pandemic.
- **Exposure to COVID-19.** If you have definitely been exposed, how, and when.
- **Your questions.** If there is anything specific you want to know about your health or the health of other people in your home.

IF YOU HAVE COVID-19 SYMPTOMS FOUR OR MORE WEEKS AFTER INFECTION

Some COVID-19 patients continue to have symptoms four or more weeks after they are diagnosed. They have what is called "long COVID" or "post-acute sequelae of SARS-CoV-2 infection" (PASC). Even people who did not have symptoms in the first days or weeks after they were infected can have a post-COVID-19 condition.

Post-COVID-19 health symptoms include:

- Tiredness or fatigue
- Difficulty concentrating or "brain fog"
- Headache
- Loss of smell or taste

Virtual Health-Care Services

- Dizziness on standing
- Fast-beating or pounding heart
- Chest pain
- Difficulty breathing or shortness of breath
- Cough
- Joint or muscle pain
- Depression or anxiety
- Fever
- Symptoms that get worse after physical or mental activities

How Telehealth Helps People with Long-Haul COVID-19

Telehealth can help you get the care and monitoring you need without having to leave the comfort of your own home.

The following are a few among several ways you may be able to receive care for long-term COVID-19 symptoms:

- Talk to your health-care provider about telehealth options for follow-up care after leaving the hospital or their office.
- Use remote patient monitoring (RPM) devices so your health-care provider can check on you at home. For example, these devices might check your blood sugar or blood pressure.
- Get support for specialty care faster via telehealth than waiting to see a health-care provider in person.
- Meet with your health-care provider during a telehealth appointment to discuss lab test results to clearly understand how your symptoms are affecting your body.
- Take time during your telehealth appointment to ask your health-care provider about medications or treatments that can help manage your symptoms.
- Use telehealth as a bridge between your in-person appointments. While telehealth is a convenient way to access fast, quality health care, your health-care provider may want to examine you in person from time to time.

IF YOU HAVE A HEALTH ISSUE THAT IS NOT RELATED TO COVID-19

It is important to take care of yourself, especially during a pandemic. Stress and anxiety can make other health problems even harder to manage.

Do not ignore health concerns. Contact your health-care provider for their advice.

Section 9.5 | Telehealth for HIV Care

This section includes text excerpted from "Introduction to Telehealth for HIV Care," U.S. Department of Health and Human Services (HHS), March 25, 2022.

Regular appointment attendance can help patients with human immunodeficiency virus (HIV) slow the progression of the disease, reduce the risk of transmission, and improve health outcomes.

But factors such as time and transportation challenges, the stigma surrounding HIV, and a shortage of HIV care providers can make following a care plan difficult.

Incorporating telehealth into a primary care practice can overcome these barriers by giving patients a safe and convenient way to access HIV prevention and care services.

TYPES OF HIV AND TELEHEALTH
Telehealth and HIV Diagnosis

Testing for HIV is a necessary first step in any patient's care plan and can be completed without an in-person visit.

SCREENING FOR HIV WITH TELEHEALTH

Any patient aged 15–65 should be screened for HIV risk during a telehealth appointment. These risk factors can help you identify potential untreated infections and prevent future transmission.

If a patient answers "yes" to any of the following questions, it is strongly recommended that they take an HIV test:
- Have you or your sexual partner(s) had other sexual partners in the past year?

Virtual Health-Care Services

- Have you ever had a sexually transmitted infection?
- Are you pregnant or considering becoming pregnant?
- Have you or your sexual partner(s) injected drugs or other substances and/or shared needles with another person?
- Have you ever had sex with a male partner who has had sex with another male?
- Have you ever had sex with a person who is HIV infected?
- Have you ever been paid for sex and/or had sex with a sex worker?
- Have you engaged in behavior resulting in blood-to-blood contact?
- Have you or your sexual partner(s) received a blood transfusion or blood products before 1985?
- Have you been the victim of rape, date rape, or sexual abuse?

HIV SELF-TESTING

There are two HIV self-testing options. These self-tests are covered by most insurance plans, and you can order them during a tele-health appointment.

A rapid self-test requires the user to swab an absorbent pad around the outer gums near the teeth. This test can produce results within 20 minutes.

Mail-in self-tests come with a collection kit containing supplies to collect a blood sample from a fingerstick. After the sample has been sent to a lab for testing, the results are delivered by the organization that produces the kit.

If a patient's rapid self-test returns a positive result, you should strongly recommend that they get retested to confirm their positive status. Mail-in self-tests are tested twice in a lab to confirm a positive sample.

If a patient has a confirmed positive test result, it is important to start their care plan as soon as possible.

Ensuring Access to HIV Self-Testing

If your practice cannot offer HIV self-testing, your patients can still get tested for little or no cost. The Center for Disease Control and Prevention (CDC; gettested.cdc.gov) offers services that connect users with testing resources in their area.

PREPARING PATIENTS FOR HIV TELEHEALTH TREATMENT

Receiving an HIV diagnosis can be a traumatic experience.

Telehealth support groups and counseling can reduce that mental burden, keep patients on track with their treatment plans, and allow them to receive care from the comfort of their own safe space.

Contact your local health department to find mental health professionals in your area who specialize in virtual HIV care.

Treating HIV through Telehealth

A comprehensive, telehealth-based approach to HIV treatment can help your patients with HIV live longer, healthier lives.

ANTIRETROVIRAL THERAPY

During telehealth appointments, signing off on multimonth antiretroviral therapy (ART) prescription refills ensures patients have short- and long-term access to the drugs they need and can sustain viral suppression.

Medication adherence is especially important during the first weeks of therapy, and current HIV treatment guidelines (clinicalinfo.hiv.gov/en/guidelines/hiv-clinical-guidelines-adult-and-adolescent-arv/adolescents-and-young-adults-hiv?view=full) recommend telehealth as an approach to support medication adherence then and during all phases of treatment.

If your patient struggles with access to ART, the Ryan White HIV/AIDS Program's AIDS Drug Assistance Program (ryanwhite.hrsa.gov/about/parts-and-initiatives/part-b-adap) provides FDA-approved medications to low-income people living with HIV who have limited or no health coverage from private insurance, Medicaid, or Medicare.

Virtual Health-Care Services

LAB TESTING

Current HIV treatment guidelines (clinicalinfo.hiv.gov/en/guidelines) recommend that most people with HIV undergo lab testing to measure viral load and CD4 levels every six months. While these tests cannot be completed virtually, you can use telehealth to order tests and coordinate appointments with your patients.

Many clinical laboratories (www.ahrq.gov/sites/default/files/wysiwyg/professionals/quality-patient-safety/quality-resources/tools/lab-testiing/lab-testing-toolkit.pdf) have integrated telehealth into their practice. If there is a lab that you work with regularly, contact them to coordinate online appointment scheduling.

TELEMENTORING

An effective telehealth HIV treatment program requires more than medication adherence. Patients need to be supported in a variety of ways.

During telementoring sessions, primary care providers collaborate with multidisciplinary specialists around individual patient cases, a format known as "case-based learning."

These live videoconference sessions serve patients by training primary care physicians on the necessary skills to provide HIV care and helping manage the complexities often associated with HIV care, including tailoring treatment to high-risk populations. Studies show improved clinical outcomes among people with HIV, including adherence to ART, when clinicians with HIV experience and training through telementoring provide care.

Preventing HIV with Telehealth

Using telehealth proactively can help prevent the spread of HIV, protecting your patients and your community.

PREP AND PEP

Pre-exposure prophylaxis (PrEP) is a medication for people who are HIV-negative and at high risk for exposure through sexual contact or injection drug use. When someone is exposed to HIV

Health Technology Sourcebook, Third Edition

through sex or injection drug use, these medicines can work to keep the virus from establishing an infection.

Post-exposure prophylaxis (PEP) refers to the use of antiretroviral drugs for people who are HIV-negative after a single high-risk exposure to stop a potential infection. PEP must be started as soon as possible to be effective—always within 72 hours of possible exposure—and continued for four weeks.

INTEGRATING TELEPREP INTO YOUR PRACTICE

Making PrEP and PEP delivery part of your telehealth practice (also known as "TelePrEP") can be beneficial for both you and your patients.

Several core activities of PrEP/PEP delivery, such as assessing the risk for HIV, counseling about the risks and benefits of the medication, and evaluating adherence, can be completed through telemedicine.

Plus, TelePrEP may increase PrEP and PEP access for people who live far from clinics or otherwise face transportation or schedule challenges. TelePrEP may also help overcome confidentiality concerns or stigma that prevent some people from seeking PrEP care in person.

Responding to HIV with Telehealth

Responding to HIV with telehealth requires a community-wide effort.

CULTURAL HUMILITY TRAINING

Providers and staff need to acknowledge the unique elements of every patient's identity to give them the best HIV telehealth care possible.

Cultural humility training helps combat stigma and misinformation related to HIV. By fully understanding the complexity of a patient's daily life, you can support them in ways that help them follow their HIV treatment plan.

Contact your local health department to find cultural humility training resources in your area.

Virtual Health-Care Services

Section 9.6 | Telehealth for Maternal Health Services

This section includes text excerpted from "Introduction to Telehealth for Maternal Health Services," U.S. Department of Health and Human Services (HHS), April 12, 2022.

Maternal health care is critical for the long-term health and success of parents and children. Health equity in maternal care has long been a struggle, especially for those in rural and underserved communities. Telehealth is one way to bridge those gaps.

This section will highlight the types and procedures for a successful maternal telehealth program.

The United States offers some of the most advanced medical technologies in the world. But its maternal morbidity rate still lags far behind other high-income countries.

According to the Centers for Disease Control and Prevention (CDC), the current maternal mortality rate is 17.4 deaths per 100,000 live births, and Black mothers are 2.5 times more likely to die from pregnancy or childbirth causes than White women. Overall, more than 65 percent of pregnancy-related deaths are preventable.

Additionally, pregnant patients are at higher risk of maternal mortality from COVID-19 infection during pregnancy. Complications associated with a COVID-19 infection during pregnancy include more severe forms of COVID-19, preterm birth, and transmission of COVID-19 to newborns.

PREPARING PATIENTS AND PROVIDERS FOR MATERNAL TELEHEALTH

Preparation is key, both for health-care providers who are new to maternal telehealth visits and for patients who are participating in telehealth care.

Health-Care Provider Preparation

There are several ways health-care providers and staff can make sure telehealth visits are successful for them and their patients.

111

Health Technology Sourcebook, Third Edition

HEALTH EQUITY TRAINING

- **Encourage health-care providers and staff members to take online training in health equity.** This will help provide the best quality care to the patients who need it the most. The populations most underserved when it comes to maternal health equity include:
  - Black women and other patients of color
  - LGBTQ+ patients
  - Low-income patients
  - Underinsured or uninsured patients
- **Book longer appointments for new patients and new parents.** This extra time is critical for patients who may be new to telehealth or for patients with connectivity or privacy issues. The extra time will help them fully understand their maternal telehealth-care plan and give them the opportunity to ask questions.

HAVE AN EMERGENCY PLAN IN PLACE

Pregnancy and postpartum complications can sometimes be severe, even life-threatening for the mother and the baby.

- **Set up an emergency plan with each telehealth patient and keep it in their file.** The emergency plan could include the following:
  - The patient's closest emergency contact and phone number
  - The patient's phone number and address in an easily accessible location if you need to call emergency medical personnel
  - The closest hospital or medical facility that can handle a maternal health emergency
- **Be flexible with your health-care provider and patient communication methods.** Many pregnant families may not always have access to reliable and stable Internet connections. This affects the very people who could benefit the most from health equity using

112

Virtual Health-Care Services

maternal telehealth care. Other forms of nonvideo communication could include:
- Phone calls
- E-mail
- Chat through a health-care portal
- **Keep up-to-date electronic health records (EHRs) and read them**. Pregnancy and maternal health care can be sensitive issues for many patients. Give yourself time to read the patient's EHR before each appointment. This will help you treat your telehealth patients who are dealing with sensitive issues, such as:
  - Miscarriage
  - Pregnancy from rape
  - Potential or known birth defects
  - Pregnancy or infant loss
  - Planned adoption
  - Fertility issues

Be prepared with follow-up plans after the appointment. Let your patient know what will come next in their maternal tele-health-care plan. Take time to answer questions and ensure they understand their next steps. You will also need to consider what staffing you will need to handle follow-up planning and instructions. Choose a nurse or staff member who will join the call to go over instructions and the next steps. You may also want a member of the front desk staff to call and book the follow-up appointment. While some follow-up plans will need to be done in person, there are several ways you can continue to provide maternal telehealth care, such as:
- **Order lab or diagnostics tests**. Set up a telehealth appointment to discuss the results.
- **Start or continue remote monitoring**. Remote patient monitoring services provide easier access to care for rural and underserved pregnant women.
- **Provide health-care references**. Refer your patient for other types of telehealth care, including lactation support or tele-behavioral health.

Health Technology Sourcebook, Third Edition

Preparation for Your Patients

Your patients will need some time to prepare for their maternal telehealth appointments, whether it is their first time or a follow-up visit.

BEFORE THE TELEHEALTH APPOINTMENT

There are several things you can do prior to your patient appointments to make sure they feel comfortable, including:

- Confirm your patient has access to the Internet. If not, share resources with them and/or consider other forms of telehealth communication.
- Ask them to write down their concerns ahead of time.
- Ask if they need assistive devices for the telehealth appointment.
- Ask that they wear loose clothing in case you need to see parts of their body.
- Make sure they receive and understand the instructions on how to get online.

DURING THE TELEHEALTH APPOINTMENT

There are also several ways to help your patient feel comfortable and confident during the appointment, including:

- Introduce yourself and ask if the patient has privacy and feels safe to speak.
- Ask what questions or concerns they may have.
- Make sure they understand the test results or diagnoses that you are giving them.
- Include the patient's spouse, partner, or other family members in the discussion if the patient includes them in the video chat.
- Follow up on remote monitoring results or concerns.
- Provide information on the Women, Infants, and Children (WIC) program or Medicaid, if needed.
- Encourage patients to get a COVID-19 vaccine and educate them on the safety of the vaccine during and after pregnancy.

Virtual Health-Care Services

AFTER THE TELEHEALTH APPOINTMENT

Maternal telehealth care does not end when your video chat is finished. Here are a few ways to follow up with your patient and continue building the relationship:

- Send your patient instructions on what to do if they go into labor or experience preterm bleeding or contractions.
- Follow up with links or mail handouts on prenatal and postpartum local, state, and federal resources.
- Schedule any testing or diagnostic imaging as soon as possible.
- Send your patients for referrals to specialists, mental health professionals, or substance abuse counselors, if needed.
- Schedule any follow-up maternal telehealth appointments.

TYPES OF MATERNAL TELEHEALTH
Telehealth and High-Risk Pregnancy

High-risk pregnancies can be treated and managed through telehealth as long as the patient and health-care provider have an emergency plan in place.

Telehealth can provide life-saving health care for pregnant patients. Some rural patients live far from high-risk specialists. Others cannot afford to take time off work or find childcare to go to the doctor's office.

There are several ways to ensure quality telehealth care for high-risk patients.

USE REMOTE PATIENT MONITORING

There are several devices that can monitor a patient's health without the patient having to come into the office for multiple checkups. Remote patient monitoring can also be used to gauge whether a patient has breached the high-risk threshold, meaning it is time to seek immediate medical care.

Pregnancy-related remote monitoring devices may include:
- Blood pressure monitors
- Blood glucose testing
- At-home fetal monitors

KNOW WHEN TO SEEK IN-PERSON CARE

Part of your telehealth workflow should include a protocol for when to send a high-risk patient to the office or hospital. Some high-risk conditions, including multiples and certain chronic conditions, need more in-person oversight than telehealth can provide.

Patients should be sent to in-person care when:
- There is decreased fetal movement.
- There are known fetal abnormalities that require multiple checkups.
- The patient is experiencing severe preeclampsia symptoms.
- The patient is experiencing signs of early labor.

PARTNER WITH LOCAL RESOURCES FOR RURAL AND UNDERSERVED PATIENTS

Telehealth can be a life-saving resource and also the first line of defense for potential pregnancy complications. This is especially true for rural and underserved patients who may delay, or entirely forgo, prenatal care.

High-risk care tends to be more hands-on than complication-free maternal health care. But there are many ways telehealth providers can make sure rural and underserved patients get the care they need when they need it.
- **Identify and partner with the patient's local clinic or hospital**. Local facilities can often provide routine testing that will help you determine the best course of care and keep an eye on potentially serious complications. This could include:
  - Baseline 24 urine collection and labs for preeclampsia

Virtual Health-Care Services

- STI panels
- Ultrasound
- COVID-19 testing and treatment
- **Work with local obstetrics and gynecologists (OB-GYNs) for in-person appointments.** Underserved patients may often feel more comfortable with health-care providers that are not local to their area. This is especially true for Black patients who have reported feeling unheard or mistreated by non-Black physicians. Telehealth providers can also help non-English speaking patients understand their local, in-person care, and birth plan if they share a native language. In these cases, telehealth providers can partner with local OB-GYNs for in-person testing and exams while still continuing monitoring and management via telehealth.
- **Research local resources and online help post-childbirth.** Rural and underserved mothers do not stop needing maternal telehealth care once the baby is born. Telehealth providers can help in those first few days and weeks with telehealth lactation consulting and mental health counseling. Other potential resources following high-risk pregnancies could include:
  - Maternal or pediatric specialists, local and online
  - Substance abuse counseling
  - Smoking cessation
  - Parenting classes

TELEHEALTH AND POSTPARTUM CARE

Your maternal telehealth program can still play an important role in the care and health of your patients even after they give birth. Patients from rural or underserved communities may have an even harder time getting to in-person appointments after childbirth.

Barriers to postpartum care could include:
- The cost associated with travel, parking, or the cost of gas

Health Technology Sourcebook, Third Edition

- Long driving distances between home and the doctor's office
- Not being able to drive for a period after childbirth per doctor's instructions
- Lack of childcare for the new baby or older siblings
- Lack of maternity leave for patients who have to begin work as soon as possible after childbirth

Postpartum Telehealth Services

In-person appointments will be necessary in some postpartum cases. In-person visits will check surgical incision sites or for hands-on lactation support.

But there are still many ways to care for postpartum patients with telehealth. A list of potential services includes:

- General health check-in to see how the patient is doing after childbirth
- Lactation support
- Screening and treatment for postpartum depression
- Therapy appointments with telehealth
- Referrals to specialists, including substance abuse programs
- Birth control counseling and prescriptions

Section 9.7 | Telehealth for Children with Special Health-Care Needs

This section includes text excerpted from "Telehealth for Families of Children with Special Health Care Needs," U.S. Department of Health and Human Services (HHS), January 5, 2022.

Health care for a child with complex medical needs can be improved through telehealth. Virtual visits give your child the same level of care with less exposure to doctors' offices and hospitals. It means less stress, less time away from home, and fewer germs. Telehealth allows you and your child to focus on their health-care needs from the comfort of your own home.

118

Virtual Health-Care Services

TELEHEALTH AND FAMILY-CENTERED CARE

Family-centered care focuses on collaboration between health-care professionals and families. This approach benefits many families, but especially those with children who have special health-care needs.

The combination of telehealth visits and family-centered care can greatly improve your family's health-care experience:

You and your child may feel more relaxed attending virtual visits from your own home. Doctor's offices can be distracting and stressful for children. This means less focus on the conversation with the doctor. Children with special health-care needs will likely feel more comfortable in familiar surroundings.

You can have more quality one-on-one time with your child's doctor. Your child may not need to attend every virtual visit. You can use these child-free virtual visits to discuss sensitive topics you may not want your child to hear. You can also take time to discuss your child's emotional and social needs.

Virtual visits fit into your schedule. Families with children who have special health-care needs often juggle many appointments every week. This could include doctor's visits, meetings at school, and therapy sessions. Choosing virtual visits means less time driving back and forth. They also cut down on germ exposure for children who are medically fragile.

WHAT TO EXPECT DURING YOUR CHILD'S TELEHEALTH EXAM

The doctor will examine your child a bit differently over telehealth than in person. Your child will still get quality health care through a virtual visit.

Family-centered care means you should feel like an equal partner in your child's health care. During the virtual visit, you should feel free to share your opinions, concerns, and questions.

- You may want to write down important thoughts before the visit.
- Keep a pen and a piece of paper handy to write down notes from the doctor.
- Ask the doctor to explain anything you or your child may not fully understand.

The doctor will ask about your child's general health and medications. You can prepare this information ahead of the virtual visit. Likely topics include:

- Your child's approximate weight and height
- Your child's current medications and dosages, including supplements
- Any medical diagnoses
- Allergies, including food and medication
- Any recent illnesses, hospitalizations, or surgeries
- Social and emotional health

Tip: Dress your child in loose clothing that is easy to move around. This is helpful if the doctor asks to see their skin or a certain part of the body. Clothing that works best includes short sleeves or a jacket that can be easily unzipped, shorts, or pull-on pants.

The doctor should address your child directly during the virtual visit. Your child deserves to be a part of their own health care. There are ways for your child to participate, even if it is difficult for them to communicate, including:

- The doctor should make eye contact with your child and address them by name.
- The doctor should include your child in the conversation, even if your child cannot make medical decisions.
- Some pediatric doctors use toys, stuffed animals, or drawings to engage your child.

Your child's doctor should discuss the next steps before you end the virtual visit. Ask for more information if you are unclear about what you need to do before your next visit. The next steps could include the following:

- Scheduling a follow-up visit, either virtual or in-person
- Lab testing or blood work
- Referral to another doctor, specialist, or therapist
- Change of medication
- A plan to address behavior, emotional regulation, or social interactions

Virtual Health-Care Services

HOW TO SUPPORT YOUR CHILD DURING A VIRTUAL VISIT

Every child reacts to a doctor's visits a little differently. Virtual visits are no exception. It is very common for your child to feel excited, nervous, scared, or even bored.

There are many ways you can help your child feel comfortable during a virtual visit.

Practice the visit ahead of time. You could use another video-conferencing platform, such as Zoom, FaceTime, Skype, or Google Hangouts. Role-play with your child and take turns playing the role of the doctor.

Ask your child what questions they have about the virtual visit. Give them any answers you may have and write down the rest for the doctor to answer.

Attend the virtual visit in a place that is comfortable for your child. This could be their bedroom, the kitchen, their playroom, or a quiet room at school.

Remove distractions for the virtual visit. This includes:

- Other people, including siblings
- Pets
- Electronics you are not using to communicate with the doctor
- Toys that make noise

A comfort item may be helpful for your child during the virtual visit. The comfort item should be small and quiet. A favorite blanket, stuffed animal, or doll is a good option.

Guide your child to participate in the virtual visit, if possible. Help your child advocate for themselves.

- Encourage them to ask questions.
- Pause to ask how they feel during the visit.
- If they feel shy or are nonverbal, encourage your child to give a thumbs-up or thumbs-down or a nod of their head, if possible.

Health Technology Sourcebook, Third Edition

Section 9.8 | **School-Based Telehealth Services**

This section includes text excerpted from "Introduction to School-Based Telehealth," U.S. Department of Health and Human Services (HHS), September 17, 2021.

School-based telehealth improves and expands a student's ability to access doctors and other caregivers. Increased access to health care helps students stay or become healthy and focus on learning. Examples of school-based telehealth appointments include:

- Students seeing a doctor for annual appointments
- Students seeing a doctor to monitor conditions, such as diabetes or asthma
- Students getting behavioral health care to help them focus on learning

Telehealth provides many benefits to student patients, including:

- **Improved access to and availability of different types of care.** Students who are already attending school will have easy access to doctors, including specialists.
- **Reduced time away from class.** Students can attend telehealth appointments in the school environment and quickly return to class.
- **Reduced time and travel costs for the parent or guardian.** Patients will have to travel to their doctor's office less frequently.

PRIMARY CARE APPOINTMENTS

Primary care doctors are the "front door" to health care. They manage a patient's care, physical examinations, and nonemergency injury or illness. They also send patients to specialists as needed.

Primary Care Physician School-Based Telehealth Benefits

- Annual physicals can be conducted in the school, so they are not a barrier to school enrollment.
- Patients can be seen immediately for things such as strep throat or ear infections, so care is not put off or ignored.
- Doctors can treat minor injuries before they get worse.

Virtual Health-Care Services

More Health-Care Services for School-Based Telehealth
- Schools can provide care for chronic health problems such as asthma.
- Schools can provide annual screening for eyesight, hearing, and other assessments.
  - Parents or guardians have been responsible for following up on the results of this testing. School-based telehealth can reduce this burden on the parents or guardians.
- Schools can provide expanded telehealth-based speech and occupational therapy to students.
  - These programs can be expanded to include additional doctors or other specialists, such as therapists, who are not available in the school or community.
- Schools can provide healthy living programs for students, such as healthy eating, activity, and weight programs.

BEHAVIORAL HEALTH APPOINTMENTS
School-based behavioral health care can help students who would not have access to behavioral health services otherwise. This can be due to the following:
- Absence of behavioral health doctor in the area
- Parents or guardians who do not always recognize that their children are having trouble

Behavioral Health School-Based Telehealth Benefits
- School-based telehealth makes regular appointments needed for behavioral health care possible.
- Teachers may notice behavior at school that parents or guardians may not see and recommend a telehealth appointment.
- Students can address behaviors in school-based telehealth appointments that could otherwise result in detention or other disciplinary action.
- Students have almost immediate access to behavioral health care in a crisis, such as threatening suicide.

Health Technology Sourcebook, Third Edition

- Behavioral health doctors and counselors are trained to recognize symptoms of suicidal thoughts and addiction. The sooner a doctor or counselor helps, the more likely the patient will receive the care they need.
- Doctors and counselors can suggest different treatments or recommend a specialist to help.
- School-based behavioral health appointments are private. Most people, including other students and teachers, will not know that patients are having a behavioral health appointment or some other type of telehealth appointment.

DIABETES CARE APPOINTMENTS

Diabetes care requires frequent communication between doctor and patient. Patients need to share important information, such as glucose levels, diet, and physical activity. Telehealth tools reduce travel and make it faster and easier for the patient and doctor to manage the patient's health together.

- Over 10 percent of the people in the United States have diabetes.
- Type 1 diabetes affects about 187,000 student-aged patients.

Patients with Diabetes School-Based Telehealth Benefits

- Almost all students with diabetes need help to manage their diabetes at times. School-based telehealth can help with ongoing diabetes education.
  - Patients learn about insulin, the food they can and cannot eat, and getting exercise.
  - Patients learn about healthy glucose levels and how to keep theirs in the correct range.
  - Patients learn how to check their blood and track their glucose levels.
  - Patients learn the signs of high or low blood glucose and know what to do.

Virtual Health-Care Services

- Proactive diabetes monitoring is when the patient and doctor talk about the patient's progress. School-based telehealth for patients with diabetes allows patients and doctors to monitor a patient's progress.
  - The patient tracks blood glucose, weight, diet, and exercise to share with the doctor.
  - Technology now allows for sharing of glucose monitoring electronically through the patient's glucometer.
  - The doctor can suggest more activity, better foods, or changes to medicine.
  - Most patients stay healthier with regular diabetes monitoring and communication with their health-care provider.
- People with diabetes typically need to see their doctor regularly. School-based telehealth makes it easier and more convenient for patients to get the care they need when they need it.
- Patients with monitored and controlled diabetes often save money by staying healthy and can prevent costly side effects.

Section 9.9 | Use of Telehealth in Emergency Departments

This section includes text excerpted from "Getting Started with Telehealth for Emergency Departments," U.S. Department of Health and Human Services (HHS), February 9, 2021.

Telehealth technology in the emergency department can help expand the quality of care to more people through increased access to medical specialists and protect providers and patients.

Telehealth can help emergency departments:
- Reduce exposure to COVID-19 and keep patients and providers safe.
- Preserve valuable personal protective equipment.
- Expand quality care to rural and underserved areas.

Consider integrating telehealth at key points of interaction:
- Before patients go to the emergency department
- As a triage point upon entering the emergency department
- Once patients are receiving care in the emergency department
- As a collaboration point between providers
- For follow-up care once released and to help prevent unnecessary return visits

Although telehealth technology in the emergency department provides many benefits—especially during public health emergencies—it is not a replacement for in-person care. Make sure to research your options for providing care to understand their impact.

TELE-EMERGENCY CARE

Tele-emergency care typically involves a provider at a spoke hospital connecting with a provider at a hub hospital. The spoke provider interacts with patients, manages the video technology, shares vitals, and executes hands-on procedures. The hub provider may consult on a diagnosis, provide a second opinion, or guide the spoke provider through a complicated procedure.

Benefits of Tele-Emergency Services
- Provide expert care for patients.
- Build confidence by ensuring patients get the best care.
- Deliver care closer to patients' homes.
- Expand the capabilities of the spoke hospital through access to providers with a wider range of experience.
- Initiate care faster by not having to wait for specialists to arrive or patients to be transferred.
- Keep small hospitals in business.

Tele-emergency is especially important during COVID-19 to help decrease the number of patients transferred to larger hospitals that may already be at or above maximum capacity.

Virtual Health-Care Services

VIRTUAL ROUNDS

Providers can use telehealth technology to check on emergency department patients virtually. This helps limit the number of providers who are physically present and exposed to contagious diseases. It also saves time and conserves personal protective equipment.

Virtual rounds typically involve a patient's care team using video technology installed in the patient's room to talk with the patient from another location.

Benefits of Virtual Rounds

- Ability to include the patient's family if they cannot be there in person
- Providing care from multiple specialists during a single exam if needed
- Opportunity to expand participation to pharmacists, care coordinators, students, and other staff to help with documentation

Virtual rounding is especially important during COVID-19 to help:

- Preserve limited personal protective equipment.
- Build trust between patient and provider because it can allow patients to see their provider's face without a protective mask.
- Allow providers who are in self-isolation to continue to provide care.

E-CONSULTS

E-consults, also known as "electronic consultations" or "interprofessional consults," are communications between health-care providers. Providers can use e-consults in the emergency department to get recommendations for complicated conditions from providers in other locations with additional expertise, for example, in specialty areas, such as acute care for stroke, trauma, intensive care unit (ICU), or behavioral health.

Benefits of E-consults

- Increase care coordination.
- Increase access to high-quality, specialty care.
- Accelerate consultation response time.
- Reduce the need for unnecessary referrals.
- Increase provider knowledge by learning from specialty experts.

TELEHEALTH FOR FOLLOW-UP CARE

Telehealth technology can be used for simple follow-up communication for patients who were triaged but not sent to the emergency department or for patients after they are discharged from the emergency department through audio, video, e-mail, text messages, and even chatbots. You may also choose to use remote patient monitoring (RPM) devices. Some RPM devices record patient vitals automatically through a wearable device, while others require patients to report their readings through an online tool or by talking with their provider.

Including follow-up care services in your telehealth program is especially important because patients who do not follow emergency department guidance are more likely to be readmitted, putting them at higher risk of health complications. This can result in increased utilization and cost burden on the emergency department.

Benefits of Telehealth for Follow-Up Care

- Provide an opportunity to further engage with the patient to perform more assessments, talk to family members, ensure they understand their follow-up instructions about medications, and encourage them to schedule any referral appointments.
- Provide additional care to patients who need observation but are not so sick that they need constant care.
- Detect potential problems and treat them before they warrant a return visit to the emergency room.
- Provide emotional support, especially for patients in isolation.

Virtual Health-Care Services

- Provide a training opportunity for resident physicians.
- Reduce hospital costs associated with unnecessary readmissions and CMS penalties for readmission for certain conditions.

Using telehealth for follow-up care is especially important during COVID-19 to help:
- Follow up with lower-acuity COVID-19 patients, allowing them to stay in the comfort of their home and not take up beds or other emergency department resources.
- Encourage patients to stay up-to-date with routine vaccinations and COVID-19 vaccinations.

Part 3 | Health Information Technology

Chapter 10 | Understanding Health Information Technology

Chapter Contents

Section 10.1—Information and Communication
Technology...135
Section 10.2—Benefits of Health Information
Technology...138

Section 10.1 | Information and Communication Technology

This section includes text excerpted from "Health Communication and Health Information Technology," Office of Disease Prevention and Health Promotion (ODPHP), U.S. Department of Health and Human Services (HHS), February 6, 2022.

Ideas about health and behaviors are shaped by the communication, information, and technology that people interact with every day. Health communication and health information technology (health IT) are central to health care, public health, and the way society views health. These processes make up the ways and the context in which professionals and the public search for, understand, and use health information, significantly impacting their health decisions and actions.

The objectives in this topic area describe many ways health communication and health IT can have a positive impact on health, health care, and health equity. They include:

- Supporting shared decision-making between patients and providers.
- Providing personalized self-management tools and resources.
- Building social support networks.
- Delivering accurate, accessible, and actionable health information that is targeted or tailored.
- Facilitating the meaningful use of health IT and the exchange of health information among health-care and public health professionals.
- Enabling quick and informed responses to health risks and public health emergencies.
- Increasing health literacy skills.
- Providing new opportunities to connect with culturally diverse and hard-to-reach populations.
- Providing sound principles in the design of programs and interventions that result in healthier behaviors.
- Increasing Internet and mobile access.

WHY ARE HEALTH COMMUNICATION AND HEALTH INFORMATION TECHNOLOGY IMPORTANT?

Effective use of communication and technology by health-care and public health professionals can bring about an age of patient- and public-centered health information and services. By strategically combining health IT tools and effective health communication processes, there is the potential to:

- Improve health-care quality and safety.
- Increase the efficiency of health-care and public health service delivery.
- Improve the public health information infrastructure.
- Support care in the community and at home.
- Facilitate clinical and consumer decision-making.
- Build health skills and knowledge.

UNDERSTANDING HEALTH COMMUNICATION AND HEALTH INFORMATION TECHNOLOGY

All people have some ability to manage their health and the health of those they care for. However, with the increasing complexity of health information and health-care settings, most people need additional information, skills, and supportive relationships to meet their health needs.

Disparities in access to health information, services, and technology can result in lower usage rates of preventive services, less knowledge of chronic disease management, higher rates of hospitalization, and poorer reported health status.

Both public and private institutions are increasingly using the Internet and other technologies to streamline the delivery of health information and services. This results in an even greater need for health professionals to develop additional skills in the understanding and use of consumer health information.

The increase in online health information and services challenges users with limited literacy skills or limited experience using the Internet. For many of these users, the Internet is stressful and overwhelming—even inaccessible. Much of this stress can be reduced through the application of evidence-based best practices in user-centered design.

Understanding Health Information Technology

In addition, despite increased access to technology, other forms of communication are essential to ensuring that everyone, including nonweb users, is able to obtain, process, and understand health information to make good health decisions. These include printed materials, media campaigns, community outreach, and interpersonal communication.

EMERGING ISSUES IN HEALTH COMMUNICATION AND HEALTH INFORMATION TECHNOLOGY

During the coming decade, the speed, scope, and scale of the adoption of health IT will only increase. Social media and emerging technologies promise to blur the line between expert and peer health information. Monitoring and assessing the impact of these new media, including mobile health, on public health will be challenging.

Equally challenging will be helping health professionals and the public adapt to the changes in health-care quality and efficiency due to the creative use of health communication and health IT. Continual feedback, productive interactions, and access to evidence on the effectiveness of treatments and interventions will likely transform the traditional patient–provider relationship. It will also change the way people receive, process, and evaluate health information. Capturing the scope and impact of these changes—and the role of health communication and health IT in facilitating them—will require multidisciplinary models and data systems.

Such systems will be critical to expanding the collection of data to better understand the effects of health communication and health IT on population health outcomes, health-care quality, and health disparities.

Health Technology Sourcebook, Third Edition

Section 10.2 | Benefits of Health Information Technology

This section includes text excerpted from "Benefits of Health IT," HealthIT.gov, Office of the National Coordinator for Health Information Technology (ONC), September 15, 2017. Reviewed November 2022.

INFORMATION TECHNOLOGY IN HEALTH CARE: THE NEXT CONSUMER REVOLUTION

Over the past 20 years, the nation has undergone a major transformation due to information technology (IT). Access to a variety of information and services is at your fingertips to help manage relationships with the organizations that are part of your lives: banks, utilities, and government offices—even entertainment companies.

Until now, relatively few Americans have had the opportunity to use this kind of technology to enhance some of the most important relationships: those related to your health. Relationships with your doctors, your pharmacy, your hospital, and other organizations that make up your circle of care are now about to benefit from the next transformation in IT: health IT.

For patients and consumers, this transformation will enhance both their relationships with providers and providers' relationships with each other. This change will place you at the center of your care.

Although it will take years for health care to realize all these improvements and fully address any pitfalls, the first changes in this transformation are already underway. At the same time, numerous technology tools are becoming available to improve health for you, your family, and your community.

Most consumers will first encounter the benefits of health IT through an electronic health record (EHR), at their doctor's office or at a hospital.

BENEFITS OF HEALTH INFORMATION TECHNOLOGY FOR YOU AND YOUR FAMILY

On a basic level, an EHR provides a digitized version of the "paper chart" you often see doctors, nurses, and others using. But, when an EHR is connected to all of your health-care providers (and, often, to you as a patient), it can offer so much more.

Understanding Health Information Technology

- **EHRs reduce your paperwork.** The clipboard and new patient questionnaire may remain a feature of your doctor's office for some time to come. But, as more information gets added to your EHR, your doctor and hospital will have more of that data available as soon as you arrive. This means fewer and shorter forms for you to complete, reducing the health-care "hassle factor."
- **EHRs get your information accurately into the hands of people who need it.** Even if you have relatively simple health-care needs, coordinating information among care providers can be a daunting task and one that can lead to medical mistakes if done incorrectly. When all of your providers can share your health information via EHRs, each of them has access to more accurate and up-to-date information about your care. It enables your providers to make the best possible decisions, particularly in a crisis.
- **EHRs help your doctors coordinate your care and protect your safety.** Suppose you see three specialists in addition to your primary care physician. Each of them may prescribe different drugs, and sometimes, these drugs may interact in harmful ways. EHRs can warn your care providers if they try to prescribe a drug that could cause that kind of interaction. An EHR may also alert one of your doctors if another doctor has already prescribed a drug that did not work out for you, saving you from the risks and costs of taking ineffective medication.
- **EHRs reduce unnecessary tests and procedures.** Have you ever had to repeat medical tests ordered by one doctor because the results were not readily available to another doctor? Those tests may have been uncomfortable and inconvenient or have posed some risk, and they also cost money. Repeating tests— whether a $20 blood test or a $2,000 MRI—results in higher costs to you in the form of bigger bills and increased insurance premiums. With EHRs, all of your care providers can have access to all your test

Health Technology Sourcebook, Third Edition

results and records at once, reducing the potential for unnecessary repeat tests.

- **EHRs give you direct access to your health records.** In the United States, you already have a federally guaranteed right to see your health records, identify wrong and missing information, and make additions or corrections as needed. Some health-care providers with EHR systems give their patients direct access to their health information online in ways that help preserve privacy and security. This access enables you to keep better track of your care and, in some cases, answer your questions immediately rather than waiting hours or days for a returned phone call. This access may also allow you to communicate directly and securely with your health-care provider.

Chapter 11 | **Integrating Technology and Health Care**

Chapter Contents

Section 11.1—Implementation and Integration
of Health Information Technology 143
Section 11.2—Basics of Health Information Exchange
Technology 145
Section 11.3—E-prescription 148

Section 11.1 | Implementation and Integration of Health Information Technology

This section contains text excerpted from the following sources: Text in this section begins with excerpts from "Implementing Health IT," HealthIT.gov, Office of the National Coordinator for Health Information Technology (ONC), September 15, 2017. Reviewed November 2022; Text beginning with the heading "Health Information Technology Integration" is excerpted from "Health Information Technology Integration," Agency for Healthcare Research and Quality (AHRQ), U.S. Department of Health and Human Services (HHS), February 15, 2013. Reviewed November 2022.

The successful implementation of a health information technology (IT) system is essential to delivering safe care for patients and a more satisfying work experience for clinicians and staff.

The implementation process is complex, including components such as tailoring the system to support safe, high-quality patient care and ensuring contingency plans are established to address system downtimes.

Health IT system implementation is a multistage process. When implementing a health IT system, it is critical to consider first what care processes it needs to support and how the hardware and software should be set up to support them in patient- and clinician-friendly ways. Configuring the system can be complex and requires a team that includes practicing clinicians to ensure the technology properly supports safe, effective clinical processes and complements efficient workflows.

Successful implementation involves assessing multiple aspects of communication within and outside the health IT system, the integration of its components with one another, and its interaction not only with other technology but also with the people, processes, and culture of the organization. Early resolution of potential integration issues can reduce future patient safety risks.

Patient identification processes are also important to consider during implementation. A well-planned configuration alone does not ensure accurate patient identification. An organization implementing a health IT system should consider how its new technology will handle generating new patient records, patient registration, and retrieval of information. Defining and mapping these processes may detect, mitigate, and prevent problems caused by duplicate records, patient mix-ups, and comingled records.

HEALTH INFORMATION TECHNOLOGY INTEGRATION

The integration of health IT into primary care includes a variety of electronic methods that are used to manage information about people's health and health care for both individual patients and groups of patients. The use of health IT can improve the quality of care and can make health care more cost-effective.

The health IT initiative of the Agency for Healthcare Research and Quality (AHRQ) is part of the nation's strategy to put IT to work in health care. The integration of health IT into primary care includes a variety of electronic methods that are used to manage information about people's health and health care for both individual patients and groups of patients.

In primary care, examples of health IT include the following:

- Clinical decision support (CDS)
- Computerized disease registries
- Computerized provider order entry
- Consumer health IT applications
- Electronic medical record systems (electronic medical records (EMRs), electronic health records (EHRs), and personal health records (PHRs))
- Electronic prescribing
- Telehealth

The AHRQ's National Resource Center for Health IT serves as the link between the health-care community and the researchers and experts who are on the front lines of health IT. The National Resource Center encourages the adoption of health IT by providing the latest tools, best practices, and research results from this unique real-world laboratory. These health IT resources include:

- Workflow Assessment for Health IT Toolkit
- Health IT Tools and Resources
- Health IT Literacy Guide

WHY IS HEALTH INFORMATION TECHNOLOGY IMPORTANT?

Health IT makes it possible for health-care providers to better manage patient care through the secure use and sharing of health information. By developing secure and private EHRs for most

Integrating Technology and Health Care

Americans and making health information available electronically when and where it is needed, health IT can improve the quality of care and can make health care more cost-effective.

With the help of health IT, health-care providers will have the following:

- **Accurate and complete information about a patient's health**. That way, providers can give the best possible care, whether during a routine visit or a medical emergency.
- **The ability to better coordinate the care given**. This is especially important if a patient has a serious medical condition.
- **A way to share information securely**. Patients who opt for health IT can share their information with health-care providers and family caregivers securely. This means patients and their families can more fully take part in decisions about their health care.
- **Complete patient information**. It helps health-care providers diagnose health problems sooner, reduce medical errors, and provide safer care at lower costs.

Section 11.2 | Basics of Health Information Exchange Technology

This section includes text excerpted from "What Is HIE?" HealthIT.gov, Office of the National Coordinator for Health Information Technology (ONC), July 24, 2020.

Electronic health information exchange (HIE) allows doctors, nurses, pharmacists, other health-care providers, and patients to appropriately access and securely share a patient's vital medical information electronically—improving the speed, quality, safety, and cost of patient care.

Despite the widespread availability of secure electronic data transfer, most Americans' medical information is stored on paper—in filing cabinets at various medical offices or in boxes and folders in patients' homes. When that medical information is shared

Health Technology Sourcebook, Third Edition

between health-care providers, it happens by mail, by fax, or—most likely—by patients themselves, who frequently carry their records from appointment to appointment. While electronic health information exchange cannot replace provider–patient communication, it can greatly improve the completeness of patient's records (which can have a big effect on care), as past history, current medications, and other information are jointly reviewed during visits.

Appropriate, timely sharing of vital patient information can better inform decision-making at the point of care and allow health-care providers to:

- Avoid readmissions.
- Avoid medication errors.
- Improve diagnoses.
- Decrease duplicate testing.

If a practice has successfully incorporated faxing patient information into their business process flow, they might question why they should transition to electronic health information exchange. Many benefits exist with information exchange, regardless of the means by which it is transferred. However, the value of the electronic exchange is the standardization of data. Once standardized, the data transferred can seamlessly integrate into the recipients' electronic health record (EHR), further improving patient care. For example:

- If laboratory results are received electronically and incorporated into a provider's EHR, a list of patients with diabetes can be generated. The health-care provider can then determine which of these patients have uncontrolled blood sugar and schedule necessary follow-up appointments.

There are currently three key forms of health information exchange.

DIRECTED EXCHANGE

This is used by health-care providers to easily and securely send patient information—such as laboratory orders and results, patient

Integrating Technology and Health Care

referrals, or discharge summaries—directly to another health-care professional. This information is sent over the Internet in an encrypted, secure, and reliable way among health-care professionals who already know and trust each other and is commonly compared to sending a secured e-mail. This form of information exchange enables coordinated care, benefitting both health-care providers and patients. For example:

- A primary care provider can directly send electronic care summaries that include medications, problems, and lab results to a specialist when referring their patients. This information helps inform the visit and prevents the duplication of tests, redundant collection of information from the patient, wasted visits, and medication errors.

Directed exchange is also being used to send immunization data to public health organizations or to report quality measures to the Centers for Medicare & Medicaid Services (CMS).

QUERY-BASED EXCHANGE

It is used by health-care providers to search and discover accessible clinical sources on a patient. This type of exchange is often used when delivering unplanned care. For example:

- Emergency room physicians who can utilize the query-based exchange to access patient information—such as medications, recent radiology images, and problem lists—might adjust treatment plans to avoid adverse medication reactions or duplicative testing.
- If a pregnant patient goes to the hospital, the query-based exchange can assist a health-care provider in obtaining her pregnancy care record, allowing them to make safer decisions about the care of the patient and her unborn baby.

CONSUMER-MEDIATED EXCHANGE

It provides patients with access to their health information, allowing them to manage their health care online in a similar fashion to how they might manage their finances through online banking. When in control of their own health information, patients can actively participate in their care coordination by:

- Providing other health-care providers with their health information.
- Identifying and correcting wrong or missing health information.
- Identifying and correcting incorrect billing information.
- Tracking and monitoring their own health.

The foundation of standards, policies, and technology required to initiate all three forms of health information exchange are complete, tested, and available today.

Section 11.3 | E-prescription

This section includes text excerpted from "E-Prescribing," Centers for Medicare & Medicaid Services (CMS), August 22, 2022.

E-prescribing is a prescriber's ability to send electronically an accurate, error-free, and understandable prescription directly to a pharmacy from the point of care and is an important element in improving the quality of patient care. The inclusion of electronic prescribing in the Medicare Modernization Act (MMA) of 2003 gave momentum to the movement, and the July 2006 Institute of Medicine report on the role of e-prescribing in reducing medication errors received widespread publicity, helping to build awareness of e-prescribing's role in enhancing patient safety. Adopting the standards to facilitate e-prescribing is one of the key action items in the federal government's plan to expedite the adoption of electronic medical records and build a national electronic health information infrastructure in the United States.

Integrating Technology and Health Care

ELECTRONIC PRESCRIBING FOR CONTROLLED SUBSTANCES

Electronic prescribing for controlled substances (EPCS) is the process of electronically transmitting prescriptions using an electronic format. Practitioners issuing electronic prescriptions for controlled substances must use a software application that meets all Drug Enforcement Administration (DEA) requirements. EPCS has many benefits, such as improved patient safety and workflow efficiencies, fraud deterrence, adherence management, and reduced burden.

In October 2018, the Substance Use-Disorder Prevention that Promotes Opioid Recovery and Treatment for Patients and Communities (SUPPORT) Act was enacted into law to address the opioid crisis. Section 2003 of the SUPPORT Act generally mandates that Schedule II–V controlled substances under Medicare Part D prescription drug plans (Medicare Part D) be electronically prescribed. The CMS EPCS Program is separate from any state EPCS program requirements.

Section 2003 of the SUPPORT Act provides the Secretary of the Department of Health and Human Services (HHS) with discretion on whether to grant waivers or exceptions to the EPCS requirement and gives the secretary of the Department of Health and Human Services authority to enforce noncompliance with the requirement and to specify appropriate penalties for noncompliance through rulemaking. In November 2021, the Centers for Medicare & Medicaid Services (CMS) released the Calendar Year 2022 Physician Fee Schedule Final Rule, which implements phase 2 of Section 2003 of the SUPPORT Act.

2023 MEASUREMENT YEAR EPCS PROGRAM OVERVIEW
EPCS Program Prescribers

Prescribers issue prescriptions for controlled substances to Medicare Part D beneficiaries.

EPCS Program Compliance Determination

The threshold is the percentage of prescription drug claims for Schedule II–V controlled substances under Medicare Part D that are electronically prescribed after exceptions are applied at the end of the calendar year. The threshold for compliance is 70 percent.

EPCS Program Exceptions

- Prescriptions for controlled substances issued when the prescriber and dispensing pharmacy are the same entity
- Prescribers who issue 100 or fewer qualifying Medicare Part D controlled substance prescriptions per calendar year
- Prescribers who the CMS determines are in the geographic area of an emergency or disaster as declared by a federal, state, or local government entity
- Prescribers who have received a CMS-approved waiver because the prescriber is unable to conduct electronic prescribing of controlled substances due to circumstances beyond the prescriber's control

Compliance actions for prescriptions for beneficiaries in a long-term care (LTC) facility will begin on January 1, 2025.

Waivers

Prescribers may request a waiver when circumstances beyond their control prevent them from electronically prescribing controlled substances. The waiver application period for the 2023 EPCS measurement year will open in the calendar year 2024.

Penalty

For the 2023 EPCS measurement year, the CMS will enforce compliance by sending notifications of noncompliance to prescribers violating the EPCS mandate.

Chapter 12 | Digital Health Records

Chapter Contents
Section 12.1—Electronic Health Records and Electronic
               Medical Records..153
Section 12.2—Blue Button 157
Section 12.3—Medical Scribes and Patient Safety 160

Section 12.1 | Electronic Health Records and Electronic Medical Records

This section includes text excerpted from "Electronic Medical Records in Healthcare," U.S. Department of Health and Human Services (HHS), July 26, 2022.

WHAT IS AN EMR, AND HOW IS IT USED IN HEALTH CARE?

Electronic medical records (EMRs) and electronic health records (EHRs) are often used interchangeably. An EMR allows the electronic entry, storage, and maintenance of digital medical data. EHR contains the patient's records from doctors and includes demographics, test results, medical history, history of present illness (HPI), and medications. EMRs are part of EHRs and contain the following:

- Patient registration, billing, preventive screenings, or checkups
- Patient appointment and scheduling
- Tracking patient data over time
- Monitoring and improving the overall quality of care

BENEFITS AND RISKS OF USING EMR/EHR

Some benefits of using EMRs and EHRs are as follows:

- Comprehensive patient-history records
- Making patient data shareable
- Improved quality of care
- Convenience and efficiency

Some risks of using electronic medical records/electronic health records are as follows.

The risks to EHRs relate primarily to a range of factors that include user-related issues, financial issues, and design flaws that create barriers to using them as effective tools to deliver health-care services. EMR is also a top target in health-care breaches. Additional risks are as follows:

- Security or privacy issues
- Potentially vulnerable to hacking

Health Technology Sourcebook, Third Edition

- Chances of data getting lost or destroyed
- Inaccurate paper-to-computer transmission
- Cause of treatment error

TOP THREATS AGAINST ELECTRONIC MEDICAL AND HEALTH RECORDS
Phishing Attacks

A phishing attack is a type of social engineering attack where the threat actor pretends to be a trusted source and tricks their target into opening an e-mail or clicking a link, revealing their login credentials, and depositing malware.

You can protect EMRs/EHRs by doing the following:
- Educate health-care professionals.
- Do not click links within an e-mail that do not match or have a top-level domain (TLD) associated with suspicious sites.
- Physicians should verify all EHR file-share requests before sending any data.

Malware and Ransomware Attacks

Malware enters a health-care system's computer network through software vulnerabilities, encrypted traffic, downloads, and phishing attacks. The effect of each type of malware attack ranges from data theft to harming host computers and networks.

Ransomware is a type of malware that locks users out of their network system or computer until the threat actor or hacker who launched the attack is paid for regained access to data, information, and files.

This could be dangerous for hospitals, health-care facilities, and others who rely on EHRs or EMRs for up-to-date information to provide patient care.

Encryption Blind Spots

Data encryption protects and secures EMR/EHR data while it is being transferred between on-site users and external cloud applications. Blind spots in encrypted traffic could pose a threat

154

Digital Health Records

to IT health care because threat actors or hackers are able to use encrypted blind spots to avoid detection, hide, and execute their targeted attack.

Cloud Threats

More health-care organizations are using cloud services to improve patient care, so there is an increasing need to keep private data secure while complying with Health Insurance Portability and Accountability Act (HIPAA).

Employees: Insider Threats

Insider threats apply across industries, including the health sector. It is recommended that your health-care organization has a cybersecurity strategy and policy that is not only understood but followed and enforced. An effective strategy involves:

- Educating all health-care partners and staff.
- Enhancing administrative controls.
- Monitoring physical and system access.
- Creating workstation usage policies.
- Auditing and monitoring system users.
- Employing device and media controls.
- Applying data encryption.

PROTECTING EMR AND EHR DATA

Here are a few strategies that health-care leaders should consider to strengthen their organization's cyber posture:

- **Evaluate risk before an attack**. Health-care leaders should understand where operational vulnerabilities exist in their organization, from marketing all the way down to critical health records. By understanding the scope of the task at hand, management and other health-care leaders can create a preparedness plan to address any weaknesses in digital infrastructure.
- **Use a virtual private network (VPN) with multifactor authentication**. Leaders in the health-care industry

should consider developing a strategy to combat ransomware that targets Remote Desktop Protocol (RDP) and other applications that face the Internet. Health-care leaders should also consider adding a VPN with multifactor authentication to avoid exposing their RDP and prioritize patching for vulnerabilities in the VPN platform and other applications.

- **Develop endpoint hardening strategy with EDR.** Developing an endpoint hardening strategy provides health-care leaders the ability to harden their digital infrastructure with multiple defense layers at various endpoints. This strategy also detects and contains an attack before it can reach patient medical records or other sensitive information. Endpoint detection and response (EDR) should also be added to detect and mitigate cyber threats.
- **E-mails and patient health records.** It is imperative that patient health records and e-mails are protected. In addition to threat actors using RDP to gain access, HIVE ransomware attacks malicious files attached to phishing emails to gain access to health records and company systems. E-mail security software with URL filtering and attachment sandboxing is recommended as a mitigation strategy.
- **Engage cyber threat hunters.** Threat hunting is a proactive practice that finds threat actors or hackers who have infiltrated a network's initial endpoint security defenses.

This type of human threat detection capability operates as an extension of the organization's cyber team that will track, prevent, or even stop potential cyberattacks on an organization.

- **Conduct red/blue team exercises.** Red and blue team exercises are essentially a face-off between two teams of highly trained cybersecurity professionals.
  - **Red team.** It uses real-world adversary tradecraft to compromise the environment.

Digital Health Records

- **Blue team**. It consists of incident responders who work within the security unit to identify, assess, and respond to the intrusion.
  These exercises are imperative to understanding issues with an organization's network, vulnerabilities, and other possible security gaps.
- **Moving beyond prevention**. It is recommended that health-care leaders shift their focus by moving beyond a prevention strategy and creating a proactive preparedness plan.

This helps understand vulnerabilities in the current network landscape and provides the guidance needed for a framework that will be effective in identifying and preventing attacks, which is key to protecting EMRs/EHRs, along with access to vital patient data.

Section 12.2 | Blue Button

This section contains text excerpted from the following sources: Text in this section begins excerpts from "Mission" is excerpted from "Blue Button® 2.0: Improving Medicare Beneficiary Access to Their Health Information," Centers for Medicare & Medicaid Services (CMS), December 1, 2021; Text beginning with the heading "What Is Blue Button?" is excerpted from "Blue Button," HealthIT.gov, Office of the National Coordinator for Health Information Technology (ONC), April 8, 2019.

The Blue Button service was established in 2010 as a joint effort of the Centers for Medicare & Medicaid Services (CMS) and the U.S. Department of Veterans Affairs (VA). Since that time, Blue Button has been used by more than one million beneficiaries.

As digital health care evolves, data becomes an important resource that patients can use to improve health outcomes for themselves and as part of research groups. This drives the need for easier data interoperability.

Health Technology Sourcebook, Third Edition

Blue Button; the slogan, "Download My Data"; the Blue Button Logo; and the Blue Button combined logo are registered service marks owned by the U.S. Department of Health and Human Services (HHS).

WHAT IS BLUE BUTTON?

The Blue Button symbol signifies that a site has functionality for customers to download health records. You can use your health data to improve your health and to have more control over your personal health information and your family's health care.

- Do you want to feel more in control of your health and your personal health information?
- Do you have a health issue?
- Are you caring for an elderly parent?
- Are you changing doctors?
- Do you need to find the results of a medical test or a complete and current list of your medications?

Blue Button May Be Able to Help

Look for the Blue Button symbol and take action using your personal health information.

YOUR HEALTH RECORDS

Health information about you may be stored in many places, such as doctors' offices, hospitals, drug stores, and health insurance companies. The Blue Button symbol signifies that an organization has a way for you to access your health records electronically so you can:

- Share them with your doctor or trusted family members or caregivers.
- Check to make sure the information, such as your medication list, is accurate and complete.
- Keep track of when your child had her/his last vaccination.
- Have your medical history available in case of emergency, when traveling, seeking a second opinion, or switching health insurance companies.

158

Digital Health Records

- Plug your health information into apps and tools that help you set and reach personalized health goals.

You have a legal right to receive your personal health information. Blue Button is one of the ways this information may be made available to you. Look for the Blue Button symbol and ask your health-care providers or health insurance company if they offer you the ability to view online, download, and share your health records.

WHAT KIND OF INFORMATION IS AVAILABLE TO YOU?

It depends on whether you are getting information from your health-care provider (doctor, hospital, nursing home, etc.), your health insurance company, or another source, such as a drug store or a lab, since each has different kinds of information. In general, you may expect to be able to electronically access important information, such as:

- Current medications you are taking
- Any allergies you have
- Medical treatment information from your doctor or hospital visits
- Your lab test results
- Your health insurance claims information (financial information, clinical information, and more)

Until recently, many health records were stored in paper files, so it was not very easy for you to access or use this information. But it is changing as more doctors and hospitals adopt electronic health records (EHRs) and other health information technologies, including mobile health apps.

Medicare beneficiaries can view and download their Medicare claims data in a more timely and user-friendly format than ever before. That information now covers three years of your health history, including claims information on services covered under Medicare Parts A and B and a list of medications that were purchased under Part D. Look for the Blue Button symbol on the MyMedicare website (www.medicare.gov).

Veterans can find the Blue Button symbol on the MyHealtheVet website (www.myhealth.va.gov/mhv-portal-web/home) and download demographic information (age, gender, ethnicity, and more), emergency contacts, a list of their prescription medications, clinical notes, and wellness reminders.

You may want to check back often as more and more organizations join the Blue Button movement. Online health records are not yet available to everyone, but access is rapidly growing, and if you ask for access, you can help grow it faster.

YOUR RIGHTS

As Americans, each one of you has the legal right to access your own health records held by doctors, hospitals, and others who provide health-care services for you. And you have the option of getting your records on paper or electronically, depending on how they are stored. You can exercise your rights by downloading your health records through an online portal or by asking how to get a copy of your health records. Some doctors or hospitals may not be familiar with your rights to access your information about your own health. You can print out and share with them a letter that explains these rights.

Section 12.3 | Medical Scribes and Patient Safety

This section includes text excerpted from "Medical Scribes and Patient Safety," Agency for Healthcare Research and Quality (AHRQ), U.S. Department of Health and Human Services (HHS), August 1, 2019.

ROLE OF MEDICAL SCRIBES

Under pressure to treat more patients while completing time-intensive electronic health record (EHR) documentation, physicians and licensed independent practitioners have increasingly turned to medical scribes for documentation assistance during patient encounters. In this sense, the use of scribes can be viewed as a work-around or unintended consequence of EHR use.

Digital Health Records

Simply by virtue of their presence, scribes—silent though they may be—make the patient encounter more complex. Interposed between a provider and an EHR, a scribe is uniquely positioned to affect not only how and what information is captured but also how health-care providers think about and seek information during an encounter. They may also affect how patients interact with health-care providers.

There are significant practice variations that can affect the quality of scribe work and ultimately patient care:

- **Qualifications**. The rapidly growing medical scribe industry is unregulated: Certification is not required, nor are there training standards for scribes (although some organizations—primarily scribe service agencies—offer to train and certify scribes). As a result, scribes possess varying levels of documentation skills and clinical knowledge.
- **Responsibilities**. There is no standard job description for scribes. Depending on the organization, scribes may be unlicensed or licensed personnel; they may only provide documentation assistance or also perform clinical duties per pre-existing professional qualifications (e.g., medical assistant, licensed practical nurse, clinical technician).
- **Employment relationships**. The type of scribe employment model may affect the ability of health-care organizations to evaluate scribe performance and control scribe service quality; scribes may be health-care organization employees or contractors provided by scribe staffing agencies.

Despite these practice variations and the sensitive role scribes play in patient encounters, relatively little has been published about how the use of scribes may affect patient safety.

WHAT WE KNOW ABOUT SCRIBES

Descriptions of scribe programs in the United States using unlicensed personnel first appeared more than 35 years ago. However,

Health Technology Sourcebook, Third Edition

the number of scribe-related publications increased significantly following the enactment of the 2009 Health Information Technology for Economic and Clinical Health (HITECH) Act and the subsequent widespread implementation of EHRs.

Initially, post-HITECH studies primarily focused on the economic impact of scribe programs in emergency departments. In the late 2010s, researchers increasingly examined scribes in ambulatory settings. In addition, more published studies explored associations between scribes and patient and provider experiences, and publications began discussing the potential for "digital scribes"—artificial intelligence (AI) that goes beyond current voice-to-text technology—to further transform clinical encounters.

While many post-HITECH publications have addressed patient safety issues associated with EHRs generally, few publications have explicitly explored safety-scribe associations. The AHRQ identified only three such studies that evaluated characteristics of documentation created by scribes, and another one used a socio-technical framework to explore the scribe phenomenon within a broader context.

Studies have suggested that scribes can have a positive economic impact. Scribe America, the largest medical scribe staffing agency in the United States, has stated that using scribes can support a culture of safety by enabling health-care providers to focus on patients, improving communication between health-care providers, and reducing documentation errors. However, scribe skeptics have expressed concern that using scribes may inhibit patient communication, harm clinical reasoning, and reduce the effectiveness of clinical decision support tools.

MOVING FORWARD

In 2018, the Joint Commission conducted an analysis to identify potential quality and safety issues related to documentation assistance practices. Based on its findings, the Joint Commission provided the following guidance:

- **Definition.** Previously defined as unlicensed personnel who were not authorized to enter orders, a documentation assistant or scribe was redefined

Digital Health Records

as "an unlicensed, certified (MA, ophthalmic tech), or licensed person (RN, LPN, PA) who provides documentation assistance to a physician or other licensed independent practitioner (such as a nursing practitioner) consistent with the roles and responsibilities defined in the job description, and within the scope of her or his certification or licensure."

- **Competencies**. Organizations must provide orientation and ongoing training for the role; the amount of training required will vary depending on individual's previous training and experience. At a minimum, education or training should include medical terminology; the Health Insurance Portability and Accountability Act of 1996 (HIPAA); principles of billing, coding, and reimbursement; EHR navigation and functionality; computerized order entry, clinical decision support, and reminders; and proper methods for pending orders for authentication and submission.
- **Policy and procedure**. Each organization should have a policy/procedure regarding documentation assistance processes, including login procedures, scope of documentation assistance, requirements for provider review of information and orders, and order entry/submission.
- **Job descriptions**. These should include the minimum requirements needed to provide documentation assistance, the allowable scope of activities, and how performance and continued competence will be assessed. If contracting with an external agency for documentation assistance, health-care organizations are responsible for ensuring the quality of the services provided.
- **Orders**. Personnel meeting the documentation assistant definition above may enter orders into an EHR at the direction of a physician or other licensed individual practitioner. Order repeat-back is encouraged, particularly for new medication orders. Documentation assistants not authorized to submit

Health Technology Sourcebook, Third Edition

orders should "pend" them for certified or licensed personnel to complete. Transcribing orders into the EHR while providing documentation assistance is not considered a verbal order.

These recommendations address many of the sources of variation listed previously; a 2012 practice brief by the American Health Information Management Association (AHIMA) provides additional guidance. Based on the experience of implementing and evaluating the seven-year-old medical scribe program at Oregon Health and Science University, the AHRQ also offers the following suggestions:

- **Hiring and workflow.** It is important to hire according to the needs of individual health-care providers and clinics. Scribing is a highly interpersonal model; not all health-care providers are well-suited to using scribes, and not every scribe-provider pair will be compatible. Some clinics are better served by unlicensed, single-role scribes, while others are served by licensed, dual-role scribes.
- **Training and orientation.** In addition to the competencies listed by the Joint Commission, new scribes may need to be oriented to medical culture generally, and they should be specifically oriented to the department(s) and provider(s) they will serve. Professionalism is an important area of focus for models in which many of the scribes intend to go on to careers in health care (such as premedical or prenursing students).
- **Ethical considerations.** Situations can arise in which a provider asks a scribe to do something outside the scribe's scope of practice. Because power differentials exist between health-care providers and scribes, policies should clearly state how these types of situations should be handled, and scribes should be knowledgeable about how to report integrity and professionalism violations.

Digital Health Records

- **Health-care provider training.** Health-care providers need clear guidance and training on best practices when it comes to the use of scribes. It is particularly important for health-care providers to supervise and review their scribes' work. Clear communication and regular feedback are key elements of effective workflows.
- **Consistency.** The most successful scribe-provider pairs have consistent clinic schedules and workflows. Scribe workflows can be incredibly variable, depending on specialty and provider preferences. It is important to recognize that scribes are rarely interchangeable; substituting one scribe for another often requires significant additional training.
- **Collaboration.** Facilitating the most effective use of scribes requires collaboration among several health-care organization stakeholders: administration to determine return-on-investment focus (patient volume, chart closure, etc.), EHR specialists and billing and coding specialists to ensure optimal workflow, and provider and scribe representation to share their perspectives.

The unique position occupied by medical scribes, variations in scribe practice, and the paucity of safety data regarding scribes make it challenging for health-care organizations to develop, implement, and evaluate scribe programs, whether they are homegrown or contracted. Until there are better data, health-care organizations may want to consider informally exchanging information about scribe program successes and failures to identify practices that appear to result in safer scribe systems.

Part 4 | Technology and Preventive Health Care

Chapter 13 | Digital Innovations in Preventive Medicine

Chapter Contents

Section 13.1—Sensors..171
Section 13.2—Body Area Networks..173
Section 13.3—Wearable Devices 176
Section 13.4—Wireless Medical Devices.....................................180
Section 13.5—Mobile Medical Applications...............................186
Section 13.6—Continuous Glucose Monitoring 198
Section 13.7—Wireless Patient Monitoring...............................206

Section 13.1 | Sensors

This section includes text excerpted from "Sensors," National Institute of Biomedical Imaging and Bioengineering (NIBIB), April 2022.

WHAT ARE SENSORS, AND HOW ARE THEY USED?

Sensors are tools that detect and respond to some type of input from the physical environment.

There is a broad range of sensors used in everyday life, which are classified based on the quantities and qualities they detect.

Examples include electric current, magnetic or radio sensors, humidity sensors, fluid velocity or flow sensors, pressure sensors, thermal or temperature sensors, optical sensors, position sensors, environmental sensors, and chemical sensors.

HOW ARE SENSORS USED IN BIOMEDICAL RESEARCH AND MEDICAL CARE?

In medicine and biomedical research, there are many types of sensors that are used to detect specific biological, chemical, or physical processes that then transmit or report this data to individual users or health-care professionals.

Thermometers translate the expansion of a fluid or bending of a metal strip in response to heat into a value that corresponds to body temperature.

Wearable technologies such as smartwatches carry sensors that can track, analyze, and transmit data about heart rate and sleep patterns. Researchers are using wearables to monitor the health of individuals and even predict and potentially intervene to prevent acute health events, such as stroke or heart attack.

Pulse oximeters measure changes in the body's absorption of special types of light to measure heart rate and the amount of oxygen in the blood. These sensors are frequently used in hospitals and clinics and can also be purchased for at-home use.

While many advanced sensors are not practical for routine medical care, they allow researchers to study and learn about the basic foundations of disease, potentially facilitating the development of new technologies.

Health Technology Sourcebook, Third Edition

WHAT ARE NIBIB-FUNDED RESEARCHERS DEVELOPING IN THE AREA OF SENSORS TO IMPROVE BIOMEDICAL RESEARCH AND MEDICAL CARE?

- **Circulating nanosensors for continuous drug monitoring.** The NIBIB-funded scientists are developing sensors that circulate in the blood and continuously monitor drug concentrations to help maintain therapeutic levels and avoid high, toxic levels. The sensors send a fluorescent signal that changes with drug concentration and can be detected through the skin. To allow the sensor to remain in the blood without being eliminated from the body, the sensors are "hidden" in red blood cell (RBC) "ghosts," which are the outer shell of the RBC. In experiments in mice, sensors designed to detect lithium carried inside the RBC ghosts remained in the bloodstream for weeks sending a fluorescent signal that accurately measured the lithium levels in the blood. The circulating nanosensors could improve drug effectiveness by allowing physicians to monitor and adjust drug concentrations to maintain optimal therapeutic levels.

- **Smart textiles for prevention of deep vein thrombosis.** Deep vein thrombosis (DVT) is the formation of blood clots in the legs. Caused by limited mobility in hospital patients, the elderly, and pregnant women, DVT can result in pulmonary embolism (PE), a life-threatening condition that occurs when clots from the legs travel to the lungs and become lodged in the pulmonary arteries. The NIBIB-funded researchers are using smart textiles to prevent DVT and reduce the occurrence of PE. The smart textiles carry sensors that do not require batteries and are woven directly into socks and other garments. The smart textiles can remotely detect movement or lack of movement that would promote DVT and automatically provide mechanical stimulation to block the formation of blood clots. The approach aims to dramatically reduce the more than 200,000 cases of PE that occur in the United States each year.

Digital Innovations in Preventive Medicine

- **Inexpensive genetic sensor for zinc deficiency.** In developing countries, the lack of the micronutrient zinc in mothers' diets is associated with fetal growth retardation, impairment of learning and memory function, and increased morbidity and mortality in children. To enable widespread testing for zinc deficiency, NIBIB-funded scientists are using synthetic biology to create an inexpensive zinc sensor for use in low-resource settings. The approach involves engineering bacteria that give a color readout in response to the amount of zinc in a blood sample. Different colored readouts are based on the zinc concentration in the sample, indicating whether zinc levels are acceptable or too low (which would indicate the need for zinc supplements). The portable, minimal-equipment bacterial biosensor for blood micronutrients would enable large-scale studies on nutritional interventions to better treat millions of undernourished people in low-resource settings.

Section 13.2 | Body Area Networks

This section contains text excerpted from the following sources: Text under the heading "Visualization of Body Area Networks" is excerpted from "Visualization of Body Area Networks," National Institute of Standards and Technology (NIST), September 21, 2016. Reviewed November 2022; Text under the heading "Implant Communications in Body Area Networks" is excerpted from "Implant Communications in Body Area Networks," National Institute of Standards and Technology (NIST), November 15, 2019.

VISUALIZATION OF BODY AREA NETWORKS

The term body area network (BAN) refers to a network intended to be used in or around the human body. While this is an emerging field, networks of medical sensors are anticipated to be a primary application. Such sensors would either be attached to or implanted in the human body and would communicate wirelessly both within the body and to devices outside the body.

For this technology to develop, a greater understanding of radio frequency (RF) propagation through the human body is needed.

Health Technology Sourcebook, Third Edition

Modeling and Visualization of Body Area Networks

Because experimentation on human subjects is currently not feasible, RF propagation through the human body is being modeled in software with a three-dimensional (3D) full-wave electromagnetic field simulator. The 3D human body model includes frequency-dependent dielectric properties of 300+ parts in a male human body. The data produced by this simulation software is then brought into a 3D immersive visualization system, which enables researchers to study the modeled RF propagation through direct interactions with the data.

The simulations are being performed by members of the Advanced Network Technologies Division of ITL, and the visualization work is being done by members of the High Performance Computing and Visualization Group of the Applied and Computational Mathematics Division of ITL.

The Immersive Visualization System

The immersive system includes several important components: three orthogonal screens that provide the visual display, the motion-tracked stereoscopic glasses, and a handheld motion-tracked input device. The screens are large projection video displays that are placed edge to edge in a corner configuration. These three screens are used to display a single 3D stereo scene. The scene is updated based on the position of the user as determined by the motion tracker. This allows the system to present to the user a 3D virtual world within which the user can move and interact with the virtual objects. The main interaction device is a handheld three usa-button motion-tracked wand with a joystick.

This virtual environment allows for more natural interaction between experts with different backgrounds, such as engineering and medical sciences. The researchers can look at data representations at any scale and position, move through data, change orientation, and control the elements of the virtual world using a variety of interaction techniques, including measurement and analysis.

For example, the National Institute of Standards and Technology (NIST) researchers have implemented interactive tools for probing the 3D data fields. One tool enables the researcher to move the

Digital Innovations in Preventive Medicine

motion-tracked wand through the virtual scene, yielding a continuously updated display of the value of the data field at the position of the wand. Another tool enables the user to interactively stretch a line segment through a virtual body and to generate graphs of the 3D data fields along that path. The NIST researchers have found these to be effective tools in getting quantitative information from the 3D scene and in gaining insight into RF propagation through the human body.

IMPLANT COMMUNICATIONS IN BODY AREA NETWORKS
What Are the Issues with Body Area Networks?
Today, there are no standards for short-range wireless communication to/from an implant (or a sensor) located inside (or on the surface) of a human body. Developing such communication protocols is a difficult task since there are currently no models/data available to characterize the propagation from implanted devices. As physical experiments are nearly impossible, intricate simulation models are the only option to study this problem. Also, RF coexistence and interoperability of such body area sensors with other wireless technologies need to be thoroughly evaluated to determine their effectiveness for practical applications.

What Are the National Institute of Standards and Technology Staff Doing to Address These Issues?
The NIST staff is facilitating the development of standards for body area networks and contributing to the efforts of IEEE 802.15.6. Their efforts include building a 3D immersive visualization platform to observe RF propagation from implant devices and investigating appropriate 3D data visualization schemes for various RF-related quantities, obtaining path loss versus distance information between an implant and a body-surface node or between two implants, investigating the possibility of driving a statistical channel model for Medical Implant Communications Service (MICS) operation and incorporate the results into the channel modeling standard document IEEE 802.15.6, and studying coexistence/interoperability issues with other wireless systems/technologies.

MAJOR ACCOMPLISHMENTS

A propagation model for implant-to-implant devices and implant-to-on-body devices was provided to IEEE 802.15.6 BAN working group (as Contribution 15-08-0519-01-0006, a statistical path loss model for MICS). A 3D immersive and visualization platform was developed to display signal propagation behavior.

Section 13.3 | Wearable Devices

This section contains text excerpted from the following sources: Text in this section begins with excerpts from "Please Review and Approve Wearable Technology Report," U.S. Consumer Product Safety Commission (CPSC), April 1, 2020; Text beginning with the heading "Health Related Wearable Technology" is excerpted from "HC3 Intelligence Briefing Wearable Device Security," U.S. Department of Health and Human Services (HHS), March 5, 2020.

Wearable technology is not a new concept. Commonly used products, such as wristwatches or earbuds, are considered wearable technology. However, due to recent advances in software and hardware, including miniaturization of products, improved batteries, wireless connectivity, and increased sophistication of sensors, these technologies have become less conspicuous and have greater capabilities. This generation is witnessing introductions of new types of wearables—from e-textiles to fitness trackers to altered-reality gaming—fueled by innovations in manufacturing, sensing, energy storage, and advancements in materials. Wearables may provide consumers with myriad benefits.

In general, a wearable can be described as a product that includes a chemical, electronic, or mechanical function that is worn on, applied to, or implanted or inserted into the human body. Consumer applications of these products include activity tracking, performance enhancement, and other methods of affecting the consumer's senses and interactions.

CATEGORIZATION OF WEARABLES

The wearables are categorized by their functions, product types, and potential hazards. A specific function may be incorporated

Digital Innovations in Preventive Medicine

into various product types. Evaluating the function of wearables is the first step in identifying potential product hazards. The categorization scheme includes products for data collection and storage, communication and repulsion, monitoring and alerting, performance enhancement, and neural stimulation. Some products included in the following categorization scheme are medical devices.

Accessories

Consumers wear accessories on the body that are loosely attached and easily removed. Data collection is a primary function of most wearable accessories. Fitness trackers, for example, have become immensely popular for measuring fitness-related data, such as heart rate, distance traveled, and calories burned. Other examples of wearable accessories include alerting devices, such as wristbands that provide a warning when the user is exposed to potentially harmful levels of ultraviolet radiation (UV) from the sun. Consumers can typically transmit information from wearable accessories to a cellular phone, computer, or other data storage device. Wearable accessories may use nonionizing radiation, such as radio frequencies, which are less energetic than devices providing cellular phone transmission. Although the acute energy potentially transferred to the body from nonionizing radiation is typically relatively low, wearable accessories may be worn directly on the skin for extended periods of time.

Articles

A wearable article is any fabric, clothing, or textile that contains electronic technology and is worn on the body. Examples of articles include coats, jackets, dresses, skirts, and pants. Biomonitoring is one of the primary functions of these products. Similar to wearable accessories, many wearable articles collect information on physiologic functions, such as heart rate and neurologic activity.

Relative to accessories, articles commonly allow manufacturers a larger surface area for embedded sensors and sampling, affording these products higher measurement accuracy and increased variety of data measured. The ability of articles to be more precise in measuring data may be of particular importance in athletics. For example, sensors can monitor and assess physical performance, in addition to protecting athletes, by providing a warning when an athlete exceeds an overexertion threshold.

The human skin is the largest organ in the body and provides protection to our internal organs. Light-emitting fabrics use light to enhance the "style" of a piece of clothing and some manufacturers' market light-emitting fabrics for therapeutic applications.

Patch

Wearable patches are applied directly to the skin, fingernails, or toenails permanently or semipermanently (such as "tattoos") and incorporate electronic circuitry. A common use of patches is for identification purposes. For example, it is used in physiological monitoring or delivery of health supplements or drugs for health and fitness. In the past, some patches have delivered compounds to the body, such as nicotine; however, new "smart" patches can include biomonitoring. Patches are attached directly to the skin, and in some cases, they are intended to be attached for long-term use. Given these factors, the likelihood of exposure to any potential harmful materials could be greater compared to other wearable products.

Imbed

Consumers apply imbed wearables beneath their skin, such as subdermal radio frequency products, for identification and entry. Although the term "imbed" is commonly used interchangeably with "insert" (discussed below), it is distinguished into two categories, based on the insertion of the device under the skin versus into an existing body portal (e.g., oral placement). The subdermal placement of imbeds allows even greater exposure to chemicals, relative to products placed on the skin due, in part, to long-term use and access to the bloodstream where potentially harmful compounds can circulate to targets within the body for physiologic effects. Furthermore, the insertion and removal of an imbed may increase infection opportunities.

Digital Innovations in Preventive Medicine

Insert

Insert wearables are placed into existing body orifices, such as the ears or mouth. Consumers have been using inserts for many years; hearing aids are one example. Technological innovations have vastly improved hearing aid performance and enhanced their capabilities. They are now being marketed to consumers without impaired hearing. For example, "augmented hearing" or "hearable" products allow users to enhance and control their sense of hearing, including blocking out user-determined background noise.

HEALTH-RELATED WEARABLE TECHNOLOGY

- **Fitness tracker**. It tracks physical activities and heart rate.
- **Electrocardiogram (ECG) monitors**. They record electric signals in the heart to monitor heart disease, anxiety, and so on.
- **Blood pressure monitors**. They can measure blood pressure and daily activity.
- **Wearable biosensors (skin patches)**. Self-adhesive patches that collect data on movement, heart rate, respiratory rate, and temperature.
- **Smart glasses**. Eyeglasses that incorporate first-person imaging, facial recognition, enhanced turn-wise directions, health sensing, and so on
- **Hearables**. Hearing aids that incorporate functions such as sleep monitoring, brain wave analysis, and virtual assistant support.

WEARABLE BENEFITS IN HEALTH CARE

- **Personalization**. A doctor, with the help of software, can quickly create a program based on the needs of the patient.
- **Early diagnosis**. Precise medical parameters in wearable devices allow early detection of symptoms.
- **Remote patient monitoring**. Health-care professionals can monitor patients remotely and in real time through the use of wearable devices.

- **Adherence to medication.** Wearable devices help the patient take medications on time and even inform medical professionals if the patient fails to adhere to medications.
- **Information registry.** The data are stored in real time, allowing a more exhaustive analysis of the information. This results in a more complete and precise report on the patient's medical history, which can be shared with other medical specialists.
- **Optimum decision by the doctor.** The doctor is able to compare and analyze data to make a sharper clinical decision to enhance the patient's quality of life.
- **Saving health-care cost.** Remote health care via wearable devices means saving time and mobility, as it removes the need for the patient to be continuously transferred to the medical center.

Section 13.4 | Wireless Medical Devices

This section includes text excerpted from "Wireless Medical Devices," U.S. Food and Drug Administration (FDA), September 4, 2018. Reviewed November 2022.

Radio frequency (RF) wireless medical devices perform at least one function that utilizes wireless RF communication, such as Wi-Fi, Bluetooth, and cellular/mobile phone to support health-care delivery. Examples of functions that can utilize wireless technology include controlling and programming a medical device, monitoring patients remotely, or transferring patient data from the medical device to another platform, such as a cell phone. As RF wireless technology continues to evolve, this technology will increasingly be incorporated into the design of medical devices.

Examples of areas that utilize RF wireless technology include:
- Wireless medical telemetry
- Radio frequency identification (RFID)

Digital Innovations in Preventive Medicine

WIRELESS MEDICAL TELEMETRY

Wireless medical telemetry is generally used to monitor a patient's vital signs (e.g., pulse and respiration) using RF communication. These devices have the advantage of allowing patient movement without restricting patients to a bedside monitor with a hardwired connection.

Regulations, Licenses, and Guidelines

The Federal Communications Commission (FCC) established the Wireless Medical Telemetry Service (WMTS) by allocating specific frequency bands exclusively for wireless medical telemetry. The WMTS set aside 14 MHz of spectrum in three defined frequency bands of 608–614 MHz, 1,395–1,400 MHz, and 1,427–1,432 MHz for primary or co-primary use by eligible wireless medical telemetry users. The WMTS creates frequencies where medical telemetry is protected against interference from other RF sources. A key feature of WMTS is the provision for the establishment of a frequency coordinator to maintain a database of user and equipment information to facilitate sharing of the spectrum and help prevent interference among users of the WMTS. Operating these devices within the specific frequency bands allocated exclusively for WMTS should reduce the risk of electromagnetic interference (EMI) with vital medical telemetry signals.

The FDA encourages manufacturers and users of medical telemetry devices to use this spectrum because of its protection against interference from other intentional transmitters and because frequency coordination will be provided.

Authorized Users

Eligible WMTS users are limited to authorized health-care providers, which include licensed physicians, health-care facilities, and certain trained and supervised technicians. The health-care facilities eligible for the WMTS are defined as those where services are offered for use beyond 24 hours, including hospitals and other medical providers. Ambulances and other moving vehicles are not included within this definition.

Service Rules

The service rules for the equipment and use of the WMTS include limitations on transmitter output power, out-of-band emissions, and protection of other services. Users of the WMTS are co-primary with the radio astronomy service operating in the 608–614 MHz frequency range and must not disrupt radio astronomy operations. WMTS users are required to obtain written permission to transmit within 80 km (50 miles) of some radio astronomy facilities and within 32 km (20 miles) of other radio astronomy facilities. The frequency coordinator maintains information to help the WMTS co-primary users avoid conflicts.

RADIO FREQUENCY IDENTIFICATION

Radio frequency identification refers to a wireless system comprised of two components: tags and readers. The reader is a device that has one or more antennas that emit radio waves and receive signals back from the RFID tag. Tags, which use radio waves to communicate their identity and other information to nearby readers, can be passive or active. Passive RFID tags are powered by the reader and do not have a battery. Active RFID tags are powered by batteries.

RFID tags can store a range of information from one serial number to several pages of data. Readers can be mobile so that they can be carried by hand, or they can be mounted on a post or overhead. Reader systems can also be built into the architecture of a cabinet, room, or building.

Uses of Radio Frequency Identification

Radio frequency identification systems use radio waves at several different frequencies to transfer data. In health-care and hospital settings, RFID technologies include the following applications:
- Inventory control
- Equipment tracking
- Out-of-bed detection and fall detection
- Personnel tracking
- Ensuring that patients receive the correct medications and medical devices

Digital Innovations in Preventive Medicine

- Preventing the distribution of counterfeit drugs and medical devices
- Monitoring patients
- Providing data for electronic medical records systems

The FDA is not aware of any adverse events associated with RFID. However, there is concern about the potential hazard of electromagnetic interference (EMI) to electronic medical devices from RF transmitters such as RFID. EMI is a degradation of the performance of equipment or systems (such as medical devices) caused by an electromagnetic disturbance.

Information for Health-Care Professionals

Because this technology continues to evolve and is more widely used, it is important to keep in mind its potential for interference with pacemakers, implantable cardioverter defibrillators (ICDs), and other electronic medical devices.

Physicians should stay informed about the use of RFID systems. If a patient experiences a problem with a device, ask questions that will help determine if RFID might have been a factor, such as when and where the episode occurred, what the patient was doing at the time, and whether or not the problem resolved once the patient moved away from that environment. If you suspect that RFID was a factor, device interrogation might be helpful in correlating the episode to the exposure. Report any suspected medical device malfunctions to MedWatch, FDA's voluntary adverse event reporting system.

Actions of the U.S. Food and Drug Administration

The U.S. Food and Drug Administration (FDA) has taken steps to study RFID and its potential effects on medical devices, including:

- Working with manufacturers of potentially susceptible medical devices to test their products for any adverse effects from RFID and encouraging them to consider RFID interference when developing new devices.
- Working with the RFID industry to better understand where RFID can be found, what power levels and

Health Technology Sourcebook, Third Edition

frequencies are being used in different locations, and how to best mitigate potential EMI with pacemakers and ICDs.

- Participating in and reviewing the development of RFID standards to better understand RFID's potential to affect medical devices and to mitigate potential EMI.
- Working with the Association for Automatic Identification and Mobility (AIM) to develop a way to test medical devices for their vulnerability to EMI from RFID systems.
- Collaborating with other government agencies, such as the Federal Communications Commission (FCC), the National Institute for Occupational Safety and Health (NIOSH), and the Occupational Safety and Health Administration (OSHA), to better identify places where RFID readers are in use.

BENEFITS AND RISKS OF WIRELESS MEDICAL DEVICES

Incorporation of wireless technology in medical devices can have many benefits, including increasing patient mobility by eliminating wires that tether a patient to a medical bed, providing health-care professionals the ability to remotely program devices, and providing the ability of physicians to remotely access and monitor patient data regardless of the location of the patient or physician (hospital, home, office, etc.). These benefits can greatly impact patient outcomes by allowing physicians access to real-time data on patients without the physician physically being in the hospital and allowing real-time adjustment of patient treatment. Remote monitoring can also help special populations, such as seniors, through home monitoring of chronic diseases so that changes can be detected earlier before more serious consequences occur.

INFORMATION FOR PATIENTS

The use of RF wireless technology can translate to advances in health care, and patients should be informed about the safe and effective use of these devices in the course of daily life.

Digital Innovations in Preventive Medicine

Because the airways are shared, the functioning of your wireless medical device may be affected (such as data loss or disruption) by other wireless devices near you. As with any medical device, if you have problems or questions, please consult the information provided by the manufacturer or contact your health-care provider.

INFORMATION FOR HEALTH-CARE FACILITIES: RISK MANAGEMENT

Most well-designed and maintained RF wireless medical devices perform adequately. However, the increasingly crowded RF environment and competition from nonmedical wireless technology users could impact the performance of RF wireless medical devices. The FDA recommends that health-care facilities develop appropriate processes and procedures to assess and manage risks associated with the integration of RF wireless technology into medical systems.

Health-care facilities should also consider the following:
- Selection of wireless technology
- Quality of service
- Coexistence
- Security
- Electromagnetic compatibility (EMC)

REPORTING PROBLEMS TO THE U.S. FOOD AND DRUG ADMINISTRATION

Prompt reporting of adverse events can help the FDA identify and better understand the risks associated with RF wireless medical devices. The FDA encourages health-care providers and patients who suspect a problem or hazardous event to file a voluntary report through MedWatch, the FDA Safety Information and Adverse Event Reporting Program (www.fda.gov/safety/medwatch-fda-safety-information-and-adverse-event-reporting-program).

Health-care personnel employed by facilities that are subject to Reporting Adverse Events (Medical Devices) requirements (www.fda.gov/medical-devices/postmarket-requirements-devices/mandatory-reporting-requirements-manufacturers-importers-and-device-user-facilities) should follow the reporting procedures established by their facilities.

Health Technology Sourcebook, Third Edition

Section 13.5 | Mobile Medical Applications

This section contains text excerpted from the following sources: Text beginning with the heading "What Are Mobile Medical Apps?" is excerpted from "Device Software Functions Including Mobile Medical Applications," U.S. Food and Drug Administration (FDA), September 29, 2022; Text under the heading "Examples of Mobile Apps That Are NOT Medical Devices" is excerpted from "Examples of Mobile Apps That Are NOT Medical Devices," U.S. Food and Drug Administration (FDA), September 29, 2022.

WHAT ARE MOBILE MEDICAL APPS?

Mobile apps are software programs that run on smartphones and other mobile communication devices. They can also be accessories that attach to a smartphone or other mobile communication devices or a combination of accessories and software.

Mobile medical apps are medical devices that are mobile apps, meet the definition of a medical device, and are an accessory to a regulated medical device or transform a mobile platform into a regulated medical device.

Consumers can use both mobile medical apps and mobile apps to manage their own health and wellness, such as to monitor their caloric intake for healthy weight maintenance. For example, the LactMed app of the National Institutes of Health (NIH) provides nursing mothers with information about the effects of medicines on breast milk and nursing infants.

Other apps aim to help health-care professionals improve and facilitate patient care. The Radiation Emergency Medical Management (REMM) app gives health-care providers guidance on diagnosing and treating radiation injuries. Some mobile medical apps can diagnose cancer or heart rhythm abnormalities or function as the "central command" for a glucose meter used by an insulin-dependent diabetic patient.

HOW DOES THE U.S. FOOD AND DRUG ADMINISTRATION REGULATE DEVICE SOFTWARE FUNCTIONS?

The FDA applies the same risk-based approach to device software functions as the agency uses to assure safety and effectiveness for other medical devices. The guidance document (www.fda.gov/regulatory-information/search-fda-guidance-documents/policy-device-software-functions-and-mobile-medical-applications)

Digital Innovations in Preventive Medicine

provides examples of how the FDA might regulate certain moderate-risk (Class II) and high-risk (Class III) device software functions. This section also provides examples of software functions that:

- Are not medical devices.
- Are medical devices, but those for which the FDA intends to exercise enforcement discretion.
- Are medical devices and are the focus of FDA oversight.

The FDA encourages software developers to e-mail (digitalhealth@fda.hhs.gov) the FDA as early as possible if they have any questions about their software, its level of risk, and whether a premarket application is required.

DEVICE SOFTWARE FUNCTIONS THAT ARE THE FOCUS OF THE U.S. FOOD AND DRUG ADMINISTRATION OVERSIGHT

The FDA is taking a tailored, risk-based approach that focuses on the subset of software functions that meet the regulatory definition of "device." Software functions span a wide range of health functions. While some software carries minimal risk, those that can pose a greater risk to patients will require FDA review.

The FDA's device software functions and mobile medical apps policy does not require software developers to seek the FDA re-evaluation for minor, iterative product changes.

SOFTWARE FUNCTIONS FOR WHICH THE U.S. FOOD AND DRUG ADMINISTRATION INTENDS TO EXERCISE ENFORCEMENT DISCRETION

For many software functions that meet the regulatory definition of a "device" but pose minimal risk to patients and consumers, the FDA will exercise enforcement discretion and will not expect manufacturers to submit premarket review applications or register and list their software with the FDA. This includes device software functions that:

- Help patients/users self-manage their disease or condition without providing specific treatment suggestions.
- Automate simple tasks for health-care providers.

DOES THE U.S. FOOD AND DRUG ADMINISTRATION REGULATE MOBILE DEVICES, SUCH AS SMARTPHONES OR TABLETS, AND MOBILE APP STORES?

The FDA's mobile medical apps policy does not regulate the sale or general consumer use of smartphones or tablets. The FDA's mobile medical apps policy does not consider entities that exclusively distribute mobile apps, such as the owners and operators of the "iTunes App Store" or the "Google Play Store," to be medical device manufacturers. The FDA's mobile medical apps policy does not consider mobile platform manufacturers to be medical device manufacturers just because their mobile platform could be used to run a mobile medical app regulated by the FDA.

EXAMPLES OF MOBILE APPS THAT ARE NOT MEDICAL DEVICES

This list provides examples of software functions to illustrate the types of mobile apps that could be used in a health-care environment, in clinical care, or in patient management but are not considered medical devices. Because these mobile apps are not considered medical devices, the U.S. Food and Drug Administration (FDA) does not regulate them. The FDA understands that there may be other unique and innovative mobile apps that may not be covered in this list that may also constitute health-care-related mobile apps. This list is not exhaustive; it is only intended to provide clarity and assistance in identifying when a mobile app is not considered to be a medical device.

Appendix A (www.fda.gov/regulatory-information/search-fda-guidance-documents/policy-device-software-functions-and-mobile-medical-applications) in the guidance includes examples of software functions not considered medical devices at the time the guidance was finalized. As part of the FDA's ongoing effort to provide clarity to mobile app manufacturers, this page includes all examples in Appendix A as well as updates with additional examples.

- **Software functions that are intended to provide access to electronic "copies" (e.g., e-books, audiobooks) of medical textbooks or other reference materials with generic text search capabilities.** These

Digital Innovations in Preventive Medicine

are not devices because these apps are intended to be used as reference materials and are not intended for use in the diagnosis of disease or other conditions or in the cure, mitigation, treatment, or prevention of disease by facilitating a health professional's assessment of a specific patient, replacing the judgment of clinical personnel, or performing any clinical assessment. Examples include mobile apps that are:

- Medical dictionaries
- Electronic copies of medical textbooks or literature articles such as the Physician's Desk Reference or Diagnostic and Statistical Manual of Mental Disorders (DSM)
- Library of clinical descriptions for diseases and conditions
- Encyclopedia of first-aid or emergency care information
- Medical abbreviations and definitions
- Translations of medical terms across multiple languages
- **Software functions that are intended for health-care professionals to use as educational tools for medical training or to reinforce training previously received**. These may have more functionality than providing an electronic copy of text (e.g., videos, interactive diagrams) but are not devices because they are intended generally for user education and are not intended for use in the diagnosis of disease or other conditions or in the cure, mitigation, treatment, or prevention of disease by facilitating a health professional's assessment of a specific patient, replacing the judgment of clinical personnel, or performing any clinical assessment. Examples include mobile apps that are:
  - Medical flash cards with medical images, pictures, graphs, and so on
  - Question/answer quiz apps
  - Interactive anatomy diagrams or videos

Health Technology Sourcebook, Third Edition

- Surgical training videos
- Medical board certification or recertification preparation apps
- Games that simulate various cardiac arrest scenarios to train health professionals in advanced cardiopulmonary resuscitation (CPR) skills
- **Software functions that are intended for general patient education and facilitate patient access to commonly used reference information.** These apps can be patient-specific (i.e., filters information to patient-specific characteristics) but are intended for increased patient awareness, education, and empowerment and ultimately support patient-centered health care. These are not devices because they are intended generally for patient education and are not intended for use in the diagnosis of disease or other conditions or in the cure, mitigation, treatment, or prevention of disease by aiding clinical decision-making (i.e., to facilitate a health professional's assessment of a specific patient, replace the judgment of a health professional, or perform any clinical assessment). Examples include mobile apps that:
  - Provide a portal for health-care professionals to distribute educational information (e.g., interactive diagrams, useful links and resources) to their patients regarding their disease, condition, treatment, or upcoming procedure.
  - Help guide patients to ask appropriate questions to their physician relevant to their particular disease, condition, or concern.
  - Provide information about gluten-free food products or restaurants.
  - Help match patients with potentially appropriate clinical trials and facilitate communication between the patient and clinical trial investigators.
  - Provide tutorials or training videos on how to administer first-aid or CPR.

Digital Innovations in Preventive Medicine

- Allow users to input pill shape, color, or imprint and display pictures and names of pills that match this description.
- Find the closest medical facilities and doctors to the user's location.
- Provide lists of emergency hotlines and physician/nurse advice lines.
- Provide and compare costs of drugs and medical products at pharmacies in the user's location.
- Provide access to education materials using digital media to help patients cope with stress.
- **Software functions that automate general office operations in a health-care setting** and are not intended for use in the diagnosis of disease or other conditions or in the cure, mitigation, treatment, or prevention of disease. Examples include mobile apps that:
  - Determine billing codes such as International Statistical Classification of Diseases (ICD-9).
  - Enable insurance claims data collection and processing and other apps that are similarly administrative in nature.
  - Analyze insurance claims for fraud or abuse.
  - Perform medical business accounting functions or track and trend billable hours and procedures.
  - Generate reminders for scheduled medical appointments or blood donation appointments.
  - Help patients track, review, and pay medical claims and bills online.
  - Manage shifts for doctors.
  - Manage or schedule hospital rooms or bed spaces.
  - Provide wait times and electronic check-in for hospital emergency rooms and urgent care facilities.
  - Allow health-care professionals or staff in health-care setting to process payments (e.g., a HIPAA-compliant app).
  - Track or perform a patient satisfaction survey after an encounter or a clinical visit.

Health Technology Sourcebook, Third Edition

- **Software functions that are generic aids or general-purpose products.** These apps are not considered devices because they are not intended for use in the diagnosis of disease or other conditions or in the cure, mitigation, treatment, or prevention of disease. Examples include mobile apps that:
  - Use the mobile platform as a magnifying glass (but are not specifically intended for medical purposes).
  - Use the mobile platform for recording audio, note-taking, replaying audio with amplification, or other similar functionalities.
  - Allow patients or health-care professionals to interact through e-mail, web-based platforms, video, or other communication mechanisms (but are not specifically intended for medical purposes).
  - Provide maps and turn-by-turn directions to medical facilities.
  - Allow health-care professionals to communicate in a secure and protected method (e.g., HIPAA-compliant app to send messages between health-care professionals in a hospital).
- **Software functions that are intended for individuals to log, record, track, evaluate, or make decisions or behavioral suggestions related to developing or maintaining general fitness, health, or wellness,** such as those that:
  - Provide tools to promote or encourage healthy eating, exercise, weight loss, or other activities generally related to a healthy lifestyle or wellness.
  - Provide dietary logs and calorie counters or make dietary suggestions.
  - Provide meal planners and recipes.
  - Track general daily activities or make exercise or posture suggestions.
  - Track a normal baby's sleeping and feeding habits.
  - Actively monitor and trend exercise activity.
  - Help healthy people track the quantity or quality of their normal sleep patterns.

Digital Innovations in Preventive Medicine

- Provide and track scores from mind-challenging games or generic "brain age" tests.
- Provide daily motivational tips (e.g., via text or other types of messaging) to reduce stress and promote a positive mental outlook.
- Use social gaming to encourage healthy lifestyle habits.
- Calculate calories burned in a workout.
- **Software functions that enable individuals to interact with electronic health record (EHR) software certified under the ONC Health IT Certification Program.** These are software functions that provide individuals with access to health record systems or enable them to gain electronic access to health information stored within an EHR system. Software functions that only allow individuals to view, transfer, or download EHR data are also included in this category. These software functions are generally meant to facilitate general patient health information management and health record-keeping activities:
  - Software functions for health-care professionals certified under the ONC Health IT Certification Program, such as those that help track or manage patient immunizations by documenting the need for immunization, consent form, and immunization lot number
  - Software functions certified under the ONC Health IT Certification Program that prompt the health-care professional to manually enter symptomatic, behavioral, or environmental information, the specifics of which are predefined by a health-care professional, and store the information for later review
- **Software functions that enable patients or health-care professionals to interact with (e.g., transfer, store, convert formats, display data) EHR systems** that are certified under the ONC Health IT Certification Program or interact with personal health record (PHR) systems.

Health Technology Sourcebook, Third Edition

- **Software functions that allow a user to record (i.e., collect and log) data**, such as blood glucose, blood pressure, heart rate, weight, or other data from a device to eventually share with a health-care professional, upload it to an EHR that is certified under the ONC Health IT Certification Program, upload it to an online (cloud) database, or upload it to a PHR.
- **Software functions that provide a list of appropriate cholesterol-lowering drugs to a health-care professional** to consider based on a patient's cholesterol levels and demographics found in the EHR, and the basis for the recommendations is provided to the health-care professional, so the health-care professional does not rely primarily on the recommendations in making a clinical decision about a patient.
- **Software functions that provide health-care professionals easy access to information related to patients' health conditions or treatments (beyond providing an electronic "copy" of a medical reference) and enable the health-care professional to independently review the basis of the information provided by the software function**, such that the health-care professional does not rely primarily on the information to make a clinical decision about an individual patient:
  - These software functions match patient-specific medical information (e.g., diagnosis, treatments, allergies, signs, or symptoms) to reference information routinely used in clinical practice (e.g., practice guidelines) to facilitate assessments of specific patients. The software function matches patient-specific medical information to peer-reviewed literature publications on related topics and enables the health-care professional to independently review the basis for the information, for example, a software function that uses a patient's diagnosis and other medical information to provide

Digital Innovations in Preventive Medicine

an HCP with current practice treatment guidelines for common illnesses or conditions such as influenza, hypertension, and hypercholesterolemia.

- Drug–drug interaction and drug–allergy contraindication notifications to avert adverse drug reactions. These software functions identify drug–drug interactions and drug–allergy contraindications based on the current version of FDA-approved drug or device labeling or other up-to-date and peer-reviewed sources and patient-specific information to attempt to prevent adverse drug reactions, and the software functions enable the health-care professional to independently review the basis for the information. For example, a software function that identifies drug–disease interactions and contraindications, such as notifying an HCP that a patient with asthma should not be prescribed a nonselective beta-blocking drug.

- **Software functions that provide patients with simple tools to organize and record their health information**. These software functions do this without providing recommendations to alter or change a previously prescribed treatment or therapy. Examples include:

  - Software functions that provide simple tools for patients with specific conditions or chronic diseases (e.g., obesity, anorexia, arthritis, diabetes, heart disease) to record their events or measurements (e.g., blood pressure measurements, drug intake times, diet, daily routine, or emotional state) and share this information with their health-care professional as part of a disease-management plan.

- **Software functions that are specifically marketed to help patients document, show, or communicate to health-care professionals regarding potential medical conditions**. These products either pose little

Health Technology Sourcebook, Third Edition

or no risk or are the sole responsibility of the health-care professionals who have used them in medical applications. Examples include:

- Software that serves as a videoconferencing portal specifically intended for medical use and to enhance communications between patients, health-care professionals, and caregivers.
- **Software functions that help asthmatics record (i.e., collect and log) inhaler usage, asthma episodes experienced, location of the user at the time of an attack, or environmental triggers of asthma attacks.**
- **Software functions that record the clinical conversation a clinician has with a patient and sends it (or a link) to the patient to access after the visit.**
- **Software functions that meet the definition of Non-Device-MDDS6.** These are software functions that are solely intended to transfer, store, convert formats, and display medical device data or results without controlling or altering the functions or parameters of any connected medical devices. These do not include software functions intended to generate alarms or alerts or prioritize patient-related information on multi-patient displays, which are typically used for active patient monitoring to enable immediate awareness for potential clinical intervention and are considered device software functions because these functions involve analysis or interpretation of laboratory test or other device data and results.
- **Software functions that display patient-specific medical device data.** These include software functions that display medical images directly from a picture archiving and communication system (PACS) server.
- **Software functions that are intended for transferring, storing, converting formats, or displaying clinical laboratory test or other device data and results,** findings by a health-care professional with respect to such data and results, general information about

196

Digital Innovations in Preventive Medicine

such findings, and general background information about such laboratory test or other devices unless such function is intended to interpret or analyze clinical laboratory test or other device data, results, and findings. Examples include:

- Software functions that transfer, store, convert formats, and display medical device data without modifying the data and do not control or alter the functions or parameters of any connected medical devices (i.e., software functions that meet the definition of Non-Device-MDDS)
- Software functions that meet the definition of Non-Device-MDDS and connect to a nursing central station and display (but do not analyze or interpret) medical device data to a physician's mobile platform for review
- Software functions that are not intended for diagnostic image review, such as image display for multidisciplinary patient management meetings (e.g., rounds) or patient consultation (and include a persistent on-screen notice, such as "for informational purposes only and not intended for diagnostic use")

Health Technology Sourcebook, Third Edition

Section 13.6 | Continuous Glucose Monitoring

This section contains text excerpted from the following sources: Text under the heading "Blood Glucose Monitoring Devices" is excerpted from "Blood Glucose Monitoring Devices," U.S. Food and Drug Administration (FDA), April 4, 2019; Text beginning with the heading "What Is Continuous Glucose Monitoring?" is excerpted from "Continuous Glucose Monitoring," National Institute of Diabetes and Digestive and Kidney Diseases (NIDDK), June 2017. Reviewed November 2022; Text under the heading "FreeStyle Libre Flash Glucose Monitoring System" is excerpted from "FDA Approves First Continuous Glucose Monitoring System for Adults Not Requiring Blood Sample Calibration," U.S. Food and Drug Administration (FDA), March 23, 2018. Reviewed November 2022.

BLOOD GLUCOSE MONITORING DEVICES
What Does This Test Do?

This is a test system for use at home or in health-care settings to measure the amount of sugar (glucose) in your blood.

What Is Glucose?

Glucose is a sugar that your body uses as a source of energy. Unless you have diabetes, your body regulates the amount of glucose in your blood. People with diabetes may need special diets and medications to control blood glucose.

What Type of Test Is This?

This is a quantitative test, which means that you will find out the amount of glucose present in your blood sample.

Why Should You Take This Test?

You should take this test if you have diabetes and you need to monitor your blood sugar (glucose) levels. You and your doctor can use the results to:
- Determine your daily adjustments in treatment.
- Know if you have dangerously high or low levels of glucose.
- Understand how your diet and exercise change your glucose levels.

The Diabetes Control and Complications Trial (1993) showed that good glucose control using home monitors led to fewer disease complications.

Digital Innovations in Preventive Medicine

How Often Should You Test Your Glucose?

Follow your doctor's recommendations about how often you test your glucose. You may need to test yourself several times each day to determine adjustments in your diet or treatment.

What Should Your Glucose Levels Be?

According to the American Diabetes Association, the blood glucose levels for an adult without diabetes are below 100 mg/dL before meals and fasting and are less than 140 mg/dL two hours after meals.

People with diabetes should consult their doctor or health-care provider to set appropriate blood glucose goals. You should treat your low or high blood glucose as recommended by your health-care provider.

How Accurate Is This Test?

The accuracy of this test depends on many factors, including:

- **The quality of your meter.**
- **The quality of your test strips**.
    - Always use new test strips that are authorized for sale in the United States. The FDA has issued a safety communication warning about the risks of using previously owned test strips or test strips that are not authorized for sale in the United States.
- **How well you perform the test**. For example, you should wash and dry your hands before testing and closely follow the instructions for operating your meter.
- **Your hematocrit** (the amount of red blood cells in the blood). If you are severely dehydrated or anemic, your test results may be less accurate. Your health-care provider can tell you if your hematocrit is low or high and can discuss with you how it may affect your glucose testing.
- **Interfering substances** (some substances, such as vitamin C, Tylenol, and uric acid, may interfere with your glucose testing). Check the instructions for your meter and test strips to find out what substances may affect the testing accuracy.

Health Technology Sourcebook, Third Edition

- **Altitude, temperature, and humidity** (high altitude, low and high temperatures, and humidity can cause unpredictable effects on glucose results).
  - Store and handle the meter and strips according to the manufacturer's instructions. It is important to store test strip vials closed.

How Do You Take This Test?

Before you test your blood glucose, you must read and understand the instructions for your meter. In general, you prick your finger with a lancet to get a drop of blood. Then you place the blood on a disposable "test strip" that is inserted in your meter. The test strip contains chemicals that react with glucose. Some meters measure the amount of electricity that passes through the test strip. Others measure how much light reflects from it. In the United States, meters report results in milligrams of glucose per deciliter of blood or mg/dl.

You can get information about your meter and test strips from several different sources, including the toll-free number in the manual that comes with your meter or on the manufacturer's website. If you have an urgent problem, always contact your health-care provider or a local emergency room for advice.

How Do You Choose a Glucose Meter?

There are many different types of meters available for purchase that differ in several ways, including:

- Accuracy
- Amount of blood needed for each test
- How easy it is to use
- Pain associated with using the product
- Testing speed
- Overall size
- Ability to store test results in memory
- Likelihood of interferences
- Ability to transmit data to a computer
- Cost of the meter

Digital Innovations in Preventive Medicine

- Cost of the test strips used
- Doctor's recommendation
- Technical support provided by the manufacturer
- Special features such as automatic timing, error codes, large display screen, or spoken instructions or results

Talk to your health-care provider about the right glucose meter for you and how to use it.

How can you check your meter's performance? There are three ways to make sure your meter works properly:

- **Use liquid control solutions:**
  - Every time you open a new container of test strips
  - Occasionally as you use the container of test strips
  - If you drop the meter
  - Whenever you get unusual results

  To test a liquid control solution, you test a drop of these solutions just like you test a drop of your blood. The value you get should match the value written on the test strip vial label.
- **Use electronic checks**. Every time you turn on your meter, it does an electronic check. If it detects a problem, it will give you an error code. Look in your meter's manual to see what the error codes mean and how to fix the problem. If you are unsure if your meter is working properly, call the toll-free number in your meter's manual or contact your health-care provider.
- **Compare your meter with a blood glucose test performed in a laboratory**. Take your meter with you to your next appointment with your health-care provider. Ask your provider to watch your testing technique to make sure you are using the meter correctly. Ask your health-care provider to have your blood tested with a laboratory method. If the values you obtain on your glucose meter match the laboratory values, then your meter is working well, and you are using good technique.

What Should You Do If Your Meter Malfunctions?

If your meter malfunctions, you should tell your health-care provider and contact the company that made your meter and strips.

Can You Test Blood Glucose from Sites Other Than Your Fingers?

Some meters allow you to test blood from sites other than the fingertip. Examples of such alternative sampling sites are your palm, upper arm, forearm, thigh, or calf. Alternative site testing (AST) should not be performed at times when your blood glucose may be changing rapidly, as these alternative sampling sites may provide inaccurate results at those times. You should use only blood from your fingertip to test if any of the following applies:

- You have just taken insulin.
- You think your blood sugar is low.
- You are not aware of symptoms when you become hypoglycemic.
- The results do not agree with the way you feel.
- You have just eaten.
- You have just exercised.
- You are ill.
- You are under stress.

Also, you should never use results from an alternative sampling site to calibrate a continuous glucose monitor (CGM) or in insulin dosing calculations.

WHAT IS CONTINUOUS GLUCOSE MONITORING?

Continuous glucose monitoring automatically tracks blood glucose levels, also called "blood sugar," throughout the day and night. You can see your glucose level anytime at a glance. You can also review how your glucose changes over a few hours or days to see trends. Seeing glucose levels in real time can help you make more informed decisions throughout the day about how to balance your food, physical activity, and medicines.

Digital Innovations in Preventive Medicine

HOW DOES A CONTINUOUS GLUCOSE MONITOR WORK?
A CGM works through a tiny sensor inserted under your skin, usually on your belly or arm. The sensor measures your interstitial glucose level, which is the glucose found in the fluid between the cells. The sensor tests glucose every few minutes. A transmitter wirelessly sends the information to a monitor.

Figure 13.1 shows the monitor that may be part of an insulin pump or a separate device, that you might carry in a pocket or purse. Some CGMs send information directly to a smartphone or tablet.

Special Features of a Continuous Glucose Monitor
Continuous glucose monitors are always on and recording glucose levels—whether you are showering, working, exercising, or sleeping. Many CGMs have special features that work with information from your glucose readings:
- An alarm can sound when your glucose level goes too low or too high.
- You can note your meals, physical activity, and medicines in a CGM device, too, alongside your glucose levels.

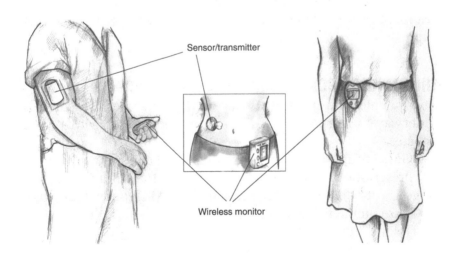

Figure 13.1. Continuous Glucose Monitoring

Health Technology Sourcebook, Third Edition

- You can download data to a computer or smart device to see your glucose trends more easily.

Some models can send information right away to a second person's smartphone—perhaps a parent, partner, or caregiver. For example, if a child's glucose drops dangerously low overnight, the CGM could be set to wake a parent in the next room.

Currently, one CGM model is approved for treatment decisions, the Dexcom G5 Mobile. It means you can make changes to your diabetes care plan based on CGM results alone. With other models, you must first confirm a CGM reading with a finger-stick blood glucose test before you take insulin or treat hypoglycemia.

Special Requirements Needed to Use a Continuous Glucose Monitor

Twice a day, you may need to check the CGM itself. You will test a drop of blood on a standard glucose meter. The glucose reading should be similar on both devices.

You will also need to replace the CGM sensor every 3–7 days, depending on the model.

For safety, it is important to take action when a CGM alarm sounds about high or low blood glucose. You should follow your treatment plan to bring your glucose into the target range or get help.

WHO CAN USE A CONTINUOUS GLUCOSE MONITOR?

Most people who use CGMs have type 1 diabetes. Research is underway to learn how CGMs might help people with type 2 diabetes.

CGMs are approved for use by adults and children with a doctor's prescription. Some models may be used for children as young as age 2. Your doctor may recommend a CGM if you or your child:

- Are on intensive insulin therapy, also called "tight blood sugar control."
- Have hypoglycemia unawareness.
- Often have high or low blood glucose.

Digital Innovations in Preventive Medicine

Your doctor may suggest using a CGM system all the time or only for a few days to help adjust your diabetes care plan.

WHAT ARE THE BENEFITS OF A CONTINUOUS GLUCOSE MONITOR?

Compared with a standard blood glucose meter, using a CGM system can help you with the following:

- Better manage your glucose levels every day.
- Have fewer low blood glucose emergencies.
- Need fewer finger sticks.

A graphic on the CGM screen shows whether your glucose is rising or dropping—and how quickly—so you can choose the best way to reach your target glucose level.

Over time, good management of glucose greatly helps people with diabetes stay healthy and prevent complications of the disease. People who gain the largest benefit from a CGM are those who use it every day or nearly every day.

WHAT ARE THE LIMITS OF A CONTINUOUS GLUCOSE MONITOR?

Researchers are working to make CGMs more accurate and easier to use. But you still need a finger-stick glucose test twice a day to check the accuracy of your CGM against a standard blood glucose meter.

With most CGM models, you cannot yet rely on the CGM alone to make treatment decisions. For example, before changing your insulin dose, you must first confirm a CGM reading by doing a finger-stick glucose test.

A CGM system is more expensive than using a standard glucose meter. Check with your health insurance plan or Medicare (medlineplus.gov/medicare.html) to see whether the costs will be covered.

WHAT IS AN ARTIFICIAL PANCREAS?

A CGM is one part of the "artificial pancreas" systems that are beginning to reach people with diabetes.

The National Institute of Diabetes and Digestive and Kidney Diseases (NIDDK) has played an important role in developing artificial pancreas technology. An artificial pancreas replaces manual blood glucose testing and the use of insulin shots. A single system monitors blood glucose levels around the clock and provides insulin or both insulin and a second hormone, glucagon, automatically. The system can also be monitored remotely, for example, by parents or medical staff.

In 2016, the U.S. Food and Drug Administration (FDA) approved a type of artificial pancreas system called a "hybrid closed-loop system." This system tests your glucose level every five minutes throughout the day and night through a CGM and automatically gives you the right amount of basal insulin, long-acting insulin, through a separate insulin pump. You will still need to test your blood with a glucose meter a few times a day. And you will manually adjust the amount of insulin the pump delivers at mealtimes and when you need a correction dose.

The hybrid closed-loop system may free you from some of the daily tasks needed to keep your blood glucose stable—or help you sleep through the night without the need to wake and test your glucose or take medicine. Talk with your health-care provider about whether this system might be right for you.

The NIDDK has funded—and continues to fund—several important studies on different types of artificial pancreas devices to better help people with type 1 diabetes manage their disease. The devices may also help people with type 2 diabetes and gestational diabetes.

Section 13.7 | **Wireless Patient Monitoring**

This section includes text excerpted from "Wireless Patient Monitoring," U.S. Department of Homeland Security (DHS), June 15, 2016. Reviewed November 2022.

Wireless patient monitoring technology provides paramedics, clinicians, and other medical personnel with a hands-free, wireless device to monitor a patient's vital signs, creating a safer environment for both emergency medical services (EMS) personnel and

Digital Innovations in Preventive Medicine

patients. No longer will first responders have to worry about entangled wires and a heavy monitor to transport with the patient. If patients require movement downstairs or through tight doorways, this wireless monitoring device poses less snag hazards and saves valuable time and space when connecting a patient to the ViSi sensors. Reducing snag hazards with just one device and a lightweight monitor will allow paramedics to respond to emergency incidents and perform daily operations more seamlessly and effectively.

The technology also allows end-to-end, real-time connectivity between the emergency medical technician in the field and the emergency room. Data can be forwarded through a remote system from the ambulance to the hospital to give doctors, nurses, and other staff better situational awareness prior to the patient's arrival.

WHY WIRELESS PATIENT MONITORING IS NEEDED

Paramedics and other EMS providers often operate in confined spaces and/or mobile environments. They are required to manage multiple tasks, including the monitoring of a patient's vital signs.

Currently, emergency medical responders must attach numerous wires and instruments to a patient to monitor vital signs. While the information received from these instruments is displayed on one screen, the entanglement of wires and the process of connecting and disconnecting the patient can be overwhelming and take up precious time and space in confined ambulatory transports (i.e., the back of an ambulance or an aircraft). EMS personnel need a hands-free, wireless technology that monitors all required patient vital signs from one location, and the ViSi Mobile® device meets this need by providing continuous, noninvasive blood pressure (cNIBP) monitoring.

HOW WIRELESS PATIENT MONITORING WORKS

In late 2012, the U.S. Department of Homeland Security Science and Technology Directorate (DHS S&T) partnered with Sotera Wireless, Inc. to develop a ViSi Mobile® device that can monitor vital signs without connecting wired sensors from the patient to other equipment. The device monitors blood pressure, 12-lead

Health Technology Sourcebook, Third Edition

electrocardiograms, temperature, and respiration. The system works with existing devices, including traditional sensor patches attached to a patient that transmit data wirelessly back to a central monitor. The system is capable of operating in confined and "on the go" spaces (e.g., when a distressed patient is moved from the scene of an incident into an ambulance) and uses a single monitor that is lightweight and easier to transport than existing models on the market.

RAPID PROTOTYPE DEVELOPMENT TO TRANSITION

In keeping with its mission of providing first responders with solutions to fill critical technology gaps, DHS S&T's R-Tech program worked with Sotera Wireless, Inc. to address the technology requirements identified by EMS subject matter experts with backgrounds in patient transport and vital sign monitoring. The continuous surveillance monitoring capabilities developed were tested during an operational field assessment (OFA) with EMS participants in San Diego, CA, in December 2013. Technological and operational feedback from this OFA has supported transitioning this device to the emergency medical response community.

Since transitioning the product to the commercial market, Sotera Wireless, Inc. has targeted the device for use in a hospital-based setting. The U.S. Food and Drug Administration (FDA) has approved the ViSi Mobile® device for continuous, noninvasive blood pressure (cNIBP) monitoring.

Chapter 14 | **Predictive Analytics in Health Care**

Chapter Contents
Section 14.1—Big Data and Its Applications in
Health Care 211
Section 14.2—Big Data in the Age of Genomics.........................214
Section 14.3—Big Data for Infectious Disease
Surveillance..217

Section 14.1 | Big Data and Its Applications in Health Care

This section includes text excerpted from "Demystifying—Big Data," National Institute of Standards and Technology (NIST), July 21, 2022.

Big data is a term that describes large volumes of high-velocity, complex, and variable data that require advanced techniques and technologies to enable the capture, storage, distribution, management, and analysis of information.

CHARACTERISTICS OF BIG DATA

Big data is often characterized by three factors: volume, velocity, and variety. Fifteen percent of the information today is structured information, or information that is easily stored in relational databases of spreadsheets, with their ordinary columns and rows. Unstructured information, such as e-mail, video, blogs, call center conversations, and social media, makes up about 85 percent of data generated today and presents challenges in deriving meaning with conventional business intelligence tools. Information-producing devices, such as sensors, tablets, and mobile phones, continue to multiply. Social networking is also growing at an accelerated pace as the world becomes more connected. Such information-sharing options represent a fundamental shift in the way people, government, and businesses interact with each other.

The characteristics of big data will shape the way government organizations ingest, analyze, manage, store, and distribute data across the enterprise and across the ecosystem. Table 14.1 illustrates the characteristics of big data that more completely describe the difference of "big data" from the historical perspective of "normal data."

HEALTH-CARE QUALITY AND EFFICIENCY

The ability to continuously improve quality and efficiency in the delivery of health care while reducing costs remains an elusive goal for care providers and payers but also represents a significant opportunity to improve the lives of everyday Americans.

Health Technology Sourcebook, Third Edition

Table 14.1. Characteristics of Big Data

Characteristic	Description	Attribute	Driver
Volume	The sheer amount of data generated or data intensity that must be ingested, analyzed, and managed to make decisions based on complete data analysis	According to IDC's Digital Universe Study, the world's "digital universe" is in the process of generating 1.8 zettabytes of information—with continuing exponential growth.	Increase in data sources, higher resolution sensors
Velocity	How fast data is being produced and changed and the speed with which data must be received, understood, and processed	• Accessibility: information when, where, and how the user wants it, at the point of impact • Applicable: relevant, valuable information for an enterprise at a torrential pace that becomes a real-time phenomenon • Time value: real-time analysis that yields improved data-driven decisions	• Increase in data sources • Improved throughput connectivity • Enhanced computing power of data-generating devices
Variety	The rise of information coming from new sources both inside and outside the walls of the enterprise or organization that creates integration, management, governance, and architectural pressures on IT	• Structured: 15 percent of data today is structured, row, columns • Unstructured: 85 percent is unstructured or human-generated information • Semistructured: the combination of structured and unstructured data is becoming paramount • Complexity: where data sources are moving and residing	• Mobile • Social media • Videos • Chat • Genomics • Sensors
Veracity	The quality and provenance of received data	The quality of big data may be good, bad, or undefined due to data inconsistency and incompleteness, ambiguities, latency, deception, and model approximations.	Data-based decisions that require traceability and justification

Predictive Analytics in Health Care

Coupled with this rise in expenditures, certain chronic diseases, such as diabetes, are increasing in prevalence and consuming a greater percentage of health-care resources. The management of these diseases and other health-related services profoundly affects the nation's well-being. Big data can help. The increased use of electronic health records (EHRs) coupled with new analytics tools presents an opportunity to mine information for the most effective outcomes across large populations. Using de-identified information carefully, researchers can look for statistically valid trends and provide assessments based on the true quality of care.

HEALTH-CARE EARLY DETECTION

Big data in health care may involve using sensors in the hospital or home to provide continuous monitoring of key biochemical markers, performing real-time analysis on the data as it streams from individual high-risk patients to a HIPAA-compliant analysis system. The analysis system can alert specific individuals and their chosen health-care provider if the analysis detects a health anomaly requiring a visit to their provider or a "911" event about to happen. This has the potential to extend and improve the quality of millions of citizens' lives.

FRAUD DETECTION: HEALTH-CARE BENEFITS SERVICES

Big data can transform improper payment detection and fundamentally change the risk and return perceptions of individuals that currently submit improper, erroneous, or fraudulent claims. For example, a significant challenge confronting the Centers for Medicare and Medicaid Services (CMS) is managing improper payments under the Medicare Fee-For-Service (FFS) program. The FFS distributes billions of dollars in estimated improper payments. Currently, contractors and employees identify improper payments by selecting a small sample of claims, requesting medical documentation from the provider who submitted the claims, and manually reviewing the claims against the medical documentation to verify the providers' compliance with Medicare's policies.

This challenge is an opportunity to explore a use case for applying big data technologies and techniques to perform unstructured data

Health Technology Sourcebook, Third Edition

analytics on medical documents to improve efficiency in mitigating improper payments. Automating the improper payment process and utilizing big data tools, techniques, and governance processes would result in greater improper payment prevention or recovery. Data management and distribution could be achieved through an image classification workflow solution to classify and route documents. Data analytics and data intelligence would be based on unstructured document analysis techniques and pattern-matching expertise.

The benefit is that the culture of submitting improper payments will be changed. Big data tools, techniques, and governance processes would increase the prevention and recovery dollar value by evaluating the entire data set and dramatically increasing the speed of identification and detection of compliance patterns.

Section 14.2 | Big Data in the Age of Genomics

This section includes text excerpted from "Public Health Approach to Big Data in the Age of Genomics: How Can We Separate Signal from Noise?" Centers for Disease Control and Prevention (CDC), October 30, 2014. Reviewed November 2022.

It turns out that big data is all around us! As Leroy Hood once commented, "We predict that in 5 to 10 years each person will be surrounded by a virtual cloud of billions of data points." Genome sequencing of humans and other organisms has been a leading contributor to big data, but other types of data are increasingly larger, more diverse, and more complex, exceeding the abilities of currently used approaches to store, manage, share, analyze, and interpret it effectively. We have all heard claims that big data will revolutionize everything, including health and health care.

Today, there are several promising applications of big data in improving health involving the use of genome sequencing technologies. For example:

- Diagnosis of rare and mysterious diseases
- Improved classification of cancer based on tumor genomes rather than anatomic locations

214

Predictive Analytics in Health Care

- Genomically driven personalized cancer treatment (precision medicine)
- Using whole genome sequencing to improve public health detection and response to outbreaks of infectious diseases

Big data today is often noisier than signal! Sorting through all of the data to determine what is a real signal and what is noise does not always work as expected. For example, in 2013, when influenza hit the United States hard and early, Google attempted to monitor the outbreak using analysis of flu-related Internet searches, drastically overestimating peak flu levels compared with traditional public health surveillance efforts. Even more problematic could be the potential for many false alarms by mindless examination on a large scale, leading to putative associations between big data points and disease outcomes. This process may falsely infer causality and could potentially lead to ineffective or harmful interventions. The field of genomics has recognized this problem and addressed it by requiring replication of study findings and for signals to be much stronger to be picked. To appropriately analyze big data, the field of genomics requires the use of epidemiologic studies, animal models, and other work in addition to big data analysis. Big data's strength is in finding associations, but its weakness is in not showing whether these associations have meaning. Finding a signal is only the first step.

- **Epidemiologic foundation**. We need a strong epidemiologic foundation for studying big data in health and disease. The associations found using big data need to be studied and replicated in ways that confirm the findings and make them generalizable. By that, we mean the study of well-characterized and representative populations such as the cohort consortium sponsored by the National Cancer Institute (NCI) that has been collecting information on more than four million people over multiple decades. Big data analysis is currently based on convenient samples of people or data available on the Internet. Both sources may be fraught with all sorts of biases, such

Health Technology Sourcebook, Third Edition

as selection, confounding, and lack of generalizability. For more than a decade, we have promoted an epidemiologic approach to the human genome, and now, it is time to extend this approach to all big data.

- **Knowledge integration**. We need to develop a robust "knowledge integration" (KI) enterprise to make sense of big data. In a recent article titled "Knowledge Integration at the Center of Genomic Medicine," the definition of KI and its three components, such as knowledge management, knowledge synthesis, and knowledge translation in genomics, have been elaborated. A similar evidence-based knowledge integration process applies to all big data beyond genomics. It is believed that the recently launched National Institutes of Health (NIH) Biomedical Data to Knowledge (BD2K) awards will support the development of new approaches, software, tools, and training programs to improve access, analysis, synthesis, and interpretation of genomic big data and improve the ability to make and validate new discoveries.
- **Evidence-based medicine**. We should embrace (and not run away from) principles of evidence-based medicine and population screening. The authors elaborated on the relationship between genomic medicine and evidence-based medicine. They believe the same relationship applies to all big data. Big data is literally a hypothesis-generating machine that could lead to interesting, robust, and predictive associations with health outcomes. However, even after these associations are established, evidence of utility (i.e., improved health outcomes and no evidence of harm) is still needed. Documenting the health-related utility of genomics and big data information may necessitate the use of randomized clinical trials and other experimental designs.
- **Translational research**. As with genomic medicine, a robust translational research agenda is needed for

Predictive Analytics in Health Care

big data that goes beyond the initial discovery (the bench-to-bedside model). In genomics, most published research is either basic scientific discoveries or preclinical research designed to develop health-related tests and interventions. What happens after that is really the research "road less traveled." In fact, less than one percent of published research deals with validation, implementation, policy, communication, and outcomes in the real world. Reaping the benefits of using big data for genomics research will require a more expanded translational research agenda beyond the initial discoveries.

Section 14.3 | Big Data for Infectious Disease Surveillance

This section includes text excerpted from "Focus: Big Data for Infectious Disease Surveillance, Modeling," Fogarty International Center (FIC), National Institutes of Health (NIH), February 2017. Reviewed November 2022.

Big data derived from electronic health records, social media, the Internet, and other digital sources have the potential to provide more timely and detailed information on infectious disease threats or outbreaks than traditional surveillance methods, but there are challenges to overcome.

Traditional infectious disease surveillance—typically based on laboratory tests and other epidemiological data collected by public health institutions—is the gold standard. But the authors note it can include time lags, is expensive to produce, and typically lacks the local resolution needed for accurate monitoring. Furthermore, it can be cost-prohibitive in low-income countries. In contrast, big data streams from internet queries, for example, are available in real time and can track disease activity locally but have their own biases. Hybrid tools that combine traditional surveillance and big data sets may provide a way forward, the scientists suggest, serving to complement, rather than replace, existing methods.

Health Technology Sourcebook, Third Edition

"The ultimate goal is to be able to forecast the size, peak or trajectory of outbreak weeks or months in advance in order to better respond to infectious disease threats. Integrating big data in surveillance is the first step toward this long-term goal," says Fogarty senior scientist Dr. Cecile Viboud, co-editor of the supplement. "Now that we have demonstrated proof of concept by comparing data sets in high-income countries, we can examine these models in low-resource settings where traditional surveillance is sparse."

The researchers report on the opportunities and challenges associated with three types of data: medical encounter files, such as records from health-care facilities and insurance claim forms; crowdsourced data collected from volunteers who self-report symptoms in near real time (part of the "citizen science" movement); and data generated by the use of social media, the Internet, and mobile phones, which may include self-reporting of health, behavior, and travel information.

But big data's potential must be tempered with caution, the authors say. Nontraditional data streams may lack key demographic identifiers such as age and sex, and the information they provide may under-represent infants, children, and the elderly, as well as residents of developing countries. Furthermore, social media outlets may not always be stable sources of data, as they can disappear if there is a loss of interest or financing. Most importantly, any novel data stream must be validated against established infectious disease surveillance data and systems, the authors emphasize.

ENSURING DATA PRIVACY

Big data offer a "tantalizing opportunity" to provide more information for public health surveillance, but the authors say its use for that purpose is decades behind other fields, such as climatology and marketing. Electronic health records with identifying information removed, for example, may be a resource to monitor outcomes of infectious diseases, vaccine uptake, and adverse drug reactions. Applying the data to surveillance has been slow, the authors say, in part because of ethical concerns about patient privacy. There is

Predictive Analytics in Health Care

also a scarcity of academic studies demonstrating how this type of data performs against traditional surveillance methods.

HARVESTING MEDICAL INSURANCE CLAIM DATA

Medical insurance claim forms, used in the United States and other countries, document the date and location of a doctor's office visit as well as a diagnosis code, which researchers say is useful in tracking disease outbreaks, especially in large populations. Working with anonymized claim form data made available for research, investigators found "excellent alignment" between claim data for flu-like illnesses and proven influenza activity reported by the Centers for Disease Control and Prevention (CDC). The body of influenza research suggests medical claims data should be harvested to generate timely, local data on acute infections, according to the researchers.

ENGAGING THE PUBLIC TO TRACK THE FLU

A European surveillance system that began collecting crowd-sourced data on influenza-like illnesses as part of a research project is now considered an adjunct to existing surveillance activities.

Influenzanet is a system that uses standardized online surveys to gather information from volunteers who self-report their symptoms on a weekly basis. Data are analyzed in real time, and national and regional results are posted on the website. Established in 2009, the tool is now being used by a number of European countries and is being expanded to collect information on Zika, salmonella, and other diseases.

In their review, the authors note the standardization of the technological and epidemiological framework makes it easier for countries to join Influenzanet and allows for coherent surveillance. The timeliness of the reporting and the inclusion of people who may not go to the doctor for treatment of the flu are other strengths.

Downsides include the potential for misreporting and the lack of validation by a physician or lab test. But the authors point out that Influenzanet estimates of illness incidence compare well with data from traditional surveillance methods.

Health Technology Sourcebook, Third Edition

AGGREGATING ANTIBIOTIC RESISTANCE DATA

Noting that antibiotic resistance is a growing concern around the world, U.S. and Canadian scientists developed an online platform to monitor it at the regional level. ResistanceOpen aggregates publicly available online data from community health-care institutions as well as regional, national, and international bodies and displays the information on a navigable map. An analysis of the resource found that the online information compared favorably with traditional reporting systems in the United States and Canada.

The scientists who developed ResistanceOpen aim to expand the database and say the platform could help fill the gap in antimicrobial resistance surveillance in many low- and middle-income countries. ResistanceOpen is an extension of HealthMap, a project that collects and analyzes disparate online data sources to track infectious disease outbreaks around the world. HealthMap has been supported by private and public partners, including the NIH, CDC, and USAID.

DETECTING ADVERSE DRUG REACTIONS

In addition to improving infectious disease surveillance, nontraditional data streams from the Internet and social media have the potential to supplement traditional systems for reporting adverse drug reactions (ADRs). While consumers rarely use official ADR reporting systems, they do search the web for information about medications and share the word of possible adverse reactions on social media sites and online health forums.

Mining and analyzing Internet search logs and social media posts may detect ADR signals more quickly than traditional physician-based reporting systems, but there are challenges. One of the many ethical questions surrounding the use of these nontraditional sources is whether privately held data should be accessible for public health research.

COMPARING EPIDEMIC AND WEATHER FORECASTING

In a comparison of the relatively new field of epidemic forecasting to the better-established one of weather forecasting, the authors

Predictive Analytics in Health Care

note the former is much more difficult given that there is less observational data for disease and because human behavior has the potential to rapidly alter the course of an epidemic.

Internet data streams, such as search queries and social media posts, may aid epidemic forecasting by providing information in near real time and at a more local level. But internet data, the authors say, are less reliable than information collected from weather stations, and the availability can vary because of limited internet access in many developing countries.

HARNESSING SPATIAL BIG DATA

To determine where an outbreak originated or where future ones may occur, for example, epidemiologists need spatial data. Medical insurance claims, social media posts, and mobile phones have the potential to fill geographical information gaps. But the authors point out that there are technical, practical, and ethical issues that must be addressed. They note possible solutions to protect privacy, such as masking individual-level information by aggregating collected data to larger spatial resolutions.

CONNECTING MOBILITY TO INFECTIOUS DISEASES

With appropriate safeguards to ensure anonymity, call data records from mobile phones may provide researchers "an unprecedented opportunity" to determine how travel affects disease transmission. Studies of malaria and rubella in Kenya showed how call data improved the understanding of the spatial transmission of those diseases. Because mobile phone data has biases, young children are not likely to be represented, for example. The authors say more research is needed to determine if mobility patterns derived from call data records are representative of general travel patterns.

CULLING INFORMATION FROM INTERNET REPORTS

Online news articles and health bulletins from public health agencies can also be manually dissected to model the sequence of transmission chains in an outbreak. The transmission dynamics and risk factors of the Ebola epidemic in West Africa and a Middle East

Health Technology Sourcebook, Third Edition

Respiratory Syndrome outbreak in South Korea were elucidated by this approach. Internet findings were in line with traditional data, providing a proof of concept that this approach can be generalized and automated to a variety of online sources, and generate information on disease transmission. This is particularly useful to improve situational awareness and guide public health interventions during emerging infectious disease crises when traditional surveillance data are particularly scarce.

MANAGING EPIDEMIC SIMULATION DATA
Researchers also describe the benefits of a novel, publicly available epidemic simulation data management system called "epiDMS," which provides storage and indexing services for large data simulation sets, as well as search functionality and data analysis to aid decision-makers during health-care emergencies.

While the new hybrid models that combine traditional and digital disease surveillance methods show promise, the scientists agree there is still an overall scarcity of reliable surveillance information, especially compared to other fields, such as climatology, where the data sets are huge.

Chapter 15 | Screening and Detection Technologies

Chapter Contents
Section 15.1—Advanced Molecular Detection 225
Section 15.2—GI Genius in Detection of Colon Cancer 231
Section 15.3—OsteoDetect in Wrist Fracture Analysis.............233
Section 15.4—Prediction of Abdominal Aneurysm
                Using Machine Learning.....................................234

Chapter 15 | Screening and Detection Techniques

Section 15.1 | Advanced Molecular Detection

This section includes text excerpted from "Advanced Molecular Detection (AMD)," Centers for Disease Control and Prevention (CDC), January 8, 2019.

THE ADVANCED MOLECULAR DETECTION PROGRAM

The Advanced Molecular Detection (AMD) program of the Centers for Disease Control and Prevention (CDC) is helping modernize the public health system's disease-investigation capabilities by employing the latest technologies and improving AMD capacity throughout the nation.

Under the AMD program, the CDC has been working to build on the nation's existing public health infrastructure by integrating AMD technologies. These modern tools deliver a greater level of detailed information on infectious pathogens than older, slower, and less cost-effective methods. Since its inception in 2014, the AMD program has increased the availability of next-generation sequencing and other AMD technologies within the CDC and in state and local public health systems.

The AMD program works with experts across the CDC to ensure the United States has the infrastructure, including technology, needed to protect Americans from infectious disease threats. The AMD office collaborates with other CDC programs to facilitate the development and pilot testing of next-generation diagnostic tests and protocols. Other programs throughout the CDC leverage these tools against a variety of infectious pathogens and help state and local public health agencies tap into them, as well.

Advanced Molecular Detection Technologies

The AMD program is helping build and integrate laboratory, bioinformatics, and epidemiology technologies across the CDC and nationwide. Building capacity in all three areas is necessary for creating a 21st-century public health detection and surveillance system to protect the United States from disease threats.

LABORATORY TECHNOLOGIES

The AMD technologies include laboratory methods to extract and sequence the deoxyribonucleic acid (DNA) of pathogens, including next-generation genomic sequencing (NGS) and whole genome sequencing (WGS). Sequencing technologies range from portable sequencers for field-based testing to benchtop and full-sized sequencers for laboratory use.

EPIDEMIOLOGY TECHNOLOGIES

Epidemiologists help detect where data from their traditional field investigations intersect with genomic data to pinpoint disease outbreaks and clusters of human illnesses. Through training in molecular epidemiology, the CDC is helping build on the existing epidemiology workforce, so they can use genomic data generated and analyzed through bioinformatics pipelines to help solve outbreak mysteries.

BIOINFORMATICS TECHNOLOGIES

Even though infectious pathogens are small, sequencing their DNA generates a tremendous amount of genomic data. To analyze those data, experts in bioinformatics use high-performance computing systems to devise programs, often called "pipelines." Once designed and validated, these pipelines can speed up the detection and characterization of pathogens. By uploading DNA sequence data into a specific pipeline, scientists can rapidly find out which species or strain of the pathogen is involved in an outbreak and specific characteristics that can be important for fighting it, such as whether it is resistant to antimicrobials.

THE OFFICE OF ADVANCED MOLECULAR DETECTION RESPONSIBILITIES

The CDC's Office of Advanced Molecular Detection (OAMD) works with experts across the CDC to ensure the United States has the infrastructure, including technology, needed to protect Americans from infectious disease threats. OAMD collaborates

Screening and Detection Technologies

with other CDC programs to facilitate the development and pilot testing of next-generation diagnostics and protocols. Other programs throughout the CDC leverage these tools against a variety of infectious pathogens and help state and local public health agencies tap into them as well:

- Exploring new technologies.
- Enhancing surveillance.
- Developing faster tests.
- Uncovering emerging threats.
- Improving vaccines.
- Tracking global health.
- Mapping environmental threats.
- Strengthening food safety.
- Identifying vector-borne diseases.
- Combating health-care-associated infections (HAIs) and antibiotic-resistant microbes (AMRs).
- Battling human immunodeficiency virus (HIV) and sexually transmitted diseases (STDs).

HOW ADVANCED MOLECULAR DETECTION PROGRAM WORKS

Since 2014, the AMD program has worked to integrate the latest next-generation sequencing technology with bioinformatics and epidemiology expertise to improve public health. Today, pathogen genomics is part of almost every infectious disease program at the CDC and has become central to the U.S. public health system's efforts to identify, track, and stop infectious diseases.

The genome, or genetic material, of an organism is made up of a unique deoxyribonucleic acid (DNA) or ribonucleic acid (RNA) sequence. These sequences are composed of chemical building blocks known as "nucleotide bases." Determining the order of bases—"genomic sequencing" or simply "sequencing"—is a core AMD technology.

The information encoded in the genomes of disease-causing bacteria, viruses, and fungi represent unique genetic fingerprints. Whole-genome sequencing (WGS) is a laboratory procedure that determines the order of all or most of the nucleotides in the genome of these disease-causing microbes, enabling public health officials

Health Technology Sourcebook, Third Edition

to better understand how microorganisms move through populations and change over time.

Next-generation sequencing (NGS) refers to sequencing technologies that can process a large quantity of genetic material at a time. These technologies have been available since 2004, and they have largely replaced the previous method ("Sanger sequencing") and make high-throughput WGS possible. Newer sequencing platforms have revolutionized this field by generating larger volumes of data and dramatically lowering the cost of sequencing.

WHAT IS NEW IN THE ADVANCED MOLECULAR DETECTION PROGRAM?

Tracking the spread of SARS-CoV-2, the virus that causes COVID-19 continues to be vital to interrupting chains of transmission, preventing new cases of illness, and saving lives. Scientists can test community wastewater samples to detect the ribonucleic acid, or "RNA," of SARS-CoV-2. Wastewater testing is a novel approach for monitoring the virus, providing timely information about the changing prevalence of COVID-19 in different communities.

SARS-CoV-2 enters wastewater through the stool of infected people. Using genomic sequencing to monitor the concentration of SARS-CoV-2 in wastewater can detect the presence of infection in a community and suggest whether levels of infection are increasing or decreasing. When used as a complement to other surveillance methods, wastewater surveillance data can provide an important early warning signal of increasing infections. To assess whether further investigation is needed, public health officials can compare wastewater surveillance data to historic levels at the same site and among neighboring communities. Public health officials can also compare these data with trends in other surveillance systems, such as case reporting. Local circumstances, such as increased tourism or changes in prevention measures, are also considered to inform public health decisions.

In response to the COVID-19 pandemic, the CDC launched the National Wastewater Surveillance System (NWSS) in September 2020 to coordinate and support the nation's capacity to monitor SARS-CoV-2 in wastewater. NWSS started as a grassroots effort to connect

Screening and Detection Technologies

independent, local wastewater surveillance efforts to form a robust, sustainable national system. Through NWSS, health departments and public health laboratories develop their capacity to conduct wastewater surveillance, including epidemiology, data analytics, and laboratory support. This information can be a critical early warning for authorities of new outbreaks and inform local decision-making, such as where to have mobile testing and vaccination sites.

Since its launch, NWSS has made great strides and now includes more than 1,000 testing sites nationwide. As of July 2022, a total of 46 states, five cities, and two territories have wastewater surveillance systems in their communities, with samples collected from wastewater systems serving more than 130 million people in the United States. The CDC scientists continue to provide technical guidance, data analysis, and access to data visualization to jurisdictions with wastewater surveillance systems.

Detecting Variants in Wastewater

Whole-genome sequencing (WGS) technology is used to decode the genetic information of infectious disease pathogens. Genomic sequencing supports public health in multiple areas, such as improving food safety, combating antimicrobial resistance, and detecting emerging infectious disease threats.

The sequencing of wastewater samples can provide valuable information about SARS-CoV-2 variants. While WGS cannot confirm the presence of any one specific variant in wastewater—because the virus's RNA breaks into pieces in wastewater—WGS of wastewater samples can detect pieces of variant-defining mutations, which can provide strong early evidence that a variant is likely to present or may be spreading in the community before clinical case detection.

For example, a January 2022 MMWR article reports there was evidence of SARS-CoV-2 B.1.1.529 (Omicron) variant mutations in community wastewater in late November 2021, shortly before the Omicron variant had been identified in cases in these communities.

Wastewater Surveillance at the Local Level

State, tribal, local, and territorial public health laboratories work closely with wastewater treatment plants to establish wastewater surveillance sampling strategies. These strategies, which may be updated as scientific knowledge increases and public health needs change, include multiple testing methods and laboratory processes used to analyze SARS-CoV-2 in wastewater and balance available resources and testing capacity with public health data needs. Two examples of how wastewater surveillance is being used in local communities are given below.

A case study in the COVID-19 Genomic Epidemiology Toolkit describes the early detection of SARS-CoV-2 RNA in the wastewater system of Burlington, VT. Wastewater surveillance provided the city of Burlington and the state of Vermont with an additional layer of COVID-19 surveillance beyond diagnostic testing. Fast wastewater testing allowed local health officials to deploy resources to areas with higher virus levels and provide specific warnings to the public, focusing on vulnerable populations.

The Delaware Public Health Laboratory has worked to implement wastewater surveillance testing since August 2020. To date, 12 out of the 18 wastewater treatment plants in Delaware are using a surveillance system that has helped the state fill data gaps in areas where clinical testing and surveillance may be limited, including in underserved communities with limited access to testing sites. Delaware plans to expand on these investments to look for other pathogens in wastewater, such as Norovirus, Influenza, RSV, and antimicrobial-resistant pathogens.

The Future of Wastewater Surveillance

The CDC will continue to expand NWSS to better understand and respond to infectious disease threats such as antimicrobial resistance or foodborne diseases. Through an annual Epidemiology and Laboratory Capacity for Prevention and Control of Emerging Infectious Diseases (ELC) funding opportunity, NWSS resources are available to public health departments to develop wastewater surveillance programs. NWSS will be establishing Wastewater Surveillance Centers of Excellence to support the continued development of wastewater surveillance for public health.

Public health laboratories across the nation are critical to our public health infrastructure. The use of innovative applications of

Screening and Detection Technologies

sequencing and other AMD technologies will help prepare communities to detect and track disease outbreaks now and in the future.

Section 15.2 | GI Genius in Detection of Colon Cancer

This section includes text excerpted from "FDA Authorizes Marketing of First Device that Uses Artificial Intelligence to Help Detect Potential Signs of Colon Cancer," U.S. Food and Drug Administration (FDA), April 9, 2021.

The U.S. Food and Drug Administration (FDA) authorized the marketing of the GI Genius, the first device that uses artificial intelligence (AI) based on machine learning to assist clinicians in detecting lesions (such as polyps or suspected tumors) in the colon in real time during a colonoscopy.

"Artificial intelligence has the potential to transform health care to better assist health care providers and improve patient care. When AI is combined with traditional screenings or surveillance methods, it could help find problems early on, when they may be easier to treat," said Dr. Courtney H. Lias, Ph.D., acting director of the GastroRenal, ObGyn, General Hospital and Urology Devices Office in the FDA's Center for Devices and Radiological Health. "Studies show that during colorectal cancer screenings, missed lesions can be a problem even for well-trained clinicians. With the FDA's authorization of this device today, clinicians now have a tool that could help improve their ability to detect gastrointestinal lesions they may have missed otherwise."

According to the National Institutes of Health (NIH), colorectal cancer is the third leading cause of death from cancer in the United States. Colorectal cancer usually starts from polyps or other precancerous growths in the rectum or the colon (large intestine). As part of a colorectal cancer screening and surveillance plan, clinicians perform colonoscopies to detect changes or abnormalities in the lining of the colon and rectum. A colonoscopy involves threading an endoscope (thin, flexible tube with a camera at the end) through the rectum and throughout the entire length of the colon, allowing a clinician to see signs of cancer or precancerous lesions.

Health Technology Sourcebook, Third Edition

The GI Genius is composed of hardware and software designed to highlight portions of the colon where the device detects a potential lesion. The software uses artificial intelligence algorithm techniques to identify regions of interest. During a colonoscopy, the GI Genius system generates markers, which look like green squares and are accompanied by a short, low-volume sound, and superimposes them on the video from the endoscope camera when it identifies a potential lesion. These signs signal to the clinician that further assessment may be needed, such as a closer visual inspection, tissue sampling, testing or removal, or ablation of (burning) the lesion. The GI Genius is designed to be compatible with many FDA-cleared standard video endoscopy systems.

The FDA assessed the safety and effectiveness of the GI Genius through a multicenter, prospective, randomized, controlled study in Italy with 700 subjects 40–80 years old who were undergoing a colonoscopy for colorectal cancer screening, surveillance, positive results from a previous fecal immunochemical (fecal occult blood) test for blood in the stool or gastrointestinal symptoms of possible colorectal cancer. The primary analyses from the study were based on a subpopulation of 263 patients who were being screened or surveilled every three years or more. Study subjects underwent either white light standard colonoscopy with the GI Genius (136 patients) or standard white light colonoscopy alone (127 patients).

The primary endpoint of the study compared how often colonoscopy plus the GI Genius identified a patient with at least one lab-confirmed adenoma (precancerous tumor) or carcinoma (cancerous tumor) to how often standard colonoscopy made the same identifications. In the study, colonoscopy plus the GI Genius was able to identify lab-confirmed adenomas or carcinomas in 55.1 percent of patients compared to identifying them in 42 percent of patients with standard colonoscopy, an observed difference of 13 percent.

While the use of this device led to more biopsies being performed, there were no adverse events reported with the additional biopsies, such as perforations, infections, or bleeding. However, there was a slight increase in the number of lesions biopsied that were not adenomas.

Screening and Detection Technologies

The GI Genius is not intended to characterize or classify a lesion nor to replace lab sampling as a means of diagnosis. The device does not provide any diagnostic assessments of colorectal polyp pathology, nor does it suggest to the clinician how to manage suspicious polyps. The GI Genius only identifies regions of the colon within the endoscope's field of view where a colorectal polyp might be located, allowing for a more extended examination in real time during colonoscopy. It is up to the clinician to decide whether the identified region actually contains a suspected lesion and how the lesion should be managed and processed per standard clinical practice and guidelines.

Section 15.3 | OsteoDetect in Wrist Fracture Analysis

This section includes text excerpted from "FDA Permits Marketing of Artificial Intelligence Algorithm for Aiding Providers in Detecting Wrist Fractures," U.S. Food and Drug Administration (FDA), May 24, 2018. Reviewed November 2022.

The U.S. Food and Drug Administration (FDA) permitted the marketing of Imagen OsteoDetect, a type of computer-aided detection and diagnosis software designed to detect wrist fractures in adult patients.

"Artificial intelligence algorithms have tremendous potential to help health care providers diagnose and treat medical conditions," said Dr. Robert Ochs, Ph.D., acting deputy director for radiological health, Office of In Vitro Diagnostics and Radiological Health in the FDA's Center for Devices and Radiological Health. "This software can help providers detect wrist fractures more quickly and aid in the diagnosis of fractures."

The OsteoDetect software is a computer-aided detection and diagnostic software that uses an artificial intelligence algorithm to analyze two-dimensional x-ray images for signs of distal radius fracture, a common type of wrist fracture. The software marks the location of the fracture on the image to aid the provider in the detection and diagnosis.

Health Technology Sourcebook, Third Edition

OsteoDetect analyzes wrist radiographs using machine learning techniques to identify and highlight regions of distal radius fracture during the review of posterior–anterior (front and back) and medial–lateral (sides) x-ray images of adult wrists. OsteoDetect is intended to be used by clinicians in various settings, including primary care, emergency medicine, urgent care, and specialty care, such as orthopedics. It is an adjunct tool and is not intended to replace a clinician's review of the radiograph or her or his clinical judgment.

The company submitted a retrospective study of 1,000 radiograph images that assessed the independent performance of the image analysis algorithm for detecting wrist fractures and the accuracy of the fracture localization of OsteoDetect against the performance of three board-certified orthopedic hand surgeons. Imagen also submitted a retrospective study of 24 providers who reviewed 200 patient cases. Both studies demonstrated that the readers' performance in detecting wrist fractures was improved using the software, including increased sensitivity, specificity, and positive and negative predictive values, when aided by OsteoDetect, as compared with their unaided performance according to standard clinical practice.

Section 15.4 | Prediction of Abdominal Aneurysm Using Machine Learning

This section includes text excerpted from "Machine Learning Predicts Risk of Aneurysm," National Institutes of Health (NIH), September 18, 2018. Reviewed November 2022.

An abnormal bulge in a blood vessel, known as an "aneurysm," usually has no symptoms but can be deadly if it expands and bursts. An aneurysm that occurs in the main artery that leads from the heart through the belly is called an "abdominal aortic aneurysm" (AAA). Some people are lucky enough to have AAA detected during medical scans for other reasons.

Screening and Detection Technologies

Being over 65, being male, smoking, having high blood pressure, and having a buildup of plaque in the arteries are AAA risk factors. A family history of AAA is also thought to play a role. Lifestyle changes and treatments may prevent an aneurysm from expanding and bursting.

A research team led by Dr. Philip S. Tsao and Dr. Michael Snyder of Stanford University set out to develop a way to predict which people are at risk of having AAA. They used genome sequences and machine learning techniques to create an algorithm they call Hierarchical Estimate from Agnostic Learning (HEAL). The work was funded in part by the National Heart, Lung, and Blood Institute (NHLBI) and the National Human Genome Research Institute (NHGRI) of the National Institutes of Health (NIH). Results were published in *Cell* on September 6, 2018.

The scientists performed whole genome sequencing on blood samples from 133 healthy people and 268 people known to have AAA. In people with AAA, medical scans showed the artery had ballooned from a normal diameter of about 2 centimeters to at least 3 centimeters.

Genome sequencing identified nearly 24 million genetic mutations. Of these, the scientists considered about 66,000 rare mutations that were not found in previous searches for common mutations in healthy people. The machine learning system analyzed this data and identified 60 genes that were more likely to have elevated mutations in people with AAA.

When the team tested HEAL on their sample, it could correctly distinguish which people had AAA based on their genomes 69 percent of the time. When smoking history, cholesterol levels, and other data from surveys and health records were included, HEAL was able to distinguish AAA 80 percent of the time.

HEAL also identified biological processes that may be involved in the development of AAA. These include the immune response and blood vessel development.

"What's important to note about AAA is that it's irreversible, so once your aorta starts enlarging, it's not like you can un-enlarge it. And typically, the disease is discovered when the aorta bursts, and by that time it's 90% lethal," Snyder explains. "No one has ever

Health Technology Sourcebook, Third Edition

set up a predictive test for it and, just from a genome sequence, we found that we could actually predict with about 70% accuracy who is at high risk for AAA."

With further development, this work could lead to ways to identify people who are at risk for AAA. The results also suggest new research directions and potential therapeutic targets. In addition, this study is proof of the principle that machine learning can be used to predict disease risk for other genetic conditions.

Chapter 16 | Genetics

Chapter Contents
Section 16.1—Genomics 239
Section 16.2—Genetic Testing......................................245
Section 16.3—DNA Microarray Technology...............249
Section 16.4—Genome Editing and CRISPR 251
Section 16.5—Messenger RNA.....................................258
Section 16.6—Cloning..264

Section 16.1 | **Genomics**

This section contains text excerpted from the following sources: Text beginning with the heading "What Is a Genome?" is excerpted from "Introduction to Genomics," National Human Genome Research Institute (NHGRI), October 11, 2019; Text under the heading "Pharmacogenomics" is excerpted from "Pharmacogenomics," National Human Genome Research Institute (NHGRI), October 17, 2022; Text beginning with the heading "Why Is There a Need for Artificial Intelligence/Machine Learning in Genomics?" is excerpted from "Artificial Intelligence, Machine Learning and Genomics," National Human Genome Research Institute (NHGRI), January 12, 2022.

WHAT IS A GENOME?

Genome is a fancy word for all your deoxyribonucleic acid (DNA). From potatoes to puppies, all living organisms have their own genome. Each genome contains the information needed to build and maintain that organism throughout its life.

Your genome is the operating manual containing all the instructions that helped you develop from a single cell into the person you are today. It guides your growth, helps your organs do their jobs, and repairs itself when it becomes damaged. And it is unique to you. The more you know about your genome and how it works, the more you will understand your own health and make informed health decisions.

WHAT DOES YOUR GENOME LOOK LIKE?

If all the DNA from a single human cell was stretched out end to end, it would make a six-foot-long strand comprised of a six-billion-letter code. It is hard to imagine how much DNA can be packed into a cell's nucleus, which is so small it can only be seen with a specialized microscope. The secret lies in the highly structured and tightly packed nature of the genome.

The DNA Double Helix

Genomes are made of DNA, an extremely large molecule that looks like a long, twisted ladder. This is the iconic DNA double helix that you may have seen in textbooks or advertising.

DNA is read like a code. This code is made up of four types of chemical building blocks, adenine, thymine, cytosine, and guanine,

Health Technology Sourcebook, Third Edition

abbreviated with the letters A, T, C, and G. The order of the letters in this code allows DNA to function in different ways. The code changes slightly from person to person to help make you who you are.

Chromosomes

The DNA in a cell is not a single long molecule. It is divided into a number of segments of uneven lengths. At certain points in the life cycle of a cell, those segments can be tightly packed bundles known as "chromosomes." During one stage, the chromosomes appear to be X-shaped.

Every fungus, plant, and animal has a set number of chromosomes. For example, humans have 46 chromosomes (23 pairs); rice plants have 24 chromosomes; and dogs have 78 chromosomes.

HOW DOES YOUR GENOME WORK?

An instruction manual is not worth much until someone reads it. The same goes for your genome. The letters of your genome combine in different ways to spell out specific instructions.

Genes

A gene is a segment of DNA that provides the cell with instructions for making a specific protein, which then carries out a particular function in your body. Nearly all humans have the same genes arranged in roughly the same order, and more than 99.9 percent of your DNA sequence is identical to any other human.

Still, we are different. On average, a human gene will have 1–3 letters that differ from person to person. These differences are enough to change the shape and function of a protein, how much protein is made, when it is made, or where it is made. They affect the color of your eyes, hair, and skin. More importantly, variations in your genome also influence your risk of developing diseases and your responses to medications.

The Role of Your Parents

The instructions necessary for you to grow throughout your lifetime are passed down from your mother and father. Half of your

Genetics

genome comes from your biological mother and half from your biological father, making you related to each but identical to neither. Your biological parents' genes influence traits such as height, eye color, and disease risk that make you a unique person.

Does Your Genome Determine Everything about You?

Not entirely. Genomes are complicated, and while a small number of your traits are mainly controlled by one gene, most traits are influenced by multiple genes. On top of that, lifestyle and environmental factors play a critical role in your development and health. The day-to-day and long-term choices you make, such as what you eat, if you smoke, how active you are, and if you get enough sleep, all affect your health.

DNA is not your destiny. The way you live influences how your genome works.

WHAT CAUSES GENETIC DISEASES?

A genetic disease is caused by a change in the DNA sequence. Some diseases are caused by mutations that are inherited from the parents and are present in an individual at birth. Other diseases are caused by acquired mutations in a gene or group of genes that occur during a person's life.

Genetic Variants

Changes in the DNA sequence are called "genetic variants." The majority of the time, genetic variants have no effect at all. But, sometimes, the effect is harmful; just one letter missing or changed may result in a damaged protein, extra protein, or no protein at all, with serious consequences for health. Additionally, the passing of genetic variants from one generation to the next helps explain why many diseases run in families, such as sickle cell disease, cystic fibrosis, and Tay-Sachs disease. If a certain disease runs in your family, doctors say you have a family health history for that condition.

The following is a list of genetic, orphan, and rare diseases under investigation by researchers at or associated with the National Human Genome Research Institute (NHGRI).

241

Health Technology Sourcebook, Third Edition

- Autism
- Breast cancer
- Cystic fibrosis (CF)
- Down syndrome
- Parkinson disease (PD)
- Sickle cell disease (SCD)
- Wilson disease
- Attention deficit hyperactivity disorder (ADHD)

WHAT IS GENETIC TESTING?

Genetic testing consists of the processes and techniques used to determine details about your DNA. Depending on the test, it may reveal some information about your ancestry and your and your family's health.

Predictive testing is for those who have a family member with a genetic disorder. The results help determine a person's risk of developing the specific disorder being tested for. These tests are done before any symptoms present themselves.

Diagnostic testing is used to confirm or rule out a suspected genetic disorder. The results of a diagnostic test may help you make choices about how to treat or manage your health.

Pharmacogenomic testing tells you about how you will react to certain medications. It can help inform your health-care provider about how to best treat your condition and avoid side effects.

Reproductive testing is related to starting or growing your family. It includes tests for the biological father and mother to see what genetic variants they carry. The tests can help parents and health-care providers make decisions before, during, and after pregnancy.

Direct-to-consumer testing can be completed at home without a health-care provider by collecting a DNA sample (e.g., spitting saliva into a tube) and sending it to a company. The company can analyze your DNA and give information about your ancestry, kinship, lifestyle factors, and potential disease risk.

Forensic testing is carried out for legal purposes and can be used to identify biological family members, suspects, and victims of crimes and disasters.

Genetics

What Are the Benefits of Genomics?

One way genomics research can benefit you is through the emerging field of precision medicine. Specifically, characteristics of your genome can help predict how you will react to certain medications, allowing your health-care provider to choose the appropriate prevention or treatment options for you.

HOW DOES GENOMICS IMPACT EVERYDAY LIFE?

As technology advances and we learn more about how the genome works, information about our genomes is quickly becoming part of our everyday life. Emerging technologies give us the ability to read someone's genome sequence. Having this information can lead to more questions about what genomics means for ourselves, our family members, and our society.

PHARMACOGENOMICS

Pharmacogenomics (also called "pharmacogenetics") is a component of genomic medicine that involves using a patient's genomic information to tailor the selection of drugs used in their medical management. In this way, pharmacogenomics aims to provide a more individualized (or precise) approach to the use of available medication in treating patients.

Doctors and patients know that people can react to the same drug in very different ways. A drug that may be very effective in most people who take it may be totally ineffective in others or can even cause very bad reactions or death. So drug treatment is not, and really has never been, one-size-fits-all. Many things can affect the way people react to drugs, such as other drugs they may be taking or other health conditions they may have. But genetic differences measured by pharmacogenetic tests can also predict, with very high accuracy, whether certain drugs will be harmful, helpful, or without effect in a specific patient. For a growing number of drugs, this information can help doctors select the right drug at the right dose, at the right time, targeted specifically to the makeup in it of an individual patient.

WHY IS THERE A NEED FOR ARTIFICIAL INTELLIGENCE/ MACHINE LEARNING IN GENOMICS?

As of 2021, 20 years have passed since the landmark completion of the draft human genome sequence. This milestone has led to the generation of an extraordinary amount of genomic data. Estimates predict that genomics research will generate between 2 and 40 exabytes of data within the next decade.

DNA sequencing and other biological techniques will continue to increase the number and complexity of such data sets. This is why genomics researchers need AI/ML-based computational tools that can handle, extract, and interpret the valuable information hidden within this large trove of data.

WHAT ARE SOME WAYS IN WHICH ARTIFICIAL INTELLIGENCE/ MACHINE LEARNING ARE BEING USED IN GENOMICS?

Although the use of AI/ML tools in genomics is still at an early stage, researchers have already benefited from developing programs that assist in specific ways.

Some examples include:

- Examining people's faces with facial analysis AI programs to accurately identify genetic disorders.
- Using machine learning techniques to identify the primary kind of cancer from a liquid biopsy.
- Predicting how a certain kind of cancer will progress in a patient.
- Identifying disease-causing genomic variants compared to benign variants using machine learning.
- Using deep learning to improve the function of gene editing tools such as CRISPR.

These are just a few ways by which AI/ML methods are helping predict and identify hidden patterns in genomic data. Scientists are also using AI/ML to predict future variations in the genomes of influenza and SARS-CoV-2 viruses to assist public health efforts.

Genetics

WHAT IS NHGRI'S ROLE IN BRINGING ARTIFICIAL INTELLIGENCE, MACHINE LEARNING, AND GENOMICS TOGETHER?

The NHGRI's Genomic Data Science Working Group collaborates closely with the National Institutes of Health (NIH) and other academic institutes to define critical areas in genomics for AI and machine learning. The group is also helping to define the NHGRI's unique role in enabling machine learning research to assist in both genomic sciences and genomic medicine. In April 2021, the NHGRI hosted a virtual workshop on machine learning in genomics that put forth a vast array of promising advances at the intersection of artificial intelligence and genomics research.

The NHGRI is also a key part of NIH's new Common Fund program, Bridge to Artificial Intelligence (Bridge2AI). The goal of the Bridge2AI program is to act as a launchpad for the widespread adoption of AI in tackling complex biomedical and precision medicine challenges.

Apart from being part of Bridge2AI, the NHGRI also independently funds research at the intersection of AI/ML and genomics and is particularly focused on ensuring that the genomic data used in AI and deep learning programs appropriately reflect fairly and ethically on the diversity of the human species. The NHGRI also supports research on the ethical, legal, and social implications of the use of AI/ML in genomics.

Section 16.2 | Genetic Testing

This section includes text excerpted from "Genetic Testing," Centers for Disease Control and Prevention (CDC), June 24, 2022.

WHAT IS GENETIC TESTING?

Genetic testing looks for changes, sometimes called "mutations" or "variants," in your deoxyribonucleic acid (DNA). Genetic testing is useful in many areas of medicine and can change the medical care you or your family member receives. For example, genetic testing

Health Technology Sourcebook, Third Edition

can provide a diagnosis for a genetic condition, such as fragile X syndrome (FXS), or information about your risk of developing cancer. There are many different kinds of genetic tests. Genetic tests are done using a blood or spit sample, and results are usually ready in a few weeks. Because we share DNA with our family members, if you are found to have a genetic change, your family members may have the same change. Genetic counseling before and after genetic testing can help make sure that you are the right person in your family to get a genetic test, you are getting the right genetic test, and you understand your results.

REASONS FOR GENETIC TESTING

- To learn whether you have a genetic condition that runs in your family before you have symptoms.
- To learn about the chance a current or future pregnancy will have a genetic condition.
- To diagnose a genetic condition if you or your child has symptoms.
- To understand and guide your cancer prevention or treatment plan.

After learning more about genetic testing, you might decide it is not right for you. Some reasons might be that it is not relevant to you or will not change your medical care, it is too expensive, and the results may make you worried or anxious.

TYPES OF GENETIC TESTS

There are many different kinds of genetic tests. There is no single genetic test that can detect all genetic conditions. The approach to genetic testing is individualized based on your medical and family history and what condition you are being tested for.

- **Single gene testing**. These tests look for changes in only one gene. Single gene testing is done when your doctor believes you or your child have symptoms of a specific condition or syndrome. Some examples of this are Duchene muscular dystrophy (DMD) or sickle cell

Genetics

disease (SCD). Single gene testing is also used when there is a known genetic mutation in a family.

- **Panel testing**. A panel genetic test looks for changes in many genes in one test. Genetic testing panels are usually grouped into categories based on different kinds of medical concerns. Some examples of genetic panel tests are low muscle tone, short stature, or epilepsy. Panel genetic tests can also be grouped into genes that are all associated with a higher risk of developing certain kinds of cancer, such as breast or colorectal (colon) cancer.
- **Large-scale genetic or genomic testing**. There are two different kinds of large-scale genetic tests:
  - Exome sequencing looks at all the genes in the DNA (whole exome) or just the genes that are related to medical conditions (clinical exome).
  - Genome sequencing is the largest genetic test and looks at all of a person's DNA, not just the genes.

Exome and genome sequencing are ordered by doctors for people with complex medical histories. Large-scale genomic testing is also used in research to learn more about the genetic causes of conditions. Large-scale genetic tests can have findings unrelated to why the test was ordered in the first place (secondary findings). Examples of secondary findings are genes associated with a predisposition to cancer or rare heart conditions when you were looking for a genetic diagnosis to explain a child's developmental disabilities.

TESTING FOR CHANGES OTHER THAN GENE CHANGES

- **Chromosomes**. DNA is packaged into structures called "chromosomes." Some tests look for changes in chromosomes rather than gene changes. Examples of these tests are karyotype and chromosomal microarrays.
- **Gene expression**. Genes are expressed, or turned on, at different levels in different types of cells. Gene expression tests compare these levels between normal cells and

Health Technology Sourcebook, Third Edition

diseased cells because knowing about the difference can provide important information for treating the disease. For example, these tests can be used to guide chemotherapy treatment for breast cancer.

TYPES OF GENETIC TEST RESULTS

- **Positive**. The test found a genetic change known to cause disease.
- **Negative**. The test did not find a genetic change known to cause disease. Sometimes, a negative result occurs when the wrong test was ordered, or there is not a genetic cause for that person's symptoms. A "true negative" is when there is a known genetic change in the family and the person tested did not inherit it. If your test results are negative and there is no known genetic change in your family, a negative test result may not give you a definite answer. This is because you might not have been tested for the genetic change that runs in your family.
- **Uncertain**. A variant of unknown or uncertain significance means there is not enough information about that genetic change to determine whether it is benign (normal) or pathogenic (disease-causing).

A good way to think about genetic testing is as if you are asking the DNA a question. Sometimes, you do not find an answer because you were not asking the right question or science just did not have the answer yet.

NEXT STEPS

If you have a family history of a genetic condition, have symptoms of a genetic condition, or are interested in learning about your chance of having a genetic condition, talk to your doctor about whether genetic testing is right for you.

Genetics

Section 16.3 | **DNA Microarray Technology**

This section contains text excerpted from the following sources: Text in this section begins with excerpts from "Microarray Technology," National Human Genome Research Institute (NHGRI), October 17, 2022; Text beginning with the heading "What Is a DNA Microarray?" is excerpted from "DNA Microarray Technology Fact Sheet," National Human Genome Research Institute (NHGRI), August 15, 2020.

Microarray technology is a general laboratory approach that involves binding an array of thousands to millions of known nucleic acid fragments to a solid surface, referred to as a "chip." The chip is then bathed with deoxyribonucleic acid (DNA) or ribonucleic acid (RNA) isolated from a study sample (such as cells or tissue). Complementary base pairing between the sample and the chip-immobilized fragments produces light through fluorescence that can be detected using a specialized machine. Microarray technology can be used for a variety of purposes in research and clinical studies, such as measuring gene expression and detecting specific DNA sequences (e.g., single-nucleotide polymorphisms, or SNPs).

WHAT IS A DNA MICROARRAY?

Scientists know that a mutation—or alteration—in a particular gene's DNA may contribute to a certain disease. However, it can be very difficult to develop a test to detect these mutations because most large genes have many regions where mutations can occur. For example, researchers believe that mutations in the genes *BRCA1* and *BRCA2* cause as many as 60 percent of all cases of hereditary breast and ovarian cancers. But there is not one specific mutation responsible for all of these cases. Researchers have already discovered over 800 different mutations in *BRCA1* alone. The DNA microarray is a tool used to determine whether the DNA from a particular individual contains a mutation in genes such as *BRCA1* and *BRCA2*. The chip consists of a small glass plate encased in plastic. Some companies manufacture microarrays using methods similar to those used to make computer microchips. On the surface, each chip contains thousands of short, synthetic, single-stranded DNA sequences, which together add up to the normal gene in question and to variants (mutations) of that gene that have been found in the human population.

249

WHAT IS A DNA MICROARRAY USED FOR?

DNA microarrays were used only as a research tool. Scientists continue today to conduct large-scale population studies—for example, to determine how often individuals with a particular mutation actually develop breast cancer or to identify the changes in gene sequences that are most often associated with particular diseases. This has become possible because, just as is the case for computer chips, very large numbers of "features" can be put on microarray chips, representing a very large portion of the human genome.

Microarrays can also be used to study the extent to which certain genes are turned on or off in cells and tissues. In this case, instead of isolating DNA from the samples, RNA (which is a transcript of the DNA) is isolated and measured.

Today, DNA microarrays are used in clinical diagnostic tests for some diseases. Sometimes, they are also used to determine which drugs might be best prescribed for particular individuals because genes determine how our bodies handle the chemistry related to those drugs. With the advent of new DNA sequencing technologies, some of the tests for which microarrays were used in the past now use DNA sequencing instead. But microarray tests still tend to be less expensive than sequencing, so they may be used for very large studies, as well as for some clinical tests.

HOW DOES A DNA MICROARRAY WORK?

To determine whether an individual possesses a mutation for a particular disease, a scientist first obtains a sample of DNA from the patient's blood as well as a control sample—one that does not contain a mutation in the gene of interest.

The researcher then denatures the DNA in the samples—a process that separates the two complementary strands of DNA into single-stranded molecules. The next step is to cut the long strands of DNA into smaller, more manageable fragments and then label each fragment by attaching a fluorescent dye (there are other ways to do this, but this is one common method). The individual's DNA is labeled with green dye, and the control—or normal—DNA is labeled with red dye. Both sets of labeled DNA are then inserted

Genetics

into the chip and allowed to hybridize—or bind—to the synthetic DNA on the chip.

If the individual does not have a mutation for the gene, both the red and green samples will bind to the sequences on the chip that represent the sequence without the mutation (the "normal" sequence).

If the individual does possess a mutation, the individual's DNA will not bind properly to the DNA sequences on the chip that represent the "normal" sequence but instead will bind to the sequence on the chip that represents the mutated DNA.

Section 16.4 | Genome Editing and CRISPR

This chapter contains text excerpted from the following sources: Text in this chapter begins with excerpts from "What Are Genome Editing and CRISPR-Cas9?" MedlinePlus, National Institutes of Health (NIH), March 22, 2022; Text beginning with the heading "How CRISPR Is Changing Cancer Research and Treatment" is excerpted from "How CRISPR Is Changing Cancer Research and Treatment," National Cancer Institute (NCI), July 27, 2020.

Genome editing (also called "gene editing") is a group of technologies that give scientists the ability to change an organism's DNA. These technologies allow genetic material to be added, removed, or altered at particular locations in the genome. Several approaches to genome editing have been developed. A well-known one is called "CRISPR-Cas9," which is short for clustered regularly interspaced short palindromic repeats and CRISPR-associated protein 9. The CRISPR-Cas9 system has generated a lot of excitement in the scientific community because it is faster, cheaper, more accurate, and more efficient than other genome editing methods.

CRISPR-Cas9 was adapted from a naturally occurring genome editing system that bacteria use as an immune defense. When infected with viruses, bacteria capture small pieces of the viruses' DNA and insert them into their own DNA in a particular pattern to create segments known as "CRISPR arrays." The CRISPR arrays allow the bacteria to "remember" the viruses (or closely related ones). If the viruses attack again, the bacteria produce RNA

Health Technology Sourcebook, Third Edition

segments from the CRISPR arrays that recognize and attach to specific regions of the viruses' DNA. The bacteria then use Cas9 or a similar enzyme to cut the DNA apart, which disables the virus.

Researchers adapted this immune defense system to edit DNA. They create a small piece of RNA with a short "guide" sequence that attaches (binds) to a specific target sequence in a cell's DNA, much like the RNA segments bacteria produce from the CRISPR array. This guide RNA also attaches to the Cas9 enzyme. When introduced into cells, the guide RNA recognizes the intended DNA sequence, and the Cas9 enzyme cuts the DNA at the targeted location, mirroring the process in bacteria. Although Cas9 is the enzyme that is used most often, other enzymes (e.g., Cpf1) can also be used. Once the DNA is cut, researchers use the cell's own DNA repair machinery to add or delete pieces of genetic material or make changes to the DNA by replacing an existing segment with a customized DNA sequence.

Genome editing is of great interest in the prevention and treatment of human diseases. Currently, genome editing is used in cells and animal models in research labs to understand diseases. Scientists are still working to determine whether this approach is safe and effective for use in people. It is being explored in research and clinical trials for a wide variety of diseases, including single-gene disorders such as cystic fibrosis, hemophilia, and sickle cell disease. It also holds promise for the treatment and prevention of more complex diseases, such as cancer, heart disease, mental illness, and human immunodeficiency virus (HIV) infection.

Ethical concerns arise when genome editing, using technologies such as CRISPR-Cas9, is used to alter human genomes. Most of the changes introduced with genome editing are limited to somatic cells, which are cells other than egg and sperm cells (germline cells). These changes are isolated to only certain tissues and are not passed from one generation to the next. However, changes made to genes in egg or sperm cells or to the genes of an embryo could be passed to future generations. Germline cell and embryo genome editing bring up a number of ethical challenges, including whether it would be permissible to use this technology to enhance normal human traits (such as height or intelligence). Based on concerns

Genetics

about ethics and safety, germline cell and embryo genome editing are currently illegal in the United States and many other countries.

HOW CRISPR IS CHANGING CANCER RESEARCH AND TREATMENT

Ever since scientists realized that changes in DNA cause cancer, they have been searching for an easy way to correct those changes by manipulating DNA. Although several methods of gene editing have been developed over the years, none has really fit the bill for a quick, easy, and cheap technology.

But a game changer occurred in 2013 when several researchers showed that a gene-editing tool called "CRISPR" could alter the DNA of human cells like a very precise and easy-to-use pair of scissors.

The new tool has taken the research world by storm, markedly shifting the line between possible and impossible. As soon as CRISPR made its way onto the shelves and freezers of labs around the world, cancer researchers jumped at the chance to use it.

"CRISPR is becoming a mainstream methodology used in many cancer biology studies because of the convenience of the technique," said Dr. Jerry Li, M.D., Ph.D., of NCI's Division of Cancer Biology.

Now CRISPR is moving out of lab dishes and into trials of people with cancer. In a small study, for example, researchers tested a cancer treatment involving immune cells that were CRISPR-edited to better hunt down and attack cancer.

Despite all the excitement, scientists have been proceeding cautiously, feeling out the tool's strengths and pitfalls, setting best practices, and debating the social and ethical consequences of gene editing in humans.

HOW DOES CRISPR WORK?

In the laboratory, the CRISPR tool consists of two main actors: a guide RNA and a DNA-cutting enzyme, the most common one called "Cas9." Scientists design the guide RNA to mirror the DNA of the gene to be edited (called "the target"). The guide RNA partners with Cas and—true to its name—leads Cas to the target. When the guide RNA matches up with the target gene's DNA, Cas cuts the DNA.

Health Technology Sourcebook, Third Edition

What happens next depends on the type of CRISPR tool that is being used. In some cases, the target gene's DNA is scrambled while it is repaired, and the gene is inactivated. With other versions of CRISPR, scientists can manipulate genes in more precise ways, such as adding a new segment of DNA or editing single DNA letters.

Scientists have also used CRISPR to detect specific targets, such as DNA from cancer-causing viruses and RNA from cancer cells. Most recently, CRISPR has been put to use as an experimental test to detect the novel coronavirus.

WHY IS CRISPR A BIG DEAL?

CRISPR is completely customizable. It can edit virtually any segment of DNA within the three billion letters of the human genome, and it is more precise than other DNA-editing tools.

And gene editing with CRISPR is a lot faster. With older methods, "it usually (took) a year or two to generate a genetically engineered mouse model, if you're lucky," said Dr. Li. But, now with CRISPR, a scientist can create a complex mouse model within a few months, he said.

Another plus is that CRISPR can be easily scaled up. Researchers can use hundreds of guide RNAs to manipulate and evaluate hundreds or thousands of genes at a time. Cancer researchers often use this type of experiment to pick out genes that might make good drug targets.

And, as an added bonus, "it's certainly cheaper than previous methods," noted Dr. Alejandro Chavez, M.D., Ph.D., an assistant professor at Columbia University who has developed several novel CRISPR tools.

WHAT ARE CRISPR'S LIMITATIONS?

With all of its advantages over other gene-editing tools, CRISPR has become a go-to for scientists studying cancer. There is also hope that it will have a place in treating cancer, too. But CRISPR is not perfect, and its downsides have made many scientists cautious about its use in people.

A major pitfall is that CRISPR sometimes cuts DNA outside of the target gene—what is known as "off-target" editing. Scientists

Genetics

are worried that such unintended edits could be harmful and could even turn cells cancerous, as occurred in a 2002 study of a gene therapy.

"If (CRISPR) starts breaking random parts of the genome, the cell can start stitching things together in really weird ways, and there's some concern about that becoming cancer," Dr. Chavez explained. But, by tweaking the structures of Cas and the guide RNA, scientists have improved CRISPR's ability to cut only the intended target, he added.

Another potential roadblock is getting CRISPR components into cells. The most common way to do this is to co-opt a virus to do the job. Instead of ferrying genes that cause disease, the virus is modified to carry genes for the guide RNA and Cas.

Slipping CRISPR into lab-grown cells is one thing, but getting it into cells in a person's body is another story. Some viruses used to carry CRISPR can infect multiple types of cells, so, for instance, they may end up editing muscle cells when the goal is to edit liver cells.

Researchers are exploring different ways to fine-tune the delivery of CRISPR to specific organs or cells in the human body. Some are testing viruses that infect only one organ, such as the liver or brain. Others have created tiny structures called "nanocapsules" that are designed to deliver CRISPR components to specific cells.

Because CRISPR is just beginning to be tested in humans, there are also concerns about how the body—in particular, the immune system—will react to viruses carrying CRISPR or to the CRISPR components themselves.

Some wonder whether the immune system could attack Cas (a bacterial enzyme that is foreign to human bodies) and destroy CRISPR-edited cells. Twenty years ago, a patient died after his immune system launched a massive attack against the viruses carrying a gene therapy he had received. However, newer CRISPR-based approaches rely on viruses that appear to be safer than those used for older gene therapies.

Another major concern is that editing cells inside the body could accidentally make changes to sperm or egg cells that can be passed on to future generations. But, for almost all ongoing human studies involving CRISPR, patients' cells are removed and edited outside of their bodies. This "ex vivo" approach is considered safer because it is more controlled than trying to edit cells inside the body, Dr. Chavez said.

However, one ongoing study is testing CRISPR gene editing directly in the eyes of people with a genetic disease that causes blindness, called "Leber congenital amaurosis."

The First Clinical Trial of CRISPR for Cancer

The first trial in the United States to test a CRISPR-made cancer therapy was launched in 2019 at the University of Pennsylvania. The study, funded in part by NCI, is testing a type of immunotherapy in which patients' own immune cells are genetically modified to better "see" and kill their cancer.

The therapy involves making four genetic modifications to T cells, immune cells that can kill cancer. First, the addition of a synthetic gene gives the T cells a claw-like protein (called a "receptor") that "sees" NY-ESO-1, a molecule on some cancer cells.

Then CRISPR is used to remove three genes: two that can interfere with the NY-ESO-1 receptor and another that limits the cells' cancer-killing abilities. The finished product, dubbed NYCE T cells, was grown in large numbers and then infused into patients. Figure 16.1 shows a model of CRISPR with edited T cells.

MORE STUDIES OF CRISPR TREATMENTS TO COME

While the study of NYCE T cells marked the first trial of a CRISPR-based cancer treatment, there are likely more to come.

"This (trial) was really a proof-of-principle, feasibility, and safety thing that now opens up the whole world of CRISPR editing and other techniques of (gene) editing to hopefully make the next generation of therapies," said the trial's leader, Edward Stadtmauer, M.D., of the University of Pennsylvania.

Other clinical studies of CRISPR-made cancer treatments are already underway. A few trials are testing CRISPR-engineered CAR T-cell therapies, another type of immunotherapy. For example, one company is testing CRISPR-engineered CAR T cells in people with B-cell cancers and people with multiple myeloma.

Genetics

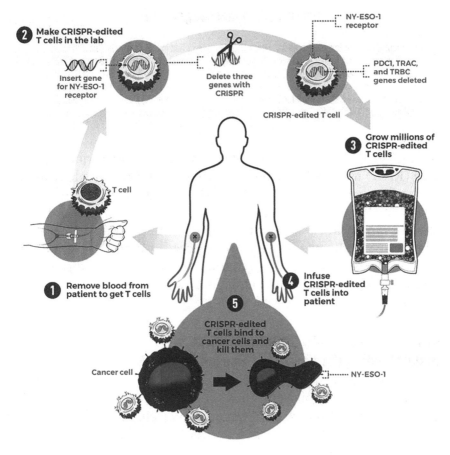

Figure 16.1. CRISPR-Edited T Cells

There are still a lot of questions about all the ways that CRISPR might be put to use in cancer research and treatment. But one thing is for certain: The field is moving incredibly fast, and new applications of the technology are constantly popping up.

"People are still improving CRISPR methods," Dr. Li said. "It's quite an active area of research and development. I'm sure that CRISPR will have even broader applications in the future."

Section 16.5 | Messenger RNA

This chapter contains text excerpted from the following sources: Text in this chapter begins with excerpts from "Messenger RNA (mRNA)," National Human Genome Research Institute (NHGRI), October 17, 2022; Text under the heading "How mRNA COVID-19 Vaccines Work" is excerpted from "How mRNA COVID-19 Vaccines Work," Centers for Disease Control and Prevention (CDC), August 16, 2022; Text under the heading "Questions and Answers for Comirnaty (COVID-19 Vaccine mRNA)" is excerpted from "Q&A for Comirnaty (COVID-19 Vaccine mRNA)," U.S. Food and Drug Administration (FDA), February 8, 2022.

Messenger RNA (mRNA) is a type of single-stranded ribonucleic acid (RNA) involved in protein synthesis. mRNA is made from a deoxyribonucleic acid (DNA) template during the process of transcription. The role of mRNA is to carry protein information from the DNA in a cell's nucleus to the cell's cytoplasm (watery interior), where the protein-making machinery reads the mRNA sequence and translates each three-base codon into its corresponding amino acid in a growing protein chain. Figure 16.2 shows the basic model of mRNA.

HOW MRNA COVID-19 VACCINES WORK
Understanding the Virus That Causes COVID-19

Coronaviruses, such as the one that causes COVID-19, are named for the crown-like spikes on their surface, called "spike proteins." These spike proteins are ideal targets for vaccines.

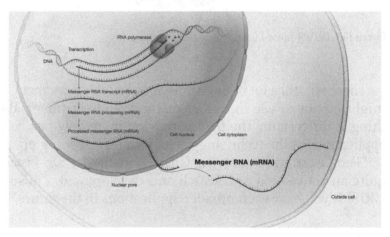

Figure 16.2. mRNA

Genetics

What Is in the Vaccine?
The vaccine is made of mRNA wrapped in a coating that makes delivery easy and keeps the body from damaging it.

How Does the Vaccine Work?
The mRNA in the vaccine teaches your cells how to make copies of the spike protein. If you are exposed to the real virus later, your body will recognize it and know how to fight it off.

QUESTIONS AND ANSWERS FOR COMIRNATY (COVID-19 VACCINE MRNA)
How Did the FDA Arrive at the Decision to Approve Comirnaty (COVID-19 Vaccine mRNA)? What Is Different Now When Compared to the December 2020 Authorization of Pfizer-BioNTech COVID-19 Vaccine?

The FDA conducted a thorough evaluation of the data and information submitted in the Biologics License Application (BLA) for Comirnaty before making a determination that the vaccine is safe and effective in preventing COVID-19 in individuals 16 years of age and older.

The EUA for the Pfizer-BioNTech COVID-19 vaccine for individuals 16 years of age and older was based on safety and effectiveness data from a randomized, controlled, blinded ongoing clinical trial in approximately 18,000 individuals who received the vaccine and approximately 18,000 who received a placebo. The vaccine was 95 percent effective in preventing COVID-19 disease among these clinical trial participants, with eight COVID-19 cases in the vaccine group and 162 in the placebo group. The duration of safety follow-up for the vaccinated and placebo participants was a median of two months after receiving the second dose.

Follow-up data from this ongoing clinical trial were analyzed by the U.S. Food and Drug Administration (FDA) to determine the safety and effectiveness of Comirnaty. The updated analysis to determine effectiveness for individuals 16 years of age and older included approximately 20,000 Comirnaty and 20,000 placebo recipients who did not have evidence of SARS-CoV-2 infection

Health Technology Sourcebook, Third Edition

through seven days after the second dose. Overall, the vaccine was 91 percent effective, with 77 cases of COVID-19 occurring in the vaccine group and 833 COVID-19 cases in the placebo group.

The safety was evaluated in approximately 22,000 Comirnaty and 22,000 placebo recipients 16 years of age and older. More than half of the vaccine and placebo recipients were followed for safety for at least four months after the second dose. After issuance of the EUA, participants were unblinded in a phased manner over a period of months to offer placebo participants Comirnaty. Overall, in blinded and unblinded follow-up, approximately 12,000 Comirnaty recipients have been followed for at least six months.

How Safe and Effective Is Comirnaty (COVID-19 Vaccine mRNA)?

Overall, the vaccine was 91 percent effective in preventing COVID-19 disease, with 77 cases of COVID-19 occurring in the vaccine group and 833 COVID-19 cases in the placebo group.

The FDA conducted a rigorous evaluation of postauthorization safety surveillance data pertaining to myocarditis and pericarditis following the administration of the Pfizer-BioNTech COVID-19 vaccine and determined that the data demonstrate increased risks, particularly within the seven days following the second dose. The observed risk is higher among males under 40 years of age compared to females and older males. The observed risk is highest in males 12–17 years of age. Available data from short-term follow-ups suggest that most individuals have had a resolution of symptoms. However, some individuals required intensive care support. Information is not yet available about potential long-term health outcomes.

What Are the Most Commonly Reported Side Effects by Those Who Received Comirnaty (COVID-19 Vaccine mRNA)?

The most commonly reported side effects by those clinical trial participants who received Comirnaty were pain, redness, and swelling at the injection site; fatigue; headache; muscle pain; chills; joint pain; and fever.

Genetics

How Long Will Comirnaty Provide Protection?
Data are not yet available to inform us about the duration of protection that the vaccine will provide.

Can People Who Have Already Had COVID-19 Get Comirnaty?
Yes. Among the participants in the study that the FDA evaluated for the December 2020 authorization, relatively few confirmed COVID-19 cases occurred overall among clinical study participants with evidence of SARS-CoV-2 infection prior to vaccination.

Current scientific evidence suggests that individuals previously infected with SARS-CoV-2, including individuals who have had COVID-19, may be at risk of reinfection and developing COVID-19 again and could benefit from vaccination. Furthermore, available data suggest that the safety profile of the vaccine in previously infected individuals is just as favorable as in previously uninfected individuals.

Does Comirnaty Protect against Asymptomatic SARS-CoV-2 Infection (i.e., the Individual Is Infected with SARS-CoV-2 but Does Not Have Signs or Symptoms of COVID-19)?
It is not known if Comirnaty protects against asymptomatic SARS-CoV-2 infection.

If a Person Has Received Comirnaty, Will the Vaccine Protect against Transmission of SARS-CoV-2 from Individuals Who Are Infected despite Vaccination?
Most vaccines that protect from viral illnesses also reduce transmission of the virus that causes the disease by those who are vaccinated. While it is hoped this will be the case, the scientific community does not yet know if Comirnaty will reduce such transmission.

Can Comirnaty Cause Infertility in Women?
There is no scientific evidence to suggest that the vaccine could cause infertility in women. In addition, infertility is not known to occur as a result of natural COVID-19 disease, further demonstrating

Health Technology Sourcebook, Third Edition

that immune responses to the virus, whether induced by infection or a vaccine, are not a cause of infertility. Reports on social media have falsely asserted that the vaccine could cause infertility in women, and the FDA is concerned that this misinformation may cause women to avoid vaccination to prevent COVID-19, which is a potentially serious and life-threatening disease. SARS-CoV-2 is the virus that causes COVID-19. The symptoms of COVID-19 vary and are unpredictable; many people have no symptoms or only mild disease, while some have severe respiratory diseases, including pneumonia and acute respiratory distress syndrome (ARDS), leading to multiorgan failure and death. Comirnaty is an mRNA vaccine. It contains a piece of the SARS-CoV-2 virus's genetic material that instructs cells in the body to make the virus's distinctive "spike" protein. After a person is vaccinated, their body produces copies of the spike protein, which does not cause disease, and triggers the immune system to learn to react defensively, producing an immune response against SARS-CoV-2. Contrary to false reports on social media, this protein is not the same as any involved in the formation of the placenta.

After FDA Granted the Emergency Use Authorization of the Pfizer-BioNTech COVID-19 Vaccine, Were Clinical Trial Participants Unblinded so That the Placebo Recipients Could Be Offered the Vaccine?

Yes. After issuance of the EUA, clinical trial participants were unblinded in a phased manner over a period of months to offer the authorized Pfizer-BioNTech COVID-19 vaccine to placebo participants. These participants were followed for safety outcomes. Overall, in blinded and unblinded follow-ups, approximately 12,000 Pfizer-BioNTech COVID-19 vaccine recipients have been followed for at least six months.

Does the Emergency Use Authorization for Pfizer-BioNTech COVID-19 Vaccine Remain in Effect after the Approval?

Yes. Pfizer-BioNTech COVID-19 vaccine is authorized for emergency use and is available under the EUA as a two-dose primary

Genetics

series in individuals five years of age and older, as a third primary series dose for individuals five years of age and older who have been determined to have certain kinds of immunocompromise, and as a single booster dose for individuals 12 years of age and older at least five months after completing a primary series of the Pfizer-BioNTech COVID-19 vaccine or Comirnaty.

The Pfizer-BioNTech COVID-19 vaccine is also authorized for use as a heterologous (or "mix and match") single booster dose for individuals 18 years of age and older following completion of primary vaccination with a different authorized COVID-19 vaccine.

How Is Comirnaty (COVID-19 Vaccine, mRNA) Related to the Pfizer-BioNTech COVID-19 Vaccine Authorized for Emergency Use?

The FDA-approved Comirnaty (COVID-19 vaccine, mRNA) and the FDA-emergency use authorized Pfizer-BioNTech COVID-19 vaccine for individuals 12 years of age and older, when prepared according to their respective instructions for use, can be used interchangeably to provide the COVID-19 vaccination series without presenting any safety or effectiveness concerns. Therefore, providers can use doses distributed under the EUA to administer the vaccination series as if the doses were the licensed vaccine. For purposes of administration, doses distributed under the EUA are interchangeable with the licensed doses.

Can Comirnaty and the Pfizer-BioNTech COVID-19 Vaccine Be Used Interchangeably?

The FDA-approved Comirnaty (COVID-19 vaccine, mRNA) and the two EUA-authorized formulations of the Pfizer-BioNTech COVID-19 vaccine for individuals 12 years of age and older when prepared according to their respective instructions for use can be used interchangeably.

The formulation of the Pfizer-BioNTech COVID-19 vaccine authorized for use in children 5–11 years of age differs from the formulations authorized for older individuals. The Pfizer-BioNTech COVID-19 vaccine authorized for use in children 5–11 years of age should not be used interchangeably with Comirnaty.

Health Technology Sourcebook, Third Edition

Section 16.6 | Cloning

This section includes text excerpted from "Cloning," National Human Genome Research Institute (NHGRI), August 15, 2020.

The term cloning describes a number of different processes that can be used to produce genetically identical copies of a biological entity. The copied material, which has the same genetic makeup as the original, is referred to as a clone. Researchers have cloned a wide range of biological materials, including genes, cells, tissues, and even entire organisms, such as sheep.

DO CLONES EVER OCCUR NATURALLY?

Yes. In nature, some plants and single-celled organisms, such as bacteria, produce genetically identical offspring through a process called "asexual reproduction." In asexual reproduction, a new individual is generated from a copy of a single cell from the parent organism.

Natural clones, also known as "identical twins," occur in humans and other mammals. These twins are produced when a fertilized egg splits, creating two or more embryos that carry almost identical DNA. Identical twins have nearly the same genetic makeup as each other, but they are genetically different from either parent.

WHAT ARE THE TYPES OF ARTIFICIAL CLONING?

There are three different types of artificial cloning: gene cloning, reproductive cloning, and therapeutic cloning.

Gene cloning produces copies of genes or segments of DNA. Reproductive cloning produces copies of whole animals. Therapeutic cloning produces embryonic stem cells for experiments aimed at creating tissues to replace injured or diseased tissues.

Gene cloning, also known as "DNA cloning," is a very different process from reproductive and therapeutic cloning. Reproductive and therapeutic cloning share many of the same techniques but are done for different purposes.

Genetics

WHAT SORT OF CLONING RESEARCH IS GOING ON AT NHGRI?

Gene cloning is the most common type of cloning done by researchers at the National Human Genome Research Institute (NHGRI). The NHGRI researchers have not cloned any mammals, and NHGRI does not clone humans.

HOW ARE GENES CLONED?

Researchers routinely use cloning techniques to make copies of genes that they wish to study. The procedure consists of inserting a gene from one organism, often referred to as "foreign DNA," into the genetic material of a carrier called a "vector." Examples of vectors include bacteria, yeast cells, viruses, or plasmids, which are small DNA circles carried by bacteria. After the gene is inserted, the vector is placed in laboratory conditions that prompt it to multiply, resulting in the gene being copied many times over.

HOW ARE ANIMALS CLONED?

In reproductive cloning, researchers remove a mature somatic cell, such as a skin cell, from an animal that they wish to copy. They then transfer the DNA of the donor animal's somatic cell into an egg cell, or oocyte, that has had its own DNA-containing nucleus removed.

Researchers can add the DNA from the somatic cell to the empty egg in two different ways. In the first method, they remove the DNA-containing nucleus of the somatic cell with a needle and inject it into the empty egg. In the second approach, they use an electrical current to fuse the entire somatic cell with the empty egg.

In both processes, the egg is allowed to develop into an early-stage embryo in the test tube and then is implanted into the womb of an adult female animal.

Ultimately, the adult female gives birth to an animal that has the same genetic makeup as the animal that donated the somatic cell. This young animal is referred to as a "clone." Reproductive cloning may require the use of a surrogate mother to allow the development of the cloned embryo, as was the case for the most famous cloned organism, Dolly the sheep.

WHAT ANIMALS HAVE BEEN CLONED?

Over the past 50 years, scientists have conducted cloning experiments on a wide range of animals using a variety of techniques. In 1979, researchers produced the first genetically identical mice by splitting mouse embryos in the test tube and then implanting the resulting embryos into the wombs of adult female mice. Shortly after that, researchers produced the first genetically identical cows, sheep, and chickens by transferring the nucleus of a cell taken from an early embryo into an egg that had been emptied of its nucleus.

It was not until 1996, however, that researchers succeeded in cloning the first mammal from a mature (somatic) cell taken from an adult animal. After 276 attempts, Scottish researchers finally produced Dolly, the lamb from the udder cell of a six-year-old sheep. Two years later, researchers in Japan cloned eight calves from a single cow, but only four survived.

Besides cattle and sheep, other mammals that have been cloned from somatic cells are as follows: cat, deer, dog, horse, mule, ox, rabbit, and rat. In addition, a rhesus monkey has been cloned by embryo splitting.

HAVE HUMANS BEEN CLONED?

Despite several highly publicized claims, human cloning still appears to be fiction. There currently is no solid scientific evidence that anyone has cloned human embryos.

In 1998, scientists in South Korea claimed to have successfully cloned a human embryo but said the experiment was interrupted very early when the clone was just a group of four cells. In 2002, Clonaid, part of a religious group that believes humans were created by extraterrestrials, held a news conference to announce the birth of what it claimed to be the first cloned human, a girl named Eve. However, despite repeated requests by the research community and the news media, Clonaid never provided any evidence to confirm the existence of this clone or the other 12 human clones it purportedly created.

In 2004, a group led by Woo-Suk Hwang of Seoul National University in South Korea published a paper in the journal *Science* in which it claimed to have created a cloned human embryo in

Genetics

a test tube. However, an independent scientific committee later found no proof to support the claim, and in January 2006, *Science* announced that Hwang's paper had been retracted.

From a technical perspective, it is more difficult to clone humans and other primates than other mammals. One reason is that two proteins essential to cell division, known as "spindle proteins," are located very close to the chromosomes in primate eggs. Consequently, the removal of the egg's nucleus to make room for the donor nucleus also removes the spindle proteins, interfering with cell division. In other mammals, such as cats, rabbits, and mice, the two spindle proteins are spread throughout the egg. So the removal of the egg's nucleus does not result in the loss of spindle proteins. In addition, some dyes and the ultraviolet light used to remove the egg's nucleus can damage the primate cell and prevent it from growing.

DO CLONED ANIMALS ALWAYS LOOK IDENTICAL?

No. Clones do not always look identical. Although clones share the same genetic material, the environment also plays a big role in how an organism turns out.

For example, the first cat to be cloned, named CC, is a female calico cat that looks very different from her mother. The explanation for the difference is that the color and pattern of the coats of cats cannot be attributed exclusively to genes. A biological phenomenon involving the inactivation of the X chromosome in every cell of the female cat (which has two X chromosomes) determines which coat color genes are switched off and which are switched on. The distribution of X inactivation, which seems to occur randomly, determines the appearance of the cat's coat.

WHAT ARE THE POTENTIAL APPLICATIONS OF CLONED ANIMALS?

Reproductive cloning may enable researchers to make copies of animals with potential benefits for the fields of medicine and agriculture.

For instance, the same Scottish researchers who cloned Dolly have cloned other sheep that have been genetically modified to produce milk that contains a human protein essential for blood

Health Technology Sourcebook, Third Edition

clotting. The hope is that someday, this protein can be purified from the milk and given to humans whose blood does not clot properly. Another possible use of cloned animals is for testing new drugs and treatment strategies. The great advantage of using cloned animals for drug testing is that they are all genetically identical, which means their responses to the drugs should be uniform rather than variable, as seen in animals with different genetic makeups.

After consulting with many independent scientists and experts in cloning, the U.S. Food and Drug Administration (FDA) decided in January 2008 that meat and milk from cloned animals, such as cattle, pigs, and goats, are as safe as those from noncloned animals. The FDA action means that researchers are now free to use cloning methods to make copies of animals with desirable agricultural traits, such as high milk production or lean meat. However, because cloning is still very expensive, it will likely take many years until food products from cloned animals actually appear in supermarkets.

Another application is to create clones to build populations of endangered, or possibly even extinct, species of animals. In 2001, researchers produced the first clone of an endangered species: a type of Asian ox known as a "guar." Sadly, the baby guar, which had developed inside a surrogate cow mother, died just a few days after its birth. In 2003, another endangered type of ox, called the "Banteg," was successfully cloned. Soon after, three African wildcats were cloned using frozen embryos as a source of DNA. Although some experts think cloning can save many species that would otherwise disappear, others argue that cloning produces a population of genetically identical individuals that lack the genetic variability necessary for species survival.

Some people also have expressed interest in having their deceased pets cloned in the hope of getting a similar animal to replace the dead one. But, as shown by CC, the cloned cat, a clone may not turn out exactly like the original pet whose DNA was used to make the clone.

WHAT ARE THE POTENTIAL DRAWBACKS OF CLONING ANIMALS?

Reproductive cloning is a very inefficient technique, and most cloned animal embryos cannot develop into healthy individuals.

Genetics

For instance, Dolly was the only clone to be born alive out of a total of 277 cloned embryos. This very low efficiency, combined with safety concerns, presents a serious obstacle to the application of reproductive cloning.

Researchers have observed some adverse health effects in sheep and other mammals that have been cloned. These include an increase in birth size and a variety of defects in vital organs, such as the liver, brain, and heart. Other consequences include premature aging and problems with the immune system. Another potential problem centers on the relative age of the cloned cell's chromosomes. As cells go through their normal rounds of division, the tips of the chromosomes, called "telomeres," shrink. Over time, the telomeres become so short that the cell can no longer divide, and consequently, the cell dies. This is part of the natural aging process that seems to happen in all cell types. As a consequence, clones created from a cell taken from an adult might have chromosomes that are already shorter than normal, which may condemn the clones' cells to a shorter life span. Indeed, Dolly, who was cloned from the cell of a six-year-old sheep, had chromosomes that were shorter than those of other sheep her age. Dolly died when she was six years old, about half the average sheep's 12-year lifespan.

WHAT IS THERAPEUTIC CLONING?

Therapeutic cloning involves creating a cloned embryo for the sole purpose of producing embryonic stem cells with the same DNA as the donor cell. These stem cells can be used in experiments aimed at understanding disease and developing new treatments for disease. To date, there is no evidence that human embryos have been produced for therapeutic cloning.

The richest source of embryonic stem cells is tissue formed during the first five days after the egg has started to divide. At this stage of development, called the "blastocyst," the embryo consists of a cluster of about 100 cells that can become any cell type. Stem cells are harvested from cloned embryos at this stage of development, resulting in the destruction of the embryo while it is still in the test tube.

Health Technology Sourcebook, Third Edition

WHAT ARE THE POTENTIAL APPLICATIONS OF THERAPEUTIC CLONING?

Researchers hope to use embryonic stem cells, which have the unique ability to generate virtually all types of cells in an organism, to grow healthy tissues in the laboratory that can be used to replace injured or diseased tissues. In addition, it may be possible to learn more about the molecular causes of disease by studying embryonic stem cell lines from cloned embryos derived from the cells of animals or humans with different diseases. Finally, differentiated tissues derived from ES cells are excellent tools for testing new therapeutic drugs.

WHAT ARE THE POTENTIAL DRAWBACKS OF THERAPEUTIC CLONING?

Many researchers think it is worthwhile to explore the use of embryonic stem cells as a path for treating human diseases. However, some experts are concerned about the striking similarities between stem cells and cancer cells. Both cell types have the ability to proliferate indefinitely, and some studies show that after 60 cycles of cell division, stem cells can accumulate mutations that could lead to cancer. Therefore, the relationship between stem cells and cancer cells needs to be more clearly understood if stem cells are to be used to treat human disease.

WHAT ARE SOME OF THE ETHICAL ISSUES RELATED TO CLONING?

Gene cloning is a carefully regulated technique that is largely accepted today and used routinely in many labs worldwide. However, both reproductive and therapeutic cloning raise important ethical issues, especially as related to the potential use of these techniques in humans.

Reproductive cloning would present the potential of creating a human that is genetically identical to another person who has previously existed or who still exists. This may conflict with long-standing religious and societal values about human dignity, possibly infringing upon principles of individual freedom, identity, and autonomy. However, some argue that reproductive cloning

Genetics

could help sterile couples fulfill their dream of parenthood. Others see human cloning as a way to avoid passing on a deleterious gene that runs in the family without having to undergo embryo screening or embryo selection.

Therapeutic cloning, while offering the potential for treating humans suffering from disease or injury, would require the destruction of human embryos in the test tube. Consequently, opponents argue that using this technique to collect embryonic stem cells is wrong, regardless of whether such cells are used to benefit sick or injured people.

Chapter 17 | **Neurotechnology**

Neurotechnology involves techniques and concepts used to study the human brain, visualize the neurological processes in the brain, and help augment, modify, or control the brain using implantable or wearable technology. Neurotechnology can be used for experimental and therapeutic purposes. It requires specialized equipment such as electrodes, intelligent prostheses, and computers that can be used to deduce the electrical pulses of the nervous system.

HOW IT WORKS

Neurotechnology uses noninvasive techniques to study and record brain activity via neural interfaces. Some standard procedures in neurotechnology include electroencephalograms (EEGs), microneedle implantation, transcranial magnetic stimulation (TMS), transcranial electrical stimulation (tES), functional magnetic resonance imaging (fMRI), and deep brain stimulation (DBS). The technology involved in neurotechnology is broadly classified into three categories, such as:

- Neuromodulation technologies and processes, such as DBS or spinal cord stimulation, use electrical or pharmaceutical methods to alter or modify the neural activity to stimulate neural processes. These neural stimulation procedures are used in treatments for epilepsy, strokes, sensory and physical rehabilitation programs, chronic pain, neurodegenerative conditions such as Parkinson disease (PD) or Alzheimer disease

"Neurotechnology," © 2023 Infobase. Reviewed November 2022.

Health Technology Sourcebook, Third Edition

(AD), and even paralysis. Some other conditions treated with neuromodulation technologies include urinary incontinence, obesity, depression, and debilitating mental illnesses such as obsessive-compulsive disorder (OCD).

- The next category, neuroprostheses, includes cochlear implants, which act as a replacement for auditory functions in people with hearing loss. Neuroprosthetic devices substitute for typical motor, sensory, and cognitive neural functions when the subject has lost sensory or mental function or their brain function is deteriorating.
- Brain–machine interfaces (BMIs) allow subjects to control external devices by feeding into or extracting information from the brain through the device. It is commonly mediated with the help of electroencephalographs (EEGs) and magnetic resonance imaging (MRI). BMIs aid in developing brain-controlled assistive devices such as wheelchairs and robotic arms.

APPLICATIONS OF NEUROTECHNOLOGY

Neurotechnology has wide-ranging applications in research, therapy, cognitive interfaces, medical industries, population studies, security, and academics. Some prominent real-world applications of neurotechnology are found in brain imaging, widely used in the medical field to diagnose tumors, strokes, developmental activity delays, and charting brain activity.

Neuropharmacology utilizes concepts of neurotechnology, where behavioral and molecular neuropharmacologies help researchers develop more proactive drugs for mental disorders and genetic disorders. One application of neuropharmacology is optogenetic implants, where neurotechnology activates or deactivates targeted genes in the neural tissue with focused beams of light. Neurotechnology in the form of EEG or fMRI is used in neuronal biofeedback techniques in cases where involuntary body functions need to be regulated.

Neurotechnology

References

Masselos, Julia. "Neurotechnology," Technology Networks, February 11, 2022.

"Neurotechnologies: The Next Technology Frontier," IEEE Brain, March 13, 2021.

"Neurotechnology, How to Reveal the Secrets of the Human Brain?" Iberdrola, August 12, 2021.

Chapter 18 | **Clinical Decision Support**

WHAT IS CLINICAL DECISION SUPPORT?

Clinical decision support (CDS) provides clinicians, staff, patients, or other individuals with knowledge and person-specific information intelligently filtered or presented at appropriate times to enhance health and health care. The CDS encompasses a variety of tools to enhance decision-making in the clinical workflow. These tools include computerized alerts and reminders to care providers and patients; clinical guidelines; condition-specific order sets; focused patient data reports and summaries; documentation templates; diagnostic support; and contextually relevant reference information, among other tools.

WHY CLINICAL DECISION SUPPORT?

Clinical decision support has a number of important benefits, including:
- Increased quality of care and enhanced health outcomes
- Avoidance of errors and adverse events
- Improved efficiency, cost benefit, and provider and patient satisfaction

This chapter contains text excerpted from the following sources: Text beginning with the heading "What is Clinical Decision Support?" is excerpted from "Clinical Decision Support," HealthIT.gov, Office of the National Coordinator for Health Information Technology (ONC), April 10, 2018; Text under the heading "Scope of Clinical Decision Support" is excerpted from "CDS—Clinical Decision Support," HealthIT.gov, Office of the National Coordinator for Health Information Technology (ONC), August 14, 2022.

Health Technology Sourcebook, Third Edition

Clinical decision support is a sophisticated health IT component. It requires computable biomedical knowledge, person-specific data, and a reasoning or inferencing mechanism that combines knowledge and data to generate and present helpful information to clinicians as care is delivered. This information must be filtered, organized, and presented in a way that supports the current workflow, allowing the user to make an informed decision quickly and take action. Different types of CDS may be ideal for different processes of care in different settings.

Health information technologies designed to improve clinical decision-making are particularly attractive for their ability to address the growing information overload clinicians face and to provide a platform for integrating evidence-based knowledge into care delivery. The majority of CDS applications operate as components of comprehensive EHR systems although stand-alone CDS systems are also used.

CLINICAL DECISION SUPPORT PROMOTES PATIENT SAFETY

Clinical decision support can significantly impact improvements in the quality, safety, efficiency, and effectiveness of health care. The Office of the National Coordinator for Health IT (ONC) supports efforts to develop, adopt, implement, and evaluate the use of CDS to improve health-care decision-making.

The ONC aims to help the health-care industry create the technical infrastructure needed to allow health systems to share data with each other electronically to provide the complete information possible to CDS systems. Complete records allow CDS systems to help with diagnoses and track for negative drug interactions by having a better view of a patient's whole health.

OPTIMIZING STRATEGIES FOR CLINICAL DECISION SUPPORT

The ONC collaborated with the National Academy of Medicine (NAM) to engage key experts and develop a series of strategies and recommendations to optimize CDS in support of improved care. The project's goals were to identify actionable opportunities to accelerate progress in CDS creation, distribution, and use; inspire

Clinical Decision Support

action on priority opportunities among diverse stakeholder groups; and drive progress toward a usable, interoperable CDS.

SCOPE OF CLINICAL DECISION SUPPORT

Clinical decision support is not intended to replace clinician judgment but rather to assist care team members in making timely, informed, and higher quality, evidence-based decisions, incorporating resources such as clinical guidelines and best practices. The Five Rights model of the CDS states improvements are achieved in desired health care outcomes if communicating:

- The right information
- To the right people
- In the right CDS intervention formats
- Through the right channels
- At the right times in the workflow

Clinical decision support and electronic clinical quality measures (eCQMs) are closely related, share many common requirements and data elements, and support health-care quality improvement. The impact of a CDS intervention may be assessed with an eCQM.

Part 5 | Diagnostic Technology

Chapter 19 | Advances in Imaging

Chapter Contents

Section 19.1—Detection of Diabetic Retinopathy 285
Section 19.2—Artificial Intelligence in Diagnostic
Imaging...286
Section 19.3—Neuroimaging Technique to Predict
Autism among High-Risk Infants 290
Section 19.4—Artificial-Intelligence-Based Analysis
of Cardiovascular Disease Risk 291
Section 19.5—Virtual Colonoscopy...293
Section 19.6—Liver Elastography 297

Section 19.1 | **Detection of Diabetic Retinopathy**

This section includes text excerpted from "Artificial Intelligence for Health and Health Care," HealthIT.gov, Office of the National Coordinator for Health Information Technology (ONC), December 2017. Reviewed November 2022.

DETECTION OF DIABETIC RETINOPATHY IN RETINAL FUNDUS IMAGES

Many diseases of the eye can be diagnosed through noninvasive imaging of the retina through the pupil. Early screening for diabetic retinopathy is important as early treatment can prevent vision loss and blindness in the rapidly growing population of patients with diabetes. Such screening also provides the opportunity to identify other eye diseases and also provide indicators of cardiovascular disease (CVD).

The increasing need for such screening and the demands for expert analysis that it creates motivate the goal of low-cost, quantitative retinal image analysis. Routine imaging for screening uses the specially designed optics of a "fundus camera," with several images taken at different orientations (fields), and can be accomplished with (mydriatic) or without (nonmydriatic) dilation of the pupil. Assessment of the image requires skilled readers and may be performed by remote specialists. With the advent of digital photography, digital recording of retinal images can be carried out routinely through picture archiving and communication systems (PACSs).

Screening using fundus photography, followed by manual image analysis, yields sensitivity and specificity rates cited as 96%/89% when two fields (angles of view) are included and 92%/97% for three fields. (For a single field, cited rates are 78%/86%.)

Recently, a transformational advance in automated retinal image analysis using deep learning algorithms has been demonstrated. The algorithm was trained against a data set of over 100,000 images, which were recorded with one field (macula-centered). Each image in the training set was evaluated by 3–7 ophthalmologists, thus allowing training with significantly reduced image analysis variability. The results from tests on two validation sets, also involving only one image per eye (fovea-centered), are striking. Selecting for high specificity (low false negatives) yielded sensitivities/specificities of 90.3%/98.1% and 87.0%/98.5%. Selecting for high sensitivity yielded values of 97.5%/93.4% and 96.1%/93.9%. These results compare favorably with manual assessments, even where those are based on images from multiple fields, as noted above. They are also a significant advance over previous automated assessments, which consistently suffered from significantly lower sensitivities.

The deep learning algorithm shows great promise to provide increased quality of outcomes with increased accessibility. Continued work to establish its use as an approved clinical protocol will be needed. Once validated, its use can be envisioned in a wide range of scenarios, including decision support in existing practice, rapid and reduced cost analysis in place of manual assessment, or enabling diagnostics in nontraditional settings able to reach underserved populations.

Section 19.2 | Artificial Intelligence in Diagnostic Imaging

This section includes text excerpted from "Artificial Intelligence and Diagnostic Errors," Agency for Healthcare Research and Quality (AHRQ), U.S. Department of Health and Human Services (HHS), January 31, 2020.

CURRENT USE OF ARTIFICIAL INTELLIGENCE IN DIAGNOSTIC IMAGING

Medical imaging is one of the most promising areas for the application and innovative use of artificial intelligence (AI). The use of AI in radiology has the potential to improve the efficiency and efficacy of medical imaging. Its use may also alleviate some of the burden and burnout experienced by radiologists who feel overwhelmed by the proliferation in the volume of imaging studies performed and are unable to devote sufficient time to provide meaningful, patient-centric care.

The use of AI in diagnostic imaging can be included in processes such as acquiring the image, processing the image, interpreting the

Advances in Imaging

findings, determining follow-up care, and selecting appropriate data storage. When conducting an imaging study, the use of AI can improve the quality of the image captured. AI systems can detect at the time of imaging whether the quality of the data acquired is optimal for analysis and then alert radiologists, should additional scans be necessary. Automated protocols can also ensure that no necessary components of the scan are overlooked by the providers during its examination and that all required images are captured. Furthermore, AI systems can learn the features of a high-quality image, apply computational strategies to increase the odds of producing that image, and automatically compensate for any distortions. As a result, AI use during image capture can optimize staffing, reduce scanner time, and decrease radiation dosing for the patient.

Once the image has been captured, AI can support imaging analysis. Approaches utilizing AI for imaging analysis have been an area of rapid growth. AI algorithms look at images to identify patterns and then use pattern recognition to identify abnormalities. It may include flagging apparent abnormal findings or actually identifying masses and fractures. AI may be particularly beneficial when using imaging devices that produce a high number of images for each study conducted, such as magnetic resonance imaging (MRI). An electronic system can efficiently review significantly more images than would be feasible for an individual provider. AI can then support the diagnosis and treatment decision-making process by facilitating the integration of the imaging results within the patient electronic medical record. Once incorporated, the image can then be used alongside patient clinical data and medical history in computer-aided diagnosis. In some instances, AI may even predict which treatment protocols are most likely to be successful.

Once the imaging study has been conducted, AI systems can help ensure continuity in provider communication and patient care. For example, AI can review patient records to ensure that an imaging diagnosis is correlated with the radiological reports and that there is an associated treatment plan. Providers can then be alerted to any discrepancies. This can ensure that findings from radiological reports are addressed expeditiously and avoid unnecessary patient return visits.

MOVING BEYOND IMAGING

As the technology supporting AI and the sophistication of its applications continues to advance, the role AI plays in imaging diagnostics will likely expand. For example, with improvements in image analysis, systems may be used to autonomously triage patients for review by a radiologist. Additionally, as predictive algorithms become more advanced and adaptive, the role of AI in the review of both pathology and radiology images will grow. AI can also be expected to play a more direct role in the recommendation of treatment protocols.

RISKS ASSOCIATED WITH THE IMPLEMENTATION OF ARTIFICIAL INTELLIGENCE

Artificial intelligence in imaging has already demonstrated a great deal of potential and opportunity to improve patient safety through enhancing imaging processes, aiding physician diagnosis, and minimizing discrepancies. However, there are several ethical concerns directly related to patient safety that must be addressed as the use of AI becomes more pervasive and plays a greater role in patient diagnosis. The first is in the evaluation of the AI technology and determining what level of accuracy is required, and conversely the percentage of misses that are acceptable, to substitute review and decision-making by a human. Establishing a standardized benchmark for what constitutes "good enough" in AI products may be beneficial both for approval processes by the U.S. Food and Drug Administration (FDA) and also for guiding its use in facilities.

This first consideration directly leads to the second question of accountability. Should the use of AI directly or indirectly lead to misdiagnosis and improper treatment recommendations who is (and who should be) held at fault? Similarly, should a physician opt not to use available AI and the patient is misdiagnosed, is the physician accountable for that decision? In either instance, is it possible to prove that using or not using AI would have ended in a different result for the patient?

Advances in Imaging

Finally, while AI is intended to reduce diagnostic errors, there is the risk that the use of AI can introduce new potential errors. New potential errors have been detailed in a 2019 analysis by Dr. Robert Challen, University of Exeter College of Engineering Mathematics and Physical Sciences, and his team. One example notes the potential for error resulting from discrepancies between the data used to train AI systems and the real-world clinical scenario due to the limited availability of high-quality training data. AI systems are not as equipped as humans to recognize when there is a relevant change in context or data that can impact the validity of learned predictive assumptions. Therefore, AI systems may unknowingly apply a programmed methodology for assessment inappropriately, resulting in error. Another example includes an insensitivity to potential impact. AI systems may not be trained in the same ways as humans to "err on the side of caution." While that can result in more false positives, this approach may be appropriate when the alternative is a serious safety outcome for the patient.

Despite the potential of AI in diagnostic imaging, in the short term, it is most likely to complement rather than replace traditional approaches used by radiologists. With many unanswered questions associated with the use of AI and concerns regarding the introduction of new patient safety risks, AI will continue to serve as an adjunct rather than an alternative to a radiologist. However, the appropriate incorporation of AI has the potential to alleviate some of the workflow burden experienced by radiologists and allow them to spend more time on other aspects of their role in caring for the patient. This includes providing emotional support and guidance, implementing interventional procedures, and participating in multidisciplinary clinical team patient safety initiatives.

Section 19.3 | Neuroimaging Technique to Predict Autism among High-Risk Infants

This section includes text excerpted from "Neuroimaging Technique May Help Predict Autism among High-Risk Infants," National Institutes of Health (NIH), June 7, 2017. Reviewed November 2022.

Functional connectivity magnetic resonance imaging (fcMRI) may predict which high-risk, six-month-old infants will develop autism spectrum disorder (ASD) by age two, according to a study funded by the *Eunice Kennedy Shriver* National Institute of Child Health and Human Development (NICHD) and the National Institute of Mental Health (NIMH), two components of the National Institutes of Health (NIH). The study is published in the June 7, 2017, issue of *Science Translational Medicine*.

Autism affects roughly one out of every 68 children in the United States. Siblings of children diagnosed with autism are at higher risk of developing the disorder. Although early diagnosis and intervention can help improve outcomes for children with autism, there is currently no method to diagnose the disease before children show symptoms.

"Previous findings suggest that brain-related changes occur in autism before behavioral symptoms emerge," said Dr. Diana Bianchi, M.D., NICHD director. "If future studies confirm these results, detecting brain differences may enable physicians to diagnose and treat autism earlier than they do today."

In the current study, a research team led by NIH-funded investigators at the University of North Carolina at Chapel Hill and Washington University School of Medicine in St. Louis focused on the brain's functional connectivity—how regions of the brain work together during different tasks and during rest. Using fcMRI, the researchers scanned 59 high-risk, six-month-old infants while they slept naturally. The children were deemed high-risk because they have older siblings with autism. At age two, 11 of the 59 infants in this group were diagnosed with autism.

The researchers used a computer-based technology called "machine learning," which trains itself to look for differences that can separate the neuroimaging results into two groups—autism or

Advances in Imaging

nonautism—and predict future diagnoses. One analysis predicted each infant's future diagnosis by using the other 58 infants' data to train the computer program. This method identified 82 percent of the infants who would go on to have autism (9 out of 11), and it correctly identified all of the infants who did not develop autism. In another analysis that tested how well the results could apply to other cases, the computer program predicted diagnoses for groups of 10 infants at an accuracy rate of 93 percent.

"Although the findings are early-stage, the study suggests that in the future, neuroimaging may be a useful tool to diagnose autism or help health-care providers evaluate a child's risk of developing the disorder," said Dr. Joshua Gordon, M.D., Ph.D., NIMH director.

Overall, the team found 974 functional connections in the brains of six-month-olds that were associated with autism-related behaviors. The authors propose that a single neuroimaging scan may accurately predict autism among high-risk infants but caution that the findings need to be replicated in a larger group.

Section 19.4 | Artificial-Intelligence-Based Analysis of Cardiovascular Disease Risk

This section includes text excerpted from "Artificial Intelligence Predicts Heart Disease Risk from CT Scans," National Institutes of Health (NIH), March 17, 2020.

Cardiovascular disease (CVD) remains the leading cause of death in the United States. If people at high risk of heart attack, stroke, and related conditions could be identified, medications and lifestyle changes may help reduce their risk of disease and death.

Traditionally, heart disease risk has been assessed using clinical measurements. These include body mass index (BMI)—a ratio of weight to height. Another commonly used measurement is the Framingham risk score (FRS), which incorporates age, sex, blood pressure, blood cholesterol, and related information. However, these tools are not precise. They can miss people at high risk and misidentify others who are not.

Health Technology Sourcebook, Third Edition

A research team led by Dr. Perry J. Pickhardt of the University of Wisconsin and Dr. Ronald Summers from the NIH Clinical Center has been developing computer programs to estimate disease risk from computed tomography (CT) scans taken for other purposes. Tens of millions of people undergo such scans every year for reasons ranging from accidents to surgical planning.

The researchers previously showed that CT scans could be reused to diagnose osteoporosis. In their new study, they tested whether artificial intelligence (AI) algorithms they would develop to reanalyze CT scans could predict the risk of heart disease better than BMI or the FRS.

The team used CT scans of the abdomen previously taken for colorectal cancer screening from more than 9,200 men and women without symptomatic heart disease. Participants had an average age of 57. The AI programs measured calcification in the aortic artery, muscle density, the ratio of fat deep in the body to that under the skin, liver fat, and bone mineral density as seen on the scans.

The researchers collected follow-up information for all participants for an average of almost nine years. They then assessed whether their AI measures correlated with the later development of heart disease or death. Results were published on March 2, 2020, in *Lancet Digital Health*.

Over the follow-up period, 20 percent of study participants experienced a heart attack or stroke, developed heart failure, or died. All five body-composition measures assessed by AI differed substantially between people who had and had not developed heart disease.

AI scores of calcification in the aortic artery alone were better than the FRS at predicting heart disease risk. All five measures alone were more predictive than BMI taken at the start of the study. In general, combining more than one of the AI measurements increased the ability to predict later heart disease risk from an abdominal scan. Adding the FRS to the AI measurements did not improve their predictive performance.

"We found that automated measures provided more accurate risk assessments than established clinical biomarkers," Summers explains.

Advances in Imaging

But, because CT imaging comes with some risks, including exposure to small amounts of radiation, the researchers do not propose taking CT scans solely for heart disease risk assessment.

"This opportunistic use of additional CT-based biomarkers provides objective value to what doctors are already doing," Pickhardt says. "This automated process requires no additional time, effort, or radiation exposure to patients."

Section 19.5 | Virtual Colonoscopy

This section includes text excerpted from "Virtual Colonoscopy," National Institute of Diabetes and Digestive and Kidney Diseases (NIDDK), August 2016. Reviewed November 2022.

WHAT IS VIRTUAL COLONOSCOPY?

Virtual colonoscopy is a procedure in which a radiologist uses x-rays and a computer to create images of your rectum and colon from outside the body. Virtual colonoscopy can show ulcers, polyps, and cancer.

Does Virtual Colonoscopy Have Another Name?

Virtual colonoscopy is also called "computerized tomography (CT) colonography."

How Is Virtual Colonoscopy Different from Colonoscopy?

Colonoscopy and virtual colonoscopy are different in several ways. Colonoscopy is a procedure in which a trained specialist uses a long, flexible, narrow tube with a light and tiny camera on one end, called a "colonoscope" or "scope," to look inside your rectum and colon. Virtual colonoscopy is an x-ray test, takes less time, and does not require a doctor to insert a scope into the entire length of your colon. Unlike colonoscopy, virtual colonoscopy does not require sedation or anesthesia.

Health Technology Sourcebook, Third Edition

However, virtual colonoscopy may not be as effective as colonoscopy at finding certain polyps. Also, doctors cannot remove polyps or treat certain other problems during virtual colonoscopy, as they can during colonoscopy. Your health insurance coverage for virtual colonoscopy and colonoscopy also may be different.

Why Do Doctors Use Virtual Colonoscopy?

Doctors mainly use virtual colonoscopy to screen for polyps or cancer. Screening may find diseases at an early stage when a doctor has a better chance of curing the disease.

Occasionally, doctors may use virtual colonoscopy when colonoscopy is incomplete or not possible due to other medical reasons.

Screening for Colon and Rectal Cancer

Your doctor will recommend screening for colon and rectal cancer at age 45 if you do not have health problems or other factors that make you more likely to develop colon cancer.

Factors that make you more likely to develop colorectal cancer include:

- Someone in your family who has had polyps or cancer of the colon or rectum
- A personal history of inflammatory bowel disease (IBD), such as ulcerative colitis or Crohn disease
- Other factors, such as if you weigh too much or smoke cigarettes

If you are more likely to develop colorectal cancer, your doctor may recommend screening at a younger age, and you may need to be tested more often.

If you are older than age 75, talk with your doctor about whether you should be screened. Government health insurance plans, such as Medicare, and private health insurance plans sometimes change whether and how often they pay for cancer screening tests. Check with your insurance plan to find out if and how often your insurance will cover a screening virtual colonoscopy.

Advances in Imaging

HOW DO YOU PREPARE FOR A VIRTUAL COLONOSCOPY?

To prepare for a virtual colonoscopy, you will need to talk with your doctor, change your diet, clean out your bowel, and drink a special liquid called "contrast medium." The contrast medium makes your rectum and colon easier to see in the x-rays.

Talk with Your Doctor

You should talk with your doctor about any medical conditions you have and all prescribed and over-the-counter (OTC) medicines, vitamins, and supplements you take, including:

- Arthritis medicines
- Aspirin or medicines that contain aspirin
- Blood thinners
- Diabetes medicines
- Nonsteroidal anti-inflammatory drugs, such as ibuprofen or naproxen
- Vitamins that contain iron or iron supplements

X-rays may interfere with personal medical devices. Tell your doctor if you have any implanted medical devices, such as a pacemaker.

Doctors do not recommend x-rays for pregnant women because x-rays may harm the fetus. Tell your doctor if you are, or may be, pregnant. Your doctor may suggest a different procedure, such as a colonoscopy.

Change Your Diet and Clean Out Your Bowel

As in colonoscopy, a health-care professional will give you written bowel prep instructions to follow at home before the procedure. A health-care professional orders a bowel prep so that little or no stool is present in your intestine. A complete bowel prep lets you pass stool that is clear and liquid. The stool inside your colon can prevent the x-ray machine from taking clear images of the lining of your intestine.

You may need to follow a clear liquid diet the day before the procedure. The instructions will provide specific directions about

Health Technology Sourcebook, Third Edition

when to start and stop the clear liquid diet. In most cases, you may drink or eat the following:

- Fat-free bouillon or broth
- Gelatin in flavors such as lemon, lime, or orange
- Plain coffee or tea without cream or milk
- Sports drinks in flavors such as lemon, lime, or orange
- Strained fruit juice, such as apple or white grape—doctors recommend avoiding orange juice and red or purple beverages
- Water

Your doctor will tell you how long before the procedure you should have nothing by mouth.

A health-care professional will ask you to follow the directions for a bowel prep before the procedure. The bowel prep will cause diarrhea, so you should stay close to a bathroom.

Different bowel preps may contain different combinations of laxatives—pills that you swallow or powders that you dissolve in water and other clear liquids and enemas. Some people will need to drink a large amount, often a gallon, of liquid laxative over a scheduled amount of time—most often the night before the procedure.

You may find this part of the bowel prep difficult; however, completing the prep is very important. The images will not be clear if the prep is incomplete.

Drink Contrast Medium

The night before the procedure, you will drink a contrast medium. Contrast medium is visible on x-rays and can help your doctor tell the difference between stool and polyps.

HOW DO HEALTH-CARE PROFESSIONALS PERFORM A VIRTUAL COLONOSCOPY?

A specially trained x-ray technician performs a virtual colonoscopy at an outpatient center or a hospital. You do not need anesthesia.

For the procedure, you will lie on a table while the technician inserts a thin tube through your anus and into your rectum. The

Advances in Imaging

tube inflates your large intestine with air for a better view. The table slides into a tunnel-shaped device where the technician takes the x-ray images. The technician may ask you to hold your breath several times during the procedure to steady the images. The technician will ask you to turn over on your side or stomach so she or he can take different images of the large intestine. The procedure lasts about 10–15 minutes.

WHAT SHOULD YOU EXPECT AFTER A VIRTUAL COLONOSCOPY?

After a virtual colonoscopy, you can expect to:
- Feel cramping or bloating during the first hour after the test.
- Resume your regular activities right after the test.
- Return to a normal diet.

After the test, a radiologist looks at the images to find any problems and sends a report to your doctor. If the radiologist finds problems, your doctor may perform a colonoscopy the same day or at a later time.

WHAT ARE THE RISKS OF A VIRTUAL COLONOSCOPY?

Inflating the colon with air has a small risk of perforating the lining of the large intestine. The doctor may need to treat perforation with surgery.

Section 19.6 | Liver Elastography

This section includes text excerpted from "Elastography," MedlinePlus, National Institutes of Health (NIH), September 9, 2021.

WHAT IS ELASTOGRAPHY?

Elastography, also known as "liver elastography," is a type of imaging test that checks the liver for fibrosis. Fibrosis is a condition that reduces blood flow to and inside the liver. This causes the buildup of scar tissue. If left untreated, fibrosis can lead to serious problems in the liver. These include cirrhosis, liver cancer, and liver failure. But early diagnosis and treatment can reduce or even reverse the effects of fibrosis.

Here are the two types of liver elastography tests:

- **Ultrasound elastography**, also known as "Fibroscan," the brand name of the ultrasound device. The test uses sound waves to measure the stiffness of liver tissue. Stiffness is a sign of fibrosis.
- **Magnetic resonance elastography (MRE)**, a test that combines ultrasound technology with magnetic resonance imaging (MRI). MRI is a procedure that uses powerful magnets and radio waves to create images of organs and structures inside the body. In an MRE test, a computer program creates a visual map that shows liver stiffness.

Elastography testing may be used in place of a liver biopsy, a more invasive test that involves removing a piece of liver tissue for testing.

Other names include liver elastography, transient elastography, FibroScan, and MRE.

WHAT IS IT USED FOR?

Elastography is used to diagnose fatty liver disease (FLD) and fibrosis. FLD is a condition in which fat builds up in the liver. This fat can lead to cell death and fibrosis.

WHY DO YOU NEED ELASTOGRAPHY?

Many people with fibrosis do not have symptoms. But, if left untreated, fibrosis will continue to scar the liver and eventually turn into cirrhosis.

Cirrhosis is a term used to describe excessive scarring of the liver. Cirrhosis is most often caused by alcohol abuse or hepatitis. In severe cases, cirrhosis can be life-threatening. Cirrhosis does cause symptoms. So you may need this test if you have symptoms of cirrhosis or another liver disease.

Advances in Imaging

Symptoms of cirrhosis and other liver diseases are similar and may include the following:
- Yellowing of the skin (known as "jaundice")
- Fatigue
- Itching
- Bruising easily
- Heavy nosebleeds
- Swelling in the legs
- Weight loss
- Confusion

WHAT HAPPENS DURING AN ELASTOGRAPHY?

During an ultrasound (FibroScan) elastography:
- You will lie on an examination table on your back, with your right abdominal area exposed.
- A radiology technician will spread the gel on your skin over the area.
- She or he will place a wand-like device, called a transducer, on the area of skin that covers your liver.
- The probe will deliver a series of sound waves. The waves will travel to your liver and bounce back. The waves are so high-pitched you cannot hear them.
- You may feel a gentle flick as this is done, but it should not hurt.
- The sound waves are recorded, measured, and displayed on a monitor.
- The measurement shows the level of stiffness in the liver.
- The procedure only takes about five minutes, but your entire appointment may take a half hour or so.

MRE is done with the same type of machine and many of the same steps as a traditional MRI test. During an MRE procedure:
- You will lie on a narrow examination table.
- A radiology technician will place a small pad on your abdomen. The pad will emit vibrations that pass through your liver.

Health Technology Sourcebook, Third Edition

- The table will slide into an MRI scanner, which is a tunnel-shaped machine that contains the magnet. You may be given earplugs or headphones before the test to help block the noise of the scanner, which is very loud.
- Once inside the scanner, the pad will activate and send measurements of vibrations from your liver. The measurements will be recorded onto a computer and turned into a visual map that shows the stiffness of your liver.
- The test takes about 30–60 minutes.

WILL YOU NEED TO DO ANYTHING TO PREPARE FOR THE TEST?

You do not need any special preparations for ultrasound elastography. If you are having an MRE, be sure to remove all metal jewelry and accessories before the test.

ARE THERE ANY RISKS TO THE TEST?

There are no known risks to having ultrasound elastography. There is little risk of having an MRE for most people. Some people feel nervous or claustrophobic inside the scanner. If you feel this way, you may be given medicine before the test to help you relax.

Also, MRE testing may not be a good choice for people who have metal devices implanted in their bodies. These include pacemakers, artificial heart valves, and infusion pumps. The magnet in the MRI can affect the operation of these devices, and in some cases, it could be dangerous. Dental braces and certain types of tattoos that contain metal may also cause problems during the procedure.

The test is also not recommended for women who are pregnant or think they might be pregnant. It is not known whether magnetic fields are harmful to unborn babies.

WHAT DO THE RESULTS MEAN?

Both types of elastography measure the stiffness of the liver. The stiffer the liver, the more fibrosis you have. Your results may range from no scarring to mild, moderate, or advanced liver scarring. Advanced scarring is known as "cirrhosis." Your health-care

Advances in Imaging

provider may order additional testing, including liver function blood tests or a liver biopsy, to confirm a diagnosis.

If you are diagnosed with mild-to-moderate fibrosis, you may be able to take steps to stop further scarring and sometimes even improve your condition. These steps include:

- Not drinking alcohol.
- Not taking illegal drugs.
- Eating a healthy diet.
- Increasing exercise.
- Taking medicine. There are medicines that are effective in treating some types of hepatitis.

If you wait too long for treatment, more and more scar tissue will build up in your liver. This can lead to cirrhosis. Sometimes, the only treatment for advanced cirrhosis is a liver transplant.

If you have questions about your results, talk to your health-care provider.

IS THERE ANYTHING ELSE YOU NEED TO KNOW ABOUT AN ELASTOGRAPHY?

While elastography is usually used to diagnose problems in the liver, it may also be used to diagnose conditions in other organs. These include the breast, thyroid, and prostate.

Chapter 20 | **Advanced Imaging in Laboratory Technology**

Chapter Contents

Section 20.1—Live Cell Imaging 305
Section 20.2—Nonlinear Optical Imaging 306
Section 20.3—Surface Plasmon Resonance Imaging 309

Section 20.1 | **Live Cell Imaging**

This section includes text excerpted from "Live Cell Imaging of Induced Pluripotent Stem Cell Populations," National Institute of Standards and Technology (NIST), December 21, 2018. Reviewed November 2022.

Induced pluripotent stem cell (iPSC) populations are complex, dynamic, and heterogeneous. Individual cells within a population are constantly changing while maintaining the capacity to differentiate into numerous possible cell types. Sophisticated measurement tools are required to adequately describe and develop predictive models for complex cellular systems such as these. The technology to record live cell images from cellular populations has been available for some time, but only recently has it become routine to derive quantitative data from these image sets using image analysis. The National Institute of Standards and Technology (NIST) has focused on developing live cell imaging tools to monitor large numbers of single cells and to quantify changes in morphology and gene expression using fluorescence protein reporters.

The NIST's live cell image program supports the advancement of iPSC technology in the following ways:

- **Identification of process control measurements.** A critical component of the translation of iPSCs into therapeutic applications is to design principles for predictably and reproducibly culturing cells and efficiently differentiating them into cell types of interest. Live cell imaging provides "high-resolution" measurements in the sense that we collect time-dependent data from large numbers of individual cells. The NIST then uses this data to discover lower-resolution measurements, such as the activity of a biomarker at a single point in time, that can serve as critical process control points during the processing of pluripotent stem cells.

- **Interpreting biomarkers.** Cells are stochastic and dynamic and may interconvert between states, and the expression of biomarkers can change over time. The predictive power of a biomarker or a set of biomarkers that indicate the differentiated state of a cell can be evaluated by examining the history of that cell by tracking forward and backward in time through a time-lapse image set.

- **Predictive modeling.** The NIST has shown that fluctuations in promoter activity can be used in combination with appropriate models to predict rates of state change in cell populations. Similar mathematical models that can inform bioprocessing decisions during scale-up will be critical to obtaining iPSC populations with a desired set of characteristics.

Over the past several years, the NIST has developed tools for measuring parameters related to size, shape, and intensity from single cells over time. They have also developed modeling tools for using temporal information to model the stochastic and deterministic components of gene expression.

They are now applying these live cell imaging tools to the study of stem cell pluripotency and differentiation. Induced pluripotent stem cell technologies are a powerful new tool for biomedical research and have the potential to revolutionize medicine.

Section 20.2 | Nonlinear Optical Imaging

This section contains text excerpted from the following sources: Text in this section begins with excerpts from "Multi-Photon Microscopy System Configured for Multiview Non-Linear Optical Imaging," Office of Technology Transfer (OTT), National Institutes of Health (NIH), June 27, 2016. Reviewed November 2022; Text under the heading "Broadband Coherent Anti-Stokes Raman Scattering (BCARS) Microscopy" is excerpted from "Broadband Coherent Anti-Stokes Raman Scattering (BCARS) Microscopy," National Institute of Standards and Technology (NIST), June 2, 2022.

Nonlinear optical imaging remains the premier technique for deep-tissue imaging in which, typically, a multiphoton arrangement may be used to illuminate and excite a sample. However, the penetration depth, signal-to-noise ratio, and resolution of this technique are ultimately limited by scattering. The present system

Advanced Imaging in Laboratory Technology

addresses these issues by sequential excitation of a sample through three or more objective lenses oriented at different axes intersecting the sample. Each objective lens is capable of focused sequential excitation that elicits fluorescence emissions from the excited sample, which is then simultaneously detected by each respective objective lens along a respective longitudinal axis. Including multiple lenses will improve the penetration depth and, at the same time, decrease the loss of detail because of scattering. The system also can overcome losses in spatial resolution because of the scattering of the excitation and emission of light.

Commercial applications of nonlinear optical imaging are:
- High-resolution multiphoton microscopy
- Deep tissue visualization

Competitive advantages of nonlinear optical imaging are:
- Improved signal-to-noise ratio
- Improved spatial resolution

BROADBAND COHERENT ANTI-STOKES RAMAN SCATTERING MICROSCOPY

There is a need for label-free chemical microscopy in medicine, biology, and materials science. Most of the current methods use chemical labels that often disturb the distribution and nature of the chemical components being investigated. The method developed by the NIST enables the noninvasive and rapid collection of Raman spectra for imaging.

Broadband coherent anti-Stokes Raman scattering can be used to track cell signaling processes and can provide functional readouts of cell differentiation, allowing researchers to obtain cell responses to biomaterials in real time and on a cell-by-cell basis.

Broadband coherent anti-Stokes Raman scattering can be used to acquire high-resolution chemical maps of pharmaceutical tablets, including information on the morphology of active ingredients, 10–100 times faster than spontaneous Raman scattering.

All researchers who use Raman imaging methods will benefit from this work, including biomedical researchers (and, potentially, clinicians), pharmaceutical industry scientists, geologists,

Health Technology Sourcebook, Third Edition

and others. Additionally, laser manufacturers have been influenced by this work; PolarOnyx, Toptica, Time-Bandwidth, and Spectra-Physics Laser have all developed and are marketing laser sources to enable BCARS.

Approach

Coherent anti-Stokes Raman scattering provides a signal that contains the Raman response of interest for performing label-free chemically sensitive microscopy. In CARS, a vibrational coherence is generated when a pair of photons (pump and Stokes) interact with the sample to excite a vibrationally resonant Raman mode at frequency $\omega vib = \omega pump - \omega Stokes$. A third (probe) photon is inelastically scattered off this coherent excitation, and anti-Stokes light ($\omega as = \omega pump - \omega Stokes + \omega probe$) is emitted from the sample.

The CARS signal has a frequency-independent nonresonant component and a frequency-dependent resonant component. The nonresonant component is entirely in phase with the driving field of the laser and gives the researchers no information about the chemical nature of the sample. The resonant component contains chemical information and has a frequency-dependent amplitude. It is out of phase with respect to the driving electric field of the laser. The resonant component contains elements with the same band shape as the spontaneous Raman signal.

A broadband vibrational spectrum is obtained at each laser shot by using broadband Stokes light. The Stokes light contains 3,000 cm^{-1} of bandwidth.

The spectra obtained from CARS include a resonant and non-resonant component, which made it difficult to extract the Raman spectrum of interest. The researchers have developed a deterministic mathematical approach to extracting the resonant (Raman) signal based on a time-domain Kramers–Kronig (TDKK) transform. The TDKK treatment makes the CARS signal linear in analyte concentration and quantitative. They show, based on imaging of a polymer blend below, that even minor components can be detected and quantitatively accounted for when the CARS signal is transformed in this way.

Advanced Imaging in Laboratory Technology

This TDKK transform allows the researchers to take advantage of intrinsic heterodyne amplification of the weak resonant signal and allows them to be the first group to obtain a full fingerprint and CH-stretch vibrational spectra simultaneously in biological cells. The chemical signatures contained in the combined CH and fingerprint spectral region allow them to discriminate differentiated cells from stem cells.

Section 20.3 | Surface Plasmon Resonance Imaging

This section includes text excerpted from "Label-Free Imaging of Cells and Their Extracellular Matrix by SPR Imaging," National Institute of Standards and Technology (NIST), March 10, 2020.

Cellular remodeling of their neighboring environment, extracellular matrix (ECM), is an important biological process from development biology to wound healing to diseases and cancers—this is a challenging process to measure and quantify.

Surface plasmon resonance imaging (SPRI) has been developed as quantitative, label-free microscopy to image real-time observation of live cell engagement with the surface and protein deposition and remodeling. The SPRI technique is an alternative to the commonly used fluorescence microscopy for examining cell–matrix interactions. This technique removes the requirement for modified biological molecules and transfected cells.

Researchers here have improved upon the spatial resolution of SPRI, enabling the ability to visualize subcellular structures near the sensor surface. Along with quantitative interpretation of the images, essentially refractive index measurements, dry mass values of subcellular components can now be measured. For example, a smooth muscle cell has been measured to have a focal adhesion dry mass of 980 ng/cm^2 and can deposit up to 120 ng/cm^2 of protein around its periphery under normal growth conditions.

Accomplishments have been:

- Measurement of ECM, protein deposition, and cell phenotype with SPRI

309

Health Technology Sourcebook, Third Edition

- Surface plasmon resonance imaging of cells and surface-associated fibronectin
- Quantification of cell areas, dynamic changes in cell-substrate, and changes in surface protein density over time
- Using surface plasmon resonance imaging to probe dynamic interactions between cells and extracellular matrix
- Improvement of spatial resolution to visualize subcellular components
- High-resolution surface plasmon resonance imaging for single cells
- Quantitative mass measurements of focal adhesions in single cells
- Mass measurements of focal adhesions in single cells using high-resolution surface plasmon resonance microscopy
- Calibration and correction strategy for quantitative analysis by optical modeling
- Surface plasmon resonance microscopy: achieving a quantitative optical response

Research here is underway to develop SPRI as an imaging biosensor that can visualize dry mass changes down to a single bacterium that is part of a bacterial biofilm. Measuring antibiotic drug response at an individual cell level in addition to the biofilm as a whole can provide insight and understanding of how biofilms contribute to antibiotic drug resistance.

Chapter 21 | Point-of-Care Diagnostic Testing

This chapter provides information on the regulatory requirements for SARS-CoV-2 rapid testing performed in point-of-care (POC) settings, collecting specimens and performing rapid tests safely and correctly and information on reporting test results.

This guidance is intended for individuals and facilities who are setting up and performing rapid testing in POC settings and is not intended for the use or reporting of self-tests performed by the individual being tested.

Point-of-care testing uses rapid diagnostic tests performed or interpreted by someone other than the individual being tested or their parent or guardian and can be performed in a variety of settings. Rapid tests used in POC settings can be nucleic acid amplification test (NAAT), antigen, or antibody tests.

These tests can be used to diagnose current or detect past SARS-CoV-2 infections in various POC settings, including but not limited to:
- Physician offices
- Urgent care facilities
- Pharmacies
- School health clinics
- Long-term care facilities and nursing homes
- Temporary locations, such as drive-through sites managed by local organizations

This chapter includes text excerpted from "Guidance for SARS-CoV-2 Rapid Testing Performed in Point-of-Care Settings," Centers for Disease Control and Prevention (CDC), April 4, 2022.

Health Technology Sourcebook, Third Edition

REGULATORY REQUIREMENTS FOR RAPID TESTING IN POINT-OF-CARE SETTINGS

There are four different types of CLIA certificates, any one of which is appropriate for POC testing. A CLIA certificate is required to perform POC testing. A CLIA Certificate of Waiver is appropriate if SARS-CoV-2 POC testing is the only testing being performed. It can be obtained as follows:

- Complete an application (Form CMS-116), available on the CMS CLIA website (www.cms.gov/Regulations-and-Guidance/Legislation/CLIA) or from a local state agency.
- Send the completed application to the address of the local state agency where testing will be performed.
- Pay the CLIA Certificate of Waiver fee, following instructions provided by the state agency.

Laboratories or POC testing sites that have applied for a CLIA Certificate of Waiver to perform SARS-CoV-2 POC testing can begin testing and reporting SARS-CoV-2 results as soon as they have submitted their application to the state agency as long as they meet any additional state licensure requirements that apply. A noncertified POC testing site will be treated as operating under a Certificate of Waiver while their application is being processed. The POC testing site must keep its certificate information current. The state agency should be notified of any changes to the laboratory or testing site ownership, name, address, or director within 30 days.

During the COVID-19 public health emergency, CMS allows a laboratory or testing site to use its existing Certificate of Waiver to operate a temporary COVID-19 testing site in an off-site location, such as a nursing home or drive-through location. A temporary COVID-19 testing site can only perform CLIA-waived or POC tests authorized by the U.S. Food and Drug Administration (FDA) for SARS-CoV-2 and must be under the direction of the existing laboratory or testing site director.

CMS has provided specific guidance for the use of FDA-authorized OTC self-tests when these tests are performed or the results are interpreted by someone other than the individual being

Point-of-Care Diagnostic Testing

tested or their parent or guardian. In these circumstances, the tests are not considered self-tests, and the POC testing site that performs the testing or interprets the test results needs a CLIA certificate and must report results as described below.

Tests That Can Be Used in Point-of-Care Settings

Refer to the FDA website for a list of the SARS-CoV-2 POC and rapid tests that have received Emergency Use Authorization (EUA; www.fda.gov/medical-devices/coronavirus-disease-2019-covid-19-emergency-use-authorizations-medical-devices/in-vitro-diagnostics-euas). Tests that have been authorized for use in a POC setting will have a W, for Waived, in the Authorized Settings column of the FDA table. The laboratory or testing site must use a test authorized for POC use by the FDA and must follow the manufacturer's instructions for each test. The instructions for use provide specific information on how to perform the test, which specimens can be used, and the people who may be tested.

OTC tests can be purchased and used in a POC setting. However, when these tests are performed or the results are interpreted by someone other than the individual being tested or their parent or guardian, then the CLIA reporting requirements for waived tests must be followed.

REPORTING REQUIREMENTS FOR RAPID TESTING IN POINT-OF-CARE SETTINGS

A CLIA-certified laboratory or testing site must report all positive SARS-CoV-2 diagnostic and screening test results to the person who was tested or that person's health-care provider. CLIA-certified laboratories or testing sites are no longer required to report negative results for non-NAAT (rapid or antigen test results) or antibody tests, positive or negative. Depending on the test manufacturer's instructions for use, which can be found on FDA's EUA website (www.fda.gov/medical-devices/coronavirus-disease-2019-covid-19-emergency-use-authorizations-medical-devices/in-vitro-diagnostics-euas), the laboratory or testing site may be required to report a negative test result as a "presumptive negative."

313

Health Technology Sourcebook, Third Edition

A CLIA-certified laboratory or testing site must also report all positive SARS-CoV-2 test results to their respective state, tribal, local, and territorial health department's website (www.cdc.gov/publichealthgateway/healthdirectories/index.html) in accordance with the Coronavirus Aid, Relief, and Economic Security (CARES) Act. CLIA-certified laboratories or testing sites are no longer required to report negative results for non-NAAT (rapid or antigen test results) or antibody tests, positive or negative.

CMS-certified long-term care (LTC) facilities can submit POC SARS-CoV-2 testing data, including antigen, antibody, and NAAT testing data, to CDC's National Healthcare Safety Network (NHSN). This CDC- and CMS-preferred pathway to submit data to CDC's NHSN applies only to CMS-certified LTC facilities. Test data submitted to NHSN will be reported to appropriate state, tribal, local, and territorial health departments using standard electronic laboratory messages. Other types of LTC facilities can also report testing data in NHSN for self-tracking or to fulfill state or local reporting requirements, if any.

SPECIMEN COLLECTION AND HANDLING OF RAPID TESTS IN POINT-OF-CARE SETTINGS

Each POC test has been authorized for use with certain specimen types and should only be used with those specimen types. Proper specimen collection and handling are critical for all COVID-19 testing, including those tests performed in POC settings. A specimen that is not collected or handled correctly can lead to an inaccurate or unreliable test result.

Personnel collecting specimens or working within six feet of patients suspected to be infected with SARS-CoV-2 should maintain proper infection control and use recommended personal protective equipment (PPE), which could include an N95 or higher-level respirator (or face mask if a respirator is not available), eye protection, gloves, and a lab coat or gown.

Personnel handling specimens but not directly involved in the collection (e.g., self-collection) and not working within six feet of the patient should follow standard precautions. It is recommended that personnel wear well-fitting cloth masks, face masks,

Point-of-Care Diagnostic Testing

or respirators at all times while at the POC site where the testing is being performed.

Disinfect surfaces within six feet of the specimen collection and handling area at these times:

- Before testing begins each day
- Between each specimen collection
- At least hourly during testing
- When visibly soiled
- In the event of a specimen spill or splash
- At the end of every testing day

The CDC recommends the following practices when performing tests in POC settings:

Before the test:

- Perform a risk assessment to identify what could go wrong, such as breathing in infectious material or touching contaminated objects and surfaces.
  - Implement appropriate control measures to prevent these potentially negative outcomes from happening.
- Use a new pair of gloves each time a specimen is collected from a different person. If specimens are tested in batches, also change gloves before putting a new specimen into a testing device. Doing so will help to avoid cross-contamination.
- Do not reuse used test devices, reagent tubes, solutions, swabs, lancets, or fingerstick collection devices.
- Store reagents, specimens, kit contents, and test devices according to the manufacturer's instructions found in the package insert.
- Discard tests and test components that have exceeded the expiration date or show signs of damage or discoloration (such as reagents showing any signs of alteration).
- Do not open reagents, test devices, and cassettes until the test process is about to occur. Refer to the manufacturer's instructions to see how long a reagent, test device, or cassette can be used after opening.

Health Technology Sourcebook, Third Edition

- Label each specimen with appropriate information to definitively connect that specimen to the correct person being tested.
- When transferring specimens from a collection area to a testing area, follow the instructions for the POC test used.

During the test:
- Follow all the manufacturer's instructions for performing the test in the exact order specified.
- Perform regular quality control and instrument calibration, as applicable, according to the manufacturer's instructions. If quality control or calibration fails, identify and correct issues before proceeding with patient testing.
- When processing multiple specimens successively in batches, ensure proper timing for each specimen and each step of the testing process, as specified by the test manufacturer. To avoid cross-contamination, change gloves before putting a new specimen into a testing device.

After the test:
- Read and record results only within the amount of time specified in the manufacturer's instructions. Do not record results from tests that have not been read within the manufacturer's specified time frame.
- Decontaminate the instrument after each use. Follow the manufacturer's recommendations for using an approved disinfectant, including proper dilution, contact time, and safe handling.
- Always discuss used and unused COVID-19 test kit waste with your facility leadership, facility waste management contractor, your state department of public health, and the test manufacturer's technical support. All waste disposal must comply with local, tribal, regional, state, national, and/or international regulations. Waste disposal regulations may vary at the state and local levels.

Part 6 | Role of Technology in Treatment

Chapter 22 | **Artificial Intelligence Tools to Augment Patient Care**

PROMISE OF ARTIFICIAL INTELLIGENCE TOOLS TO AUGMENT PATIENT CARE

Artificial intelligence (AI) in health care has the potential to deliver many benefits, according to the scientific literature and stakeholders, including industry representatives, academic researchers, and health-care providers. In general, AI tools augment rather than replace human providers. Studies have demonstrated improved results when providers and AI tools work together rather than each working independently. Examples of key areas where AI tools show promise to augment patient care include:

- **Improving treatment**. AI tools could improve provider decision-making with more accurate predictions of a patient's health trajectory. For example, providers could use AI to predict hospital length of stay, readmission, or mortality. The availability of large amounts of health data and advanced analytical tools, such as those using AI, also promises significant advances in precision medicine (i.e., the tailoring of medical treatment to the individual characteristics of each patient). The goal of precision medicine is to allow providers to select patient-specific treatments that minimize

---

This chapter includes text excerpted from "Artificial Intelligence in Health Care: Benefits and Challenges of Technologies to Augment Patient Care," U.S. Government Accountability Office (GAO), November 2020.

319

Health Technology Sourcebook, Third Edition

harmful side effects and ensure a more successful outcome. By integrating individual patient information with lessons gleaned from large volumes of data on prior patient cases and clinical trajectories, AI tools could assist provider decision-making with greater comprehensiveness and speed than would be possible without such tools.

- **Reducing the burden on providers**. By taking over routine or standardized tasks not requiring human judgment, intuition, or empathy, AI tools could also reduce stress and free providers to spend time on more complex tasks. Provider burnout—a long-term stress reaction marked by emotional exhaustion, depersonalization, and a lack of a sense of personal accomplishment—has been on the rise in recent years and can threaten patient safety or quality of care. For example, AI tools that ease the process of documenting clinical notes or automate aspects of the clinical workflow could give providers more time with their patients, thereby enhancing the patient–provider relationship.
- **Increasing resource efficiency**. AI tools could also increase the efficiency with which health-care facilities and providers use resources, potentially resulting in cost savings, health gains, or both. For example, AI tools could reduce the need for costly equipment, inform staffing decisions, or help direct resources to patients in the most need of care.

CLINICAL ARTIFICIAL INTELLIGENCE TOOLS TO AUGMENT PATIENT CARE

The Government Accountability Office (GAO) identified five categories of clinical applications in which AI tools have shown promise to augment patient care: predicting health trajectories, recommending treatments, guiding surgical care, monitoring patients, and supporting population health management. The selected tools described in these categories are at varying stages of maturity and

Artificial Intelligence Tools to Augment Patient Care

adoption. The GAO identified several tools in the design and development phase; these tools have been studied in the scientific literature but have not yet been clinically validated or tested in humans. The risk-prediction tool for supporting population health management is the only tool the GAO describes that has reached the monitoring and maintenance stage of development.

The first three categories include machine learning-enabled CDS tools. According to the scientific literature, many of these tools are described in academic journals but have not been fully integrated into or evaluated in a clinical setting, and evidence of the clinical or economic effect of these tools is limited.

Predicting Health Trajectories

Machine-learning-enabled CDS tools can help predict the likelihood that a patient's condition will deteriorate. In one example, in 2013–2014, a large integrated health system successfully piloted a machine learning model to identify patients at risk for transfer to the intensive care unit (ICU). Other applications in this category include the prediction of acute kidney injury and *Clostridium difficile* infection.

One of the most common health concerns targeted by recent machine learning models is sepsis. Machine-learning-based sepsis prediction models can predict sepsis and septic shock before onset and have demonstrated improved patient outcomes. Several studies have shown that early identification and treatment of patients with severe sepsis or septic shock can reduce morbidity, mortality, and hospital length of stay. Of the 21 case studies identified in a 2020 review, six are studies of sepsis prediction models. Developers have begun or published prospective clinical validation of three of these models, and five have received funding from either private or public sources to begin scaling adoption.

Despite promising results, there are limitations to sepsis prediction models. One researcher we spoke to pointed out that the retrospective data used to develop these models may not be representative of all patients who go on to develop sepsis. For example, a provider may treat a patient arriving at the emergency room (ER) with an early-stage infection with antibiotics, preventing the patient from

Health Technology Sourcebook, Third Edition

developing sepsis or delaying the onset. The model may then learn that this patient is low-risk for sepsis when in fact they were high-risk. Additionally, tools may not work when a new disease or other phenomenon emerges, according to an expert. For example, this expert reported having received many questions about using their sepsis prediction model and related tools during the COVID-19 pandemic. However, the protocol for ordering laboratory tests for COVID-19 patients is different than that of sepsis patients—for COVID-19, providers are ordering many different types of laboratory tests, whereas the expert's sepsis prediction model uses one specific laboratory test as a proxy for suspicion of infection. The emergence of this new virus may require changes to the way providers think about and respond to sepsis, according to this expert.

Recommending Treatments

Artificial-intelligence-enabled CDS tools can also recommend treatments to health-care providers, potentially helping them make decisions more effective and patient-specific. Machine learning makes it possible to process and use large-scale data from previous cases for clinical decision-making in a way that would have been difficult previously. For example, these tools could help personalize treatment decisions for patients by learning from the collective experience of others to identify patients with similar conditions and the outcomes of their treatment. However, when these tools are trained on retrospective data, they risk learning the prescribing habits of physicians rather than ideal practices. Examples from the scientific literature include tools used to recommend treatments for cancer, sepsis, and stroke.

Another promising area for AI-enabled CDS tools is in treating patients with mechanical ventilators. While ventilators can be life-saving, both prolonged use and premature weaning are associated with complications, increased mortality rates, and higher hospital costs. Deciding when to wean patients receiving ventilator treatment is an essential aspect of their care. However, there is uncertainty surrounding the best methods for conducting this process. For example, providers are using ventilators to treat COVID-19 patients, and the variation in mortality rates across ICUs suggests

Artificial Intelligence Tools to Augment Patient Care

that different methods for ventilator management may affect outcomes. Many commercially available ventilators contain automated weaning modes based on rules-based systems. In scientific studies, the use of these tools or clinical guidelines has outperformed the common practice of providers deciding on their own when to wean. However, these tools may produce suboptimal results in a clinical environment depending on what data are available and the assumptions of the rules-based system.

Recent research has explored the use of machine-learning-enabled CDS tools for this application, which may overcome some of the limitations of ventilators with automated weaning modes. Machine learning technology can help build models that incorporate the many factors affecting the respiratory system in the ICU. Supervised machine learning is a commonly used technique to train machine learning-enabled tools for ventilator weaning management. These tools have shown promise in predicting when to successfully wean patients, according to the scientific literature, although mostly as proof of concept rather than assessing the effectiveness of the tools in a clinical setting.

Researchers have also explored the use of reinforcement learning for this task; however, this technology is less mature. In a recent study, researchers used reinforcement learning to develop a CDS tool that would alert providers when a patient is ready to begin weaning. Using publicly available, retrospective ICU data, researchers showed that fewer patients had to be put back on a ventilator when providers followed a protocol similar to the one recommended by the CDS tool. However, using machine learning tools trained on outcomes data, such as timing and success of weaning, to guide this process can also be challenging. For example, successful weaning at a specified time does not preclude the possibility that the patient was ready to wean earlier.

Guiding Surgical Care

In the field of surgical care, planning and postoperative care are the most mature applications for machine-learning-enabled CDS tools. Other applications, including real-time CDS for surgery and AI-enabled surgical robots, are also active areas of research but are

Health Technology Sourcebook, Third Edition

more nascent. One tool for surgical planning that entered clinical trials in 2018 uses computer vision on magnetic resonance imaging (MRI) scans to identify areas for prostate cancer biopsy. In postoperative care, studies have demonstrated that AI tools can predict the risk of complications from surgery, such as surgical site infections and in-hospital mortality.

Other surgical applications of AI, such as using machine-learning-enabled CDS tools to enhance surgical decision-making, are also in development but are in their infancy, according to an expert. One application currently under study is the use of computer vision to analyze surgical video in real time to identify or predict adverse events and guide providers.

Another area of active research is AI-enabled surgical robotics; however, most current commercial surgical robots are primarily remote-controlled rather than AI-enabled. According to one expert, there are commercial surgical robots in use or coming to the U.S. market that claim to be AI-enabled, but these generally just contain certain AI-enabled features rather than actually guiding surgery. For example, these robotic tools may alert a surgeon when their surgical time is longer than average or predict how many cartridges they can use for the surgical stapler.

AI-enabled autonomous surgical robots have not yet been tested in humans, but studies in animals have demonstrated that they can match or outperform human surgeons for certain tasks. These tools could potentially increase the safety, efficiency, and access to soft tissue surgical procedures. Early attempts at autonomous robotic surgery focused on automating relatively simple tasks such as suturing or knot-tying, but recently researchers have demonstrated more complex tasks. For example, hospital researchers developed a robotic catheter that can autonomously navigate a beating heart in a pig and demonstrated that its performance was similar to that of experienced surgeons. Automating such tasks could free the surgeon to focus on other aspects of the procedure, potentially reducing the learning curve involved in mastering a new procedure. AI-enabled surgical robots might also have the effect of allowing less-experienced surgeons to perform operations safely and expanding the skills of providers in under-resourced areas.

Artificial Intelligence Tools to Augment Patient Care

An expert in this area expects to see some level of automation for soft tissue surgical robots in the next 20–30 years. This expert said researchers will need to acquire and label surgical video data to properly develop these machines before allowing them to perform surgical tasks autonomously.

Monitoring Patients

Artificial-intelligence-enabled tools can use the increasing availability of health data, including data from electronic health records (EHRs), wearables, and other sensors, to help monitor patients in health-care facilities. According to a recent review, patient monitoring is one of the areas where AI is likely to have the greatest influence. For example, providers can use AI analysis of vital signs for cardiovascular and respiratory monitoring in the ICU.

In another example, health-care facilities can use AI-enabled monitoring tools in hospitals to prevent patient falls and reduce provider burden. According to a 2015 report, hundreds of thousands of hospital patients fall each year. Thirty to 50 percent of those falls result in injury, which can increase the length and cost of the hospital stay or even result in death. One commercial AI tool aiming to help providers address these issues uses computer vision, Bluetooth, and sensors to analyze movements in the patient's room and alert the care team when a fall is predicted, according to company representatives. They stated the tool can also reduce provider burden by eliminating the need for hourly patient checks and help predict staffing needs by identifying patients who are visited most frequently. According to company materials, this company also developed new algorithms to use the device for infection control activities in response to the COVID-19 pandemic. For example, the tool can be used to automatically detect whether staff are complying with personal protective equipment (PPE) requirements and to conduct contact tracing within the health-care facility.

Supporting Population Health Management

Large health systems and payers widely use AI-enabled tools to support population health management activities. Population

Health Technology Sourcebook, Third Edition

health management involves using population-level data to identify broad health risks and treatment opportunities for a group of individuals or a community. One task where AI has the potential to improve population health management is the prioritization of clinical resources and targeting health-care services to patients who are the most likely to benefit. For example, large integrated health systems have deployed machine learning models to predict individual patients' risk of chronic diseases and associated complications and offer specialized care programs to high-risk patients.

However, one risk of using such tools is bias. For example, a commercial risk-prediction tool that large health systems and payers collectively apply to around 200 million people in the United States per year was found to have a racial bias in a recent study. According to the study, correcting algorithmic bias requires expert knowledge of the relevant field, the ability to identify and extract relevant data elements, and the capacity to iterate and experiment. However, one of the study's coauthors stated that the problems in machine learning tools can at least be fixed once identified, whereas bias among humans may not be as readily remedied.

Chapter 23 | **Technology and the Future of Mental Health Treatment**

Technology has opened a new frontier in mental health support and data collection. Mobile devices, such as cell phones, smartphones, and tablets, are giving the public, doctors, and researchers new ways to access help, monitor progress, and increase understanding of mental well-being.

Mobile mental health support can be very simple but effective. For example, anyone with the ability to send a text message can contact a crisis center. New technology can also be packaged into an extremely sophisticated app for smartphones or tablets. Such apps might use the device's built-in sensors to collect information on a user's typical behavior patterns. If the app detects a change in behavior, it may provide a signal that help is needed before a crisis occurs. Some apps are stand-alone programs that promise to improve memory or thinking skills. Others help the user connect to a peer counselor or to a health-care professional.

Excitement about the huge range of opportunities has led to a burst of app development. There are thousands of mental health apps available in iTunes and Android app stores, and the number is growing every year. However, this new technology frontier includes a lot of uncertainty. There is very little industry regulation and very little information on app effectiveness, which can lead consumers to wonder which apps they should trust.

This chapter includes text excerpted from "Technology and the Future of Mental Health Treatment," National Institute of Mental Health (NIMH), April 2021.

Before focusing on the state of the science and where it may lead, it is important to look at the advantages and disadvantages of expanding mental health treatment and research into a mobile world.

THE PROS AND CONS OF MENTAL HEALTH APPS

Experts believe that technology has a lot of potential for clients and clinicians alike. A few of the advantages of mobile care include the following:

- **Convenience**. Treatment can take place anytime and anywhere (e.g., at home in the middle of the night or on a bus on the way to work) and may be ideal for those who have trouble with in-person appointments.
- **Anonymity**. Clients can seek treatment options without involving other people.
- **An introduction to care**. Technology may be a good first step for those who have avoided mental health care in the past.
- **Lower cost**. Some apps are free or cost less than traditional care.
- **Service to more people**. Technology can help mental health providers offer treatment to people in remote areas or to many people in times of sudden need (e.g., following a natural disaster or terror attack).
- **Interest**. Some technologies might be more appealing than traditional treatment methods, which may encourage clients to continue therapy.
- **Twenty-four-hour service**. Technology can provide round-the-clock monitoring or intervention support.
- **Consistency**. Technology can offer the same treatment program to all users.
- **Support**. Technology can complement traditional therapy by extending an in-person session, reinforcing new skills, and providing support and monitoring.
- **Objective data collection**. Technology can quantitatively collect information such as location, movement, phone use, and other information.

Technology and the Future of Mental Health Treatment

This new era of mental health technology offers great opportunities but also raises a number of concerns. Tackling potential problems will be an important part of making sure new apps provide benefits without causing harm. That is why the mental health community and software developers are focusing on the following:

- **Effectiveness.** The biggest concern with technological interventions is obtaining scientific evidence that they work and that they work as well as traditional methods.
- **For whom and for what.** Another concern is understanding if apps work for all people and for all mental health conditions.
- **Privacy.** Apps deal with very sensitive personal information, so app makers need to be able to guarantee privacy for app users.
- **Guidance.** There are no industry-wide standards to help consumers know if an app or other mobile technology is proven effective.
- **Regulation.** The question of who will or should regulate mental health technology and the data it generates needs to be answered.
- **Overselling.** There is some concern that if an app or program promises more than it delivers, consumers may turn away from other, more effective therapies.

CURRENT TRENDS IN APP DEVELOPMENT

Creative research and engineering teams are combining their skills to address a wide range of mental health concerns. Some popular areas of app development include the following.

Self-Management Apps

Self-management means that the user puts information into the app so that the app can provide feedback. For example, the user might set up medication reminders or use the app to develop tools for managing stress, anxiety, or sleep problems. Some software can use additional equipment to track heart rate, breathing patterns, blood pressure, and so on and may help the user track progress and receive feedback.

Apps for Improving Thinking Skills

Apps that help the user with cognitive remediation (improved thinking skills) are promising. These apps are often targeted toward people with serious mental illnesses.

Skill-Training Apps

Skill-training apps such as games may feel more than other mental health apps as they help users learn new coping or thinking skills. The user might watch an educational video about anxiety management or the importance of social support. Next, the user might pick some new strategies to try and then use the app to track how often those new skills are practiced.

Illness Management and Supported Care

This type of app technology adds additional support by allowing the user to interact with another human being. The app may help the user connect with peer support or may send information to a trained health-care provider who can offer guidance and therapy options. Researchers are working on learning how much human interaction people need for app-based treatments to be effective.

Passive Symptom Tracking

A lot of effort is going into developing apps that can collect data using the sensors built into smartphones. These sensors can record movement patterns, social interactions (such as the number of texts and phone calls), behavior at different times of the day, vocal tone and speed, and more. In the future, apps may be able to analyze these data to determine the user's real-time state of mind. Such apps may be able to recognize changes in behavior patterns that signal a mood episode, such as mania, depression, or psychosis, before it occurs. An app may not replace a mental health professional, but it may be able to alert caregivers when a client needs additional attention. The goal is to create apps that support a range of users, including those with serious mental illnesses.

Technology and the Future of Mental Health Treatment

Data Collection

Data collection apps can gather data without any help from the user. Receiving information from a large number of individuals at the same time can increase researchers' understanding of mental health and help them develop better interventions.

RESEARCH VIA SMARTPHONE

Dr. Patricia Areán's pioneering BRIGHTEN study showed that research via smartphone apps is already a reality. The BRIGHTEN study was remarkable because it used technology to both deliver treatment interventions and also to actually conduct the research trial. In other words, the research team used technology to recruit, screen, enroll, treat, and assess participants. BRIGHTEN was especially exciting because the study showed that technology can be an efficient way to pilot test promising new treatments and that those treatments need to be engaging.

A NEW PARTNERSHIP: CLINICIANS AND ENGINEERS

Researchers have found that interventions are most effective when people like them, are engaged, and want to continue using them. Behavioral health apps will need to combine the engineers' skills to make an app easy to use and entertaining with the clinician's skills for providing effective treatment options.

Researchers and software engineers are developing and testing apps that do everything from managing medications to teaching coping skills to predict when someone may need more emotional help. Intervention apps may help someone give up smoking, manage symptoms, or overcome anxiety, depression, posttraumatic stress disorder (PTSD), or insomnia. While the apps are becoming more appealing and user-friendly, there still is not a lot of information on their effectiveness.

EVALUATING APPS

There are no review boards, checklists, or widely accepted rules for choosing a mental health app. Most apps do not have peer-reviewed

Health Technology Sourcebook, Third Edition

research to support their claims, and it is unlikely that every mental health app will go through a randomized, controlled research trial to test its effectiveness. One reason is that testing is a slow process, and technology evolves quickly. By the time an app has been put through rigorous scientific testing, the original technology may be outdated.

Currently, there are no national standards for evaluating the effectiveness of the hundreds of mental health apps that are available. Consumers should be cautious about trusting a program. However, there are a few suggestions for finding an app that may work for you:

- Ask a trusted health-care provider for a recommendation. Some larger providers may offer several apps and collect data on their use.
- Check to see if the app offers recommendations for what to do if symptoms get worse or if there is a psychiatric emergency.
- Decide if you want an app that is completely automated or an app that offers opportunities for contact with a trained person.
- Search for information on the app developer. Can you find helpful information about her or his credentials and experience?
- Beware of misleading logos. The National Institute of Mental Health (NIMH) has not developed and does not endorse any apps. However, some app developers have unlawfully used the NIMH logo to market their products.
- If there is no information about a particular app, check to see if it is based on a treatment that has been tested. For example, research has shown that Internet-based cognitive behavioral therapy (CBT) is as effective as conventional CBT for disorders such as depression, anxiety, social phobia, and panic disorders that respond well to CBT.
- Try it. If you are interested in an app, test it for a few days and decide if it is easy to use and holds your

Technology and the Future of Mental Health Treatment

attention and if you want to continue using it. An app is only effective if it keeps users engaged for weeks or months.

WHAT IS THE NATIONAL INSTITUTE OF MENTAL HEALTH'S ROLE IN MENTAL HEALTH INTERVENTION TECHNOLOGY?

Between fiscal years 2009 and 2015, the NIMH awarded 404 grants totaling 445 million for technology-enhanced mental health intervention grants. These grants were for studies of computer-based interventions designed to prevent or treat mental health disorders.

In recent years, these grants focused on the following:

- Feasibility, efficacy, and effectiveness of research
- Technology for disorders such as schizophrenia, HIV, depression, anxiety, autism, suicide, and trauma
- More interventions for cognitive issues, illness management, behavior, and health communication
- Fewer interventions for a personal computer and more interventions for mobile devices
- More engaging ways to deliver therapies or skill development (e.g., interactive formats or game-like approaches)
- Real time (users exchanging information with peers or professionals as needed)
- Active and passive mobile assessment/monitoring

A significant portion of NIMH funding of these types of technologies is through the Small Business Innovation Research (SBIR) and Small Business Technology Transfer (STTR) programs.

In addition, the NIMH created the National Advisory Mental Health Council Workgroup on Opportunities and Challenges of Developing Information Technologies on Behavioral and Social Science Research to track and guide the cutting edge of this rapidly changing area. In 2017, the workgroup released a report reviewing the opportunities for—and the challenges of—using new information technologies to study human behaviors relevant to the NIMH mission. The NIMH's interest in this area of research was further highlighted in a 2018 notice identifying research on digital health

Health Technology Sourcebook, Third Edition

technology to advance the assessment, detection, prevention, treatment, and delivery of services for mental health conditions as a high-priority area for the institute.

THE FUTURE: WHAT TYPES OF RESEARCH DOES THE NATIONAL INSTITUTE OF MENTAL HEALTH EXPECT IN THE FUTURE?

Recently, there has been increased interest in the following:
- Using mobile technology for a wider range of disorders, from mild depression or anxiety to schizophrenia, autism, and suicide.
- Developing and refining new interventions instead of adapting existing interventions to work with new technologies.
- Developing technologies that work on any device.
- Incorporating face-to-face contact or remote counseling (phone or online) to provide a balance between technology and the "human touch."

Chapter 24 | **Artificial Pancreas Device System**

WHAT IS THE PANCREAS?

The pancreas is an organ in the body that secretes several hormones, including insulin and glucagon, as well as digestive enzymes that help break down food. Insulin helps cells in the body take up glucose (sugar) from the blood to use for energy, which lowers blood glucose levels. Glucagon causes the liver to release stored glucose, which raises blood glucose levels.

Type 1 diabetes occurs when the pancreas produces little or none of the insulin needed to regulate blood glucose. Type 2 diabetes occurs when the pancreas does not produce enough insulin or the body becomes resistant to the insulin that is present. Patients with type 1 diabetes and some patients with type 2 diabetes inject insulin, and occasionally glucagon, to regulate their blood glucose, which is critical to lower their risk of long-term complications, such as blindness, kidney failure, and cardiovascular disease (CVD).

When managing diabetes, many patients must vigilantly test blood glucose with a glucose meter, calculate insulin doses, and administer necessary insulin doses with a needle or insulin infusion pump to lower blood glucose. Glucagon may be injected in an emergency to treat severe low blood glucose. Some patients benefit

This chapter contains text excerpted from the following sources: Text beginning with the heading "What Is the Pancreas?" is excerpted from "The Artificial Pancreas Device System," U.S. Food and Drug Administration (FDA), August 30, 2018. Reviewed November 2022; Text under the heading "The FDA's Efforts to Advance Artificial Pancreas Device Systems" is excerpted from "The Artificial Pancreas Device System," U.S. Food and Drug Administration (FDA), August 30, 2018. Reviewed November 2022.

Health Technology Sourcebook, Third Edition

from additional monitoring with a continuous glucose monitoring system.

WHAT IS AN ARTIFICIAL PANCREAS DEVICE SYSTEM?

The artificial pancreas device system (APDS) is a system of devices that closely mimics the glucose-regulating function of a healthy pancreas.

Most APDS consists of three types of devices already familiar to many people with diabetes: a continuous glucose monitoring (CGM) system and an insulin infusion pump. A blood glucose device (such as a glucose meter) is used to calibrate the CGM.

A computer-controlled algorithm connects the CGM and insulin infusion pump to allow continuous communication between the two devices. Sometimes, an artificial pancreas device system is referred to as a "closed-loop" system, an "automated insulin delivery" system, or an "autonomous system for glycemic control."

An APDS will not only monitor glucose levels in the body but also automatically adjust the delivery of insulin to reduce high blood glucose levels (hyperglycemia) and minimize the incidence of low blood glucose (hypoglycemia) with little or no input from the patient.

The U.S. Food and Drug Administration (FDA) is collaborating with diabetes patient groups, diabetes care providers, medical device manufacturers, researchers, and academic investigators to foster innovation by clarifying agency expectations for clinical studies and product approvals. These efforts have accelerated the development of the first hybrid closed-loop system, Medtronic's MiniMed 670G System.

The FDA's guidance, the Content of Investigational Device Exemption (IDE) and Premarket Approval (PMA) Applications for APDS, addresses requirements for clinical studies and premarket approval applications for and an artificial pancreas device system and provides a flexible regulatory approach to support the rapid, safe, and effective development of artificial pancreas device systems.

336

Artificial Pancreas Device System

THE ARTIFICIAL PANCREAS SYSTEM (AN AUTONOMOUS SYSTEM FOR GLYCEMIC CONTROL)

The illustration below describes the parts of a type of artificial pancreas device system and shows how they work together.

- **Continuous glucose monitor (CGM).** A CGM provides a steady stream of information that reflects the patient's blood glucose levels. A sensor placed under the patient's skin (subcutaneously) measures the glucose in the fluid around the cells (interstitial fluid), which is associated with blood glucose levels. A small transmitter sends information to a receiver. A CGM continuously displays both an estimate of blood glucose levels and their direction and rate of change of these estimates.
- **Blood glucose device (BGD).** Currently, to get the most accurate estimates of blood glucose possible from a CGM, the patient needs to periodically calibrate the CGM using a blood glucose measurement from a BGD; therefore, the BGD still plays a critical role in the proper management of patients with an APDS. However, over time, we anticipate that improved CGM performance may do away with the need for periodic blood glucose checks with a BGD.
- **Control algorithm.** A control algorithm is a software embedded in an external processor (controller) that receives information from the CGM and performs a series of mathematical calculations. Based on these calculations, the controller sends dosing instructions to the infusion pump. The control algorithm can be run on any number of devices, including an insulin pump, computer, or cellular phone. The FDA does not require the control algorithm to reside on the insulin pump.
- **Insulin pump.** Based on the instructions sent by the controller, an infusion pump adjusts the insulin delivery to the tissue under the skin.

Health Technology Sourcebook, Third Edition

- **The patient**. The patient is an important part of APDS. The concentration of glucose circulating in the patient's blood is constantly changing. It is affected by the patient's diet, activity level, and how her or his body metabolizes insulin and other substances.

TYPES OF ARTIFICIAL PANCREAS DEVICE SYSTEMS

Researchers and manufacturers are developing three main categories of Artificial Pancreas Delivery Systems. They differ in how the insulin pump acts on readings from the continuous glucose monitoring system.

- **Threshold suspend device system**. The goal of a threshold suspend device system is to help reverse a dangerous drop in blood glucose level (hypoglycemia) or reduce its severity by temporarily suspending insulin delivery when the glucose level falls to or approaches a low glucose threshold. These are sometimes referred to as "low glucose suspend systems." This kind of system serves as a potential backup when a patient is unable to respond to a low blood sugar (hypoglycemic) event. Patients using this system will still need to be active partners in managing their blood glucose levels by periodically checking their blood glucose levels and by giving themselves insulin or eating.

- **Insulin-only system**. An insulin-only system achieves a target glucose level by automatically increasing or decreasing the amount of insulin infused based on the CGM values. These systems could be hybrid systems that only automatically adjust basal insulin with the user manually delivering bolus insulin to cover meals, or could be fully closed loop systems, where the system can automatically adjust basal insulin and provide insulin for meals.

- **Bi-hormonal control system**. A bi-hormonal control system achieves a target glucose level by using two algorithms to instruct an infusion pump to deliver two different hormones—one hormone (insulin) to

Artificial Pancreas Device System

lower glucose levels and another (such as glucagon) to increase blood glucose levels. The bi-hormonal system mimics the glucose-regulating function of a healthy pancreas more closely than an insulin-only system.

THE FDA'S EFFORTS TO ADVANCE ARTIFICIAL PANCREAS DEVICE SYSTEMS

The FDA supports and fosters medical device innovation as it upholds its mission of ensuring that medical devices are safe and effective. The FDA is helping advance the development of an artificial pancreas device system, an innovative device that automatically monitors blood glucose and provides appropriate insulin doses in people with diabetes who use insulin.

The FDA has been working together with diabetes patient groups, diabetes care providers, medical device manufacturers, and researchers to advance the development of an artificial pancreas. The FDA's efforts include prioritizing the review of research protocol studies, providing clear guidelines to industry, setting performance and safety standards, fostering discussions between government and private researchers, sponsoring public forums, and finding ways to shorten study and review time.

There have been tremendous strides made in the research and development of an APDS. On September 28, 2016, the FDA approved the first hybrid closed-loop system, Medtronic's MiniMed 670G System, intended to automatically monitor blood sugar and adjust basal insulin doses in people with type 1 diabetes. There are also many research projects underway looking at the feasibility of these device systems in hospital settings.

Chapter 25 | Technology in Cancer Treatment

Chapter Contents

Section 25.1—Enabling New Cancer Technologies.................343
Section 25.2—Proton Beams for Cancer Therapy.....................347
Section 25.3—Nanotechnology for Cancer 350
Section 25.4—Biomarker Testing for Cancer Treatment..........370

Section 25.1 | Enabling New Cancer Technologies

This section includes text excerpted from "Develop New Enabling Cancer Technologies," National Cancer Institute (NCI), August 10, 2021.

INTEGRATION AND VALIDATION OF EMERGING TECHNOLOGIES TO ACCELERATE CANCER RESEARCH

The development and validation of new enabling technologies and tools that could lead to new capabilities in basic and clinical cancer research are advancing. These projects are focused on enhancing experimental and analytical tools to understand the complexities of cancer, developing new technologies to advance cancer diagnosis, designing predictive models of cancer progression and responses to treatment, and generating new approaches to improve cancer-related data quality. Technology is validated to ensure that new approaches could be readily adopted by the cancer research community.

Highlights from this initiative include the development of the following:

- The PennPET Explorer, a whole-body high-resolution positron emission tomography (PET) imaging system
- A new approach to advance single-cell mass spectrometry for broad protein coverage
- A three-dimensional (3D) microdevice to perform projection electrophoresis, creating a powerful high-throughput single-cell protein analysis tool

PATIENT-DERIVED XENOGRAFTS DEVELOPMENT NETWORK

Patient-derived xenografts (PDXs) are models of cancer where tissue from a cancer patient's tumor is implanted in a mouse. These models are emerging as an important approach for translational cancer research. PDXs simulate human tumor biology and can be used to identify the optimal combination therapy for groups of precisely defined cancer subtypes.

However, PDX models are often developed as isolated collections, leading to a lack of standardization as well as issues validating and replicating the results from experiments using these models. Also, isolated collections of PDX models are often too small to reflect the diversity of patient tumors found in large-scale clinical trials.

PDXNet is addressing these research challenges. PDX Development and Trial Centers (PDTCs) have engaged in collaborative research projects to show that PDX tumor models retain the genetic characteristics of the primary human tumor and that PDX drug responses and sequencing results are reproducible across diverse experimental protocols. This establishes the potential for multisite preclinical studies using PDX tumor models that could inform clinical trials.

Minority PDTCs ((M)-PDTCs) are developing PDXs that model tumors in racially and ethnically diverse populations that can be used to test cancer treatments. These (M)-PDTCs aim to advance the NCI's understanding of disparities observed in cancer treatment outcomes among racially and ethnically diverse populations.

Along with investigators developing PDX models, the Patient-Derived Models Repository (PDMR) at the Frederick National Laboratory for Cancer Research plays an important role in PDXNet. Over 270 PDX models, representing 33 different cancer types, are available by request through the repository.

DATA VISUALIZATION + CANCER MOONSHOT

In support of the broader goals of the Cancer Moonshot to accelerate the pace of discovery and share resources, a new effort was initiated to improve tools and approaches for visualizing the immense and complex data associated with Cancer Moonshot initiatives. Introducing truly novel tools should involve leveraging creative approaches developed for other fields. The National Cancer Institute (NCI) is bringing together diverse experts from a variety of fields to form interdisciplinary teams around innovative ideas and develop these ideas into novel pilot projects with strong potential.

A series of virtual workshops (apply.hub.ki/cancerplusviz) were organized to draw disparate groups together, coupled with facilitated brainstorming activities. These activities highlighted several

Technology in Cancer Treatment

areas where improved user experience, user-focused design, game design, and data visualization can aid cancer researchers, clinicians, and others in navigating complex cancer data. Key areas of need include engaging patients, providing a better patient experience, visualizing multidimensional data, visualizing data in context, and enabling collaborations.

ACTIVITIES TO PROMOTE TECHNOLOGY RESEARCH COLLABORATIONS FOR CANCER RESEARCH

There are two unique NCI programs related to activities to promote technology research collaborations (APTRC) that focus on supporting technology development for advancing cancer research. The Innovative Molecular Analysis Technologies (IMAT) program supports innovative data-generating platforms and methods, while the Informatics Technologies for Cancer Research (ITCR) program supports data processing and visualization technologies.

The NCI is accelerating the development of new enabling cancer technologies by leveraging expertise in IMAT and ITCR through multidisciplinary collaborations between investigators in these programs. These collaborative projects bring together complementary technology platforms and approaches to enhance their capabilities for studies of cancer.

For example, one collaborative team developed an integrated pipeline to identify clinically relevant genetic variants to inform precision treatment. The method, OpenCAP, is a novel approach that uses an open-source database to guide probe development for targeted sequencing to identify mutations relevant to cancer.

NOVEL TECHNOLOGIES TO FACILITATE RESEARCH USING NEXT-GENERATION PATIENT-DERIVED CANCER MODELS

Research projects in this program are developing technology tools to accelerate and enhance studies across the spectrum of cancer research using advanced next-generation human cancer models, including 3D organoids and conditionally reprogrammed cells. These projects are specifically advancing cancer models developed as part of the Human Cancer Models Initiative (HCMI).

Health Technology Sourcebook, Third Edition

The technology tools being examined by investigators of the program include new laboratory methods and reagents for screening studies and computational approaches for data analysis from experiments using next-generation cancer models.

SMALL BUSINESS INNOVATION RESEARCH AND SMALL BUSINESS TECHNOLOGY TRANSFER RESEARCH GRANTS AND CONTRACTS FOR ENABLING TECHNOLOGIES

The NCI supports grants and contracts with small businesses that are developing new enabling technologies for cancer research. The range of projects supported through these investments spans the breadth of Cancer Moonshot. For example, active projects include the development of experimental models to study cancer disparities, new cancer detection technologies, immunotherapy manufacturing, and subcellular microscopy.

EVALUATION OF PROSTATE-SPECIFIC MEMBRANE ANTIGEN-BASED PET IMAGING OF HIGH-RISK PROSTATE CANCER

At this time, there are limited ways to stratify high-risk prostate cancer patients. To address this issue, researchers with the NCI's Center for Cancer Research are investigating the clinical use of PET imaging on patients with high-risk prostate cancer. PET offers the opportunity to image prostate-specific membrane antigen (PSMA), a protein that is expressed in prostate cancer tissue and associated with aggressive cancer. By comparing the PSMA PET scans with complication-free survival outcomes, the researchers hope to understand if PSMA imaging could be used to identify subsets of patients with high-risk prostate cancer and guide treatment decisions.

Technology in Cancer Treatment

Section 25.2 | **Proton Beams for Cancer Therapy**

This section includes text excerpted from "Is Proton Therapy Safer than Traditional Radiation?" National Cancer Institute (NCI), February 11, 2020.

A type of radiation treatment called "proton beam radiation therapy" may be safer and just as effective as traditional radiation therapy for adults with advanced cancer. This finding comes from a study that used existing patient data to compare the two types of radiation.

Traditional radiation delivers x-rays, or beams of photons, to the tumor and beyond it. This can damage nearby healthy tissues and can cause significant side effects.

By contrast, proton therapy delivers a beam of proton particles that stops at the tumor, so it is less likely to damage nearby healthy tissues. Some experts believe that proton therapy is safer than traditional radiation, but there is limited research comparing the two treatments.

Plus, proton therapy is more expensive than traditional radiation, and not all insurance companies cover the cost of the treatment, given the limited evidence of its benefits. Nevertheless, 31 hospitals across the country have spent millions of dollars building proton therapy centers, and many advertise the potential, but unproven, advantages of the treatment.

In the new study, patients treated with proton therapy were much less likely to experience severe side effects than patients treated with traditional radiation therapy. There was no difference in how long the patients lived, however. The results were published on December 26 in *JAMA Oncology*.

"These results support the whole rationale for proton therapy," said the study's lead investigator, Dr. Brian Baumann, M.D., of the Washington University School of Medicine in St. Louis and the University of Pennsylvania.

But key aspects of the study limit how broadly the findings can be interpreted, said Dr. Jeffrey Buchsbaum, M.D., Ph.D., of NCI's Radiation Research Program, who was not involved in the study.

Health Technology Sourcebook, Third Edition

Because of those limitations, "the evidence needed to truly justify the expenses of proton therapy ... will need to come from phase 3 randomized clinical trials," wrote Dr. Henry Park, M.D., and Dr. James Yu, M.D., of Yale School of Medicine, in an accompanying editorial.

Several NCI-funded randomized clinical trials (RCTs) comparing proton and traditional radiation therapy are currently ongoing.

SAFETY AND EFFICACY OF PROTON THERAPY

Many people with locally advanced cancers are treated with a combination of chemotherapy and either traditional or proton radiation. For patients getting chemotherapy and radiation at the same time, finding ways to limit side effects without making the treatment less effective is a high priority, Dr. Baumann said.

He and his colleagues analyzed data from nearly 1,500 adults with 11 different types of cancer. All participants had received simultaneous chemotherapy plus radiation at the University of Pennsylvania Health System between 2011 and 2016 and had been followed to track side effects and cancer outcomes, including survival. Almost 400 had received proton therapy, and the rest received traditional radiation.

Those who received proton therapy experienced far fewer serious side effects than those who received traditional radiation, the researchers found. Within 90 days of starting treatment, 45 patients (12%) in the proton therapy group and 301 patients (28%) in the traditional radiation group experienced a severe side effect—that is, an effect severe enough to warrant hospitalization.

In addition, proton therapy did not affect people's abilities to perform routine activities, such as housework, as much as traditional radiation. Over the course of treatment, performance status scores were half as likely to decline for patients treated with proton therapy as for those who received traditional radiation.

And proton therapy appeared to work as well as traditional radiation therapy to treat cancer and preserve life. After three years, 46 percent of patients in the proton therapy group and 49 percent of those in the traditional radiation therapy group were cancer-free. Fifty-six percent of people who received proton therapy and 58

Technology in Cancer Treatment

percent of those who received traditional radiation were still alive after three years.

IDEAS FOR FUTURE STUDIES OF PROTON THERAPY

Despite the study's limitations, these "intriguing findings raise questions that should inform future prospective phase 3 trials," Dr. Buchsbaum said, although there are barriers to large studies of proton therapy.

For instance, it "is particularly encouraging" that proton therapy appeared to be safer in a group of older and sicker patients who typically experience more side effects, Dr. Baumann noted.

Dr. Buchsbaum agreed that proton therapy may be especially helpful for older and sicker patients, but he noted that ongoing phase 3 trials were not designed to analyze this group of patients.

And, because proton therapy may cause fewer side effects, future trials could also explore whether combining proton therapy with chemotherapy might be more tolerable for patients, the authors wrote.

For example, both chemotherapy and traditional radiation for lung cancer can irritate the esophagus, making it painful and difficult for patients to eat. But proton therapy might limit damage to the esophagus, making it easier for a patient to tolerate the combination, Dr. Baumann explained.

Future studies could also explore whether combining proton therapy with higher doses of chemotherapy might increase cures without causing more side effects, he added.

The study findings also raise "the tantalizing possibility that the higher up-front cost of proton therapy may be offset by cost savings from reduced hospitalizations and enhanced productivity from patients and caregivers," the study researchers wrote.

Dr. Buchsbaum agreed, saying that it would be worthwhile to explore this possibility. "Just asking the question: 'Is [proton therapy] more effective?' might not be giving it a fair opportunity to demonstrate its benefit to society," he said.

Dr. Baumann and his colleagues are currently studying the cost-effectiveness of proton therapy, considering aspects such as the costs of treating side effects and the value of preserved quality of life (QOL).

Health Technology Sourcebook, Third Edition

Section 25.3 | **Nanotechnology for Cancer**

This section includes text excerpted from "Cancer and Nanotechnology," National Cancer Institute (NCI), August 9, 2017. Reviewed November 2022.

Currently, scientists are limited in their ability to turn promising molecular discoveries into cancer patient benefits. Nanotechnology—the science and engineering of controlling matter at the molecular scale to create devices with novel chemical, physical, and/or biological properties—can provide technical control and tools to enable the development of new diagnostics, therapeutics, and preventions that keep pace with today's explosion in knowledge.

Although scientists and engineers have only recently (ca. 1980s) developed the ability to industrialize technologies at this scale, there has been good progress in translating nano-based cancer therapies and diagnostics into the clinic, and many more are in development.

Nanotechnology is the application of materials, functionalized structures, devices, or systems at the atomic, molecular, or macro-molecular scales. At these length scales, approximately the 1–100 nanometer range as defined by the U.S. National Nanotechnology Initiative (NNI), unique and specific physical properties of matter exist, which can be readily manipulated for a desired application or effect. Furthermore, the nanoscale structure can be used as individual entities or integrated into larger material components, systems, and architectures.

BENEFITS OF NANOTECHNOLOGY FOR CANCER

Nanoscale devices are 100–10,000 times smaller than human cells. They are similar in size to large biological molecules ("biomolecules"), such as enzymes and receptors. As an example, hemoglobin, the molecule that carries oxygen in red blood cells (RBCs), is approximately five nanometers in diameter. Nanoscale devices smaller than 50 nanometers can easily enter most cells, while those smaller than 20 nanometers can move out of blood vessels as they circulate through the body. Because of their small size, nanoscale devices can readily interact with biomolecules on both the surface

350

Technology in Cancer Treatment

and inside cells. By gaining access to so many areas of the body, they have the potential to detect disease and deliver treatment in ways unimagined before now.

Biological processes, including ones necessary for life and those that lead to cancer, occur at the nanoscale.

Nanotechnology provides researchers with the opportunity to study and manipulate macromolecules in real time and during the earliest stages of cancer progression. Nanotechnology can provide rapid and sensitive detection of cancer-related molecules, enabling scientists to detect molecular changes even when they occur only in a small percentage of cells. Nanotechnology also has the potential to generate entirely novel and highly effective therapeutic agents.

Ultimately and uniquely, the use of nanoscale materials for cancer comes down to its ability to be readily functionalized and easily tuned; its ability to deliver and/or act as the therapeutic, diagnostic, or both; and its ability to passively accumulate at the tumor site, to be actively targeted to cancer cells, and to be delivered across traditional biological barriers in the body such as dense stromal tissue of the pancreas or the blood-brain barrier (BBB) that highly regulates delivery of biomolecules to/from, our central nervous system (CNS).

Passive Tumor Accumulation

An effective cancer drug delivery should achieve high accumulation in tumors and spare the surrounding healthy tissues. The passive localization of many drugs and drug carriers due to their extravasation through leaky vasculature (named the enhanced permeability and retention (EPR) effect) works very well for tumors. As tumor mass grows rapidly, a network of blood vessels needs to expand quickly to accommodate tumor cells' need for oxygen and nutrient. This abnormal and poorly regulated vessel generation (i.e., angiogenesis) results in vessel walls with large pores (40 nm to 1 um); these leaky vessels allow relatively large nanoparticles to extravasate into tumor masses. As fast-growing tumor mass lacks a functioning lymphatic system, clearance of these nanoparticles is limited and further enhances the accumulation. Through the EPR effect, nanoparticles larger than 8 nm (between 8 and 100 nm) can passively target tumors by freely passing through large pores and achieving higher intratumoral accumulation. The majority of current nanomedicines for solid tumor treatment rely on the EPR effect to ensure high drug accumulation, thereby improving treatment efficacy. Without targeting cell types expressing targeting ligands of interest, this drug delivery system is called "passive targeting."

Before reaching the proximity of the tumor site for the EPR effect to take place, passive targeting requires the drug delivery system to be long-circulating to allow a sufficient level of drug to the target area. To design nano-drugs that can stay in blood longer, one can "mask" these nano-drugs by modifying the surface with water-soluble polymers, such as polyethylene glycol (PEG); PEG is often used to make water-insoluble nanoparticles to be water-soluble in many preclinical research laboratories. PEG-coated liposomal doxorubicin (Doxil) is used clinically for breast cancer, leveraging passive tumor accumulation. As in vivo surveillance system for macromolecules (i.e., scavenger receptors of the reticuloendothelial system, RES) reportedly showed faster uptake of negatively charged nanoparticles, nano-drugs with a neutral or positive charge are expected to have a longer plasma half-life.

Utilizing the EPR effect for passive tumor-targeting drug delivery is not without problems. Although the EPR effect is a unique phenomenon in solid tumors, the central region of metastatic or larger tumor mass does not exhibit the EPR effect, a result of an extreme hypoxic condition. For this reason, there are methods used in the clinics to artificially enhance the EPR effect: slow infusion of angiotensin II to increase systolic blood pressure, topical application of nitric-oxide-releasing agents to expand blood, and photodynamic therapy or hyperthermia-mediated vascular permeabilization in solid tumors.

Passive accumulation through the EPR effect is the most acceptable drug delivery system for solid tumor treatment. However, the size or molecular weight of the nanoparticles is not the sole determinant of the EPR effect; other factors such as surface charge, biocompatibility, and in vivo surveillance system for macromolecules

Technology in Cancer Treatment

should not be ignored in designing the nanomedicine for efficient passive tumor accumulation.

Active Tumor Targeting

An EPR effect, which serves as a nanoparticle "passive tumor targeting" scheme, is responsible for the accumulation of particles in the tumor region. However, EPR does not promote the uptake of nanoparticles into cells, yet nanoparticle/drug cell internalization is required for some of the treatment modalities relying on drug activation within the cell nucleus or cytosol. Similarly, delivery of nucleic acids (DNA, siRNA, and miRNA) in genetic therapies requires the escape of these molecules from endosomes so they can reach desired subcellular compartments. In addition, EPR is heterogenous, and its strength varies among different tumors and/or patients. For these reasons, active targeting is considered an essential feature of next-generation nanoparticle therapeutics. It will enable certain modalities of therapies not achievable with EPR and improve the effectiveness of treatments that can be accomplished using EPR but with less than satisfactory effect. Active targeting of nanoparticles to tumor cells, microenvironment, or vasculature, as well as directed delivery to intracellular compartments, can be attained through nanoparticle surface modification with small molecules, antibodies, affibodies, peptides, or aptamers.

Passive targeting (EPR effect) is the process of nanoparticles extravasating from the circulation through the leaky vasculature to the tumor region. The drug molecules carried by the nanoparticle are released in the extracellular matrix and diffuse throughout the tumor tissue. The particles carry surface ligands to facilitate the active targeting of particles to receptors present in the target cell or tissue. Active targeting is expected to enhance nanoparticle/drug accumulation in tumors and also promote their prospective cell uptake through receptor-mediated endocytosis. The particles, which are engineered for vascular targeting, incorporate ligands that bind to endothelial cell-surface receptors. The vascular targeting is expected to provide a synergistic strategy utilizing both targeting of vascular tissue and cells within the diseased tissue.

Health Technology Sourcebook, Third Edition

Most of the nanotechnology-based strategies that are approved for clinical use or are in advanced clinical trials rely on the EPR effect. It is expected that next-generation nanotherapies will use targeting to enable and enhance intracellular uptake, intracellular trafficking, and penetration of physiological barriers that block drug access to some tumors.

Transport across Tissue Barriers

Nanoparticle or nano-drug delivery is hampered by tissue barriers before the drug can reach the tumor site. Tissue barriers for the efficient transporting of nano-drugs to tumor sites include tumor stroma (e.g., biological barriers) and tumor endothelium barriers (e.g., functional barriers). Biological barriers are physical constructs or cell formations that restrict the movement of nanoparticles. Functional barriers can affect the transport of intact nanoparticles or nanomedicine into the tumor mass: elevated interstitial fluid pressure and an acidic environment, for example. It is important to design nanoparticles and strategies to overcome these barriers to improve cancer treatment efficacy.

A tumor microenvironment (TME) is a dynamic system composed of abnormal vasculature, fibroblasts, and immune cells, all embedded in an extracellular matrix (ECM). TME poses both biological and functional barriers to nano-drug delivery in cancer treatment. Increased cell density and abnormal vasculature elevate the interstitial fluid pressure within a tumor mass. Such a pressure gradient is unfavorable for the free diffusion of the nanoparticles and is often a limiting factor for the EPR effect. When tumor mass reaches 106 cells in number, metabolic strains ensue. Often, cells in the core of this proliferating cluster are distanced by 100–200 um from the source of nutrients: 200 um is a limiting distance for oxygen diffusion. As a result, cancer cells in the core live at pO2 levels below 2.5–10 mmHg and become hypoxic; an anoxic metabolic pathway can kick in and generate lactic acid. Nanoparticles become unstable in an acidic environment, and delivery of the drugs to target tumor cells will be unpredictable. ECM of the tumor provides nutrients for cancer cells and stromal cells. It is a collection of fibrous proteins and polysaccharides and expands rapidly

Technology in Cancer Treatment

in aggressive cancer as the result of stromal cell proliferation. The most notorious biological barrier to cancer treatment is pancreatic stroma in pancreatic ductal adenocarcinoma (PADC). Pancreatic cancer stroma has the characteristics of an abnormal and poorly functioning vasculature, altered extracellular matrix, infiltrating macrophages, and proliferation of fibroblasts. Not only have tumor-stroma interactions been shown to promote pancreatic cancer cell invasion and metastasis, but TME and tumor stroma also create an unfavorable environment for drug delivery and other forms of cancer treatments.

Because the EPR effect is a clinically relevant phenomenon for nanocarriers' tumor penetration, strategies have been developed to address the tumor endothelium barrier. Strategies to reduce interstitial fluid pressure to improve tumor penetration include ECM-targeting pharmacological interventions to normalize vasculature within TME; hypertonic solutions to shrink ECM cells; and hyperthermia, radio frequency (RF), or high-intensity focused ultrasound (HIFU) to enhance nano-drug transport and accumulation. These strategies can also alleviate hypoxic conditions in larger tumor masses. Although TME and tumor mass pose a harsh and acidic environment for nanocarrier stability, pH-responsive nanocarrier designs leveraging this unique feature are gaining interest in recent years. Many of the strategies described above are used to address the tumor-stroma barrier.

Another formidable tissue barrier for drugs and nanoparticle delivery is the BBB. BBB is a physical barrier in the central nervous system to prevent harmful substances from entering the brain. It consists of endothelial cells, which are sealed in continuous tight junctions around the capillaries. Outside the layer of the epithelial cell is covered by astrocytes that further contribute to the selectivity of substance passage. As BBB keeps harmful substances from the brain, it also restricts the delivery of therapeutics for brain diseases, such as brain tumors and other neurological diseases. There have been tremendous efforts in overcoming the BBB for drug delivery in general. The multivalent feature of nanoparticles makes nanocarriers appealing in designing BBB-crossing delivering strategies. One promising nanoparticle design has transferrin

Health Technology Sourcebook, Third Edition

receptor-targeting moiety to facilitate the transportation of these nanoparticles across the BBB.

EARLIER DETECTION AND DIAGNOSIS

In the fight against cancer, half of the battle is won based on its early detection. Nanotechnology provides new molecular contrast agents and materials to enable earlier and more accurate initial diagnosis as well as in continual monitoring of cancer patient treatment.

Although not yet deployed clinically for cancer detection or diagnosis, nanoparticles are already on the market in numerous medical screens and tests, with the most widespread use of gold nanoparticles in home pregnancy tests. Nanoparticles are also at the heart of the Verigene® system from nanosphere and the T2MR system from T2 Biosystems, currently used in hospitals for a variety of indications.

For cancer, nanodevices are being investigated for the capture of blood-borne biomarkers, including cancer-associated proteins circulating tumor cells, circulating tumor DNA, and tumor-shed exosomes. Nano-enabled sensors are capable of high sensitivity, specificity, and multiplexed measurements. Next-generation devices couple capture with genetic analysis to further elucidate a patient's cancer and potential treatments and disease course.

Already clinically established as contrast agents for anatomical structure, nanoparticles are being developed to act as molecular imaging agents, reporting on the presence of cancer-relevant genetic mutations or the functional characteristics of tumor cells. This information can be used to choose a treatment course or alter a therapeutic plan. Bioactivatable nanoparticles that change properties in response to factors or processes within the body act as dynamic reporters of in vivo states and can provide both spatial and temporal information on disease progression and therapeutic response.

Imaging in Vivo

Current imaging methods can only detect cancers once they have made a visible change to a tissue, by which time, thousands of

Technology in Cancer Treatment

cells will have proliferated and perhaps metastasized. And, even when visible, the nature of the tumor—malignant or benign—and the characteristics that might make it responsive to a particular treatment must be assessed through tissue biopsies. Furthermore, while some primary malignancies can be determined to be metastatic, tumor preseeding of metastatic sites and micrometastases are extremely difficult to detect with modern imaging modalities, even if the tissue in which they commonly occur is known a priori. Finally, surgical resection of tumor tissue remains the standard of care for many tumor types, and surgeons must weigh the consequences of removing often vital healthy tissue versus the cancerous mass, which has grown nonuniformly within. Ultimately, the removal of cancer cells at the single-cell level is not possible with current surgical techniques.

Nanotechnology-based imaging contrast agents being developed and translated today offer the ability to specifically target and greatly enhance the detection of tumors in vivo by way of conventional scanning devices, such as magnetic resonance imaging (MRI), positron emission tomography (PET), and computed tomography (CT). Moreover, current nanoscale imaging platforms are enabling novel imaging modalities not traditionally utilized for clinical cancer treatment and diagnosis, for example, photoacoustic tomography (PAT), Raman spectroscopic imaging, and multimodal imaging (i.e., contrast agents specific to several imaging modalities simultaneously). Nanotechnology enables all of these platforms by way of its ability to carry multiple components simultaneously (e.g., cancer cell-specific targeting agents or traditional imaging contrast agents) and nanoscale materials that are themselves the contrast agents that enable greatly enhanced signals.

The research funded by the National Cancer Institute (NCI) has produced many notable examples over the last several years. For example, researchers at Stanford University and Memorial Sloan Kettering Cancer Center developed multimodal nanoparticles capable of delineating the margins of brain tumors both preoperatively and intraoperatively. These MRI-PAT-Raman nanoparticles are able to be used both to track tumor growth and surgical staging by way of MRI but also in the same particle be used during surgical resection of brain tumor to give the surgeon's "eyes" down to the single cancer cell level, increasing the potential tumor-specific tissue removal.

For metastatic melanoma, researchers at MSKCC and Cornell University have developed silica-hybrid nanoparticles ("C-dots") that deliver both PET and optical imaging contrast in the same platform. These nanoparticles are actively targeted to cancer with cRGDY peptides that target this specific tumor type and have already made it successfully through initial clinical trials.

Another clinical cancer imaging problem being addressed by nanoscale solutions is prostate cancer. Researchers at Stanford University have recently been developing nanotechnologies that give both anatomical size and location of prostate cancer cells (nanobubbles for ultrasound imaging) and functional information to avoid overdiagnosis/treatment as well as to monitor progression (self-assembling nanoparticles for photoacoustic imaging). The nanoplatforms developed by this group are coupled directly to their recently approved handheld transrectal ultrasound and photoacoustic (TRUSPA) device, ultimately offering a more effective, integrated, and less invasive technique to image and biopsy prostate cancers for diagnosis and prognostication prior to performing common interventions (surgical resection, radiotherapy, etc.).

Similarly, gold nanoparticles are being used to enhance light scattering for endoscopic techniques that can be used during colonoscopies. One really powerful potential that has always been envisioned for nanotechnology in cancer has been the potential to simultaneously image and deliver therapy in vivo, and several groups have been pushing forward these "theranostic" nanoscale platforms. One group at Emory University has been developing one of these for ovarian and pancreatic cancers, which are traditionally harder to deliver therapeutics to. Their platform for pancreatic cancer can break through the fibrotic stromal tissue by which these tumors are protected in the pancreas. After traversing through this barrier, they are composed of magnetic iron cores, which allow MRI contrast for diagnosis and deliver small-molecule drugs directly to cancer cells to treat.

Technology in Cancer Treatment

Finally, nanotechnology enables the visualization of molecular markers that identify specific stages and cancer cell death induced by therapy, allowing doctors to see cells and molecules undetectable through conventional imaging. A group at Stanford has developed the Target-Enabled in Situ Ligand Assembly (TESLA) nanoparticle system. This is based on nanoparticles that form directly in the body after intravenous (IV) injection of molecular precursors. The precursors contain specific sequences of atoms that can only form larger nanoparticles after being cleaved by enzymes produced by cancer cells during apoptosis (i.e., cell death) and carry various image contrast agents to monitor (PET, MRI, etc.) local tumor response to therapies. Being able to track cancer cell death in vivo and at the molecular level is extremely important for delivering effective dosing regimens and/or precisely administering novel therapies or combinations.

Sensing in Vitro

Nanotechnology-enabled in vitro diagnostic devices offer high sensitivity, selectivity, and capability to perform simultaneous measurements of multiple targets. Well-established fabrication techniques (e.g., lithography) can be used to manufacture integrated, portable devices or point-of-care systems. A diagnostic device or biosensor contains a biological recognition element, which through biochemical reaction can detect the presence, activity, or concentration of a specific biological molecule in the solution. This reaction could be associated, for example, with the binding of antigen and antibody, hybridization of two single-stranded DNA fragments, or binding of capture ligand to the cell surface epitope. A transducer part of the detection device is used to convert the biochemical event into a quantifiable signal, which can be measured. The transduction mechanisms can rely on light, magnetic, or electronic effects.

Several devices have been designed for the detection of various biological signatures from serum or tissue. A few examples of diagnostic devices relying on nanotechnology or nanoparticles are given in this chapter. The bio-barcode assay was designed as a sandwich immunoassay in the laboratory of Chad Mirkin at Northwestern

Health Technology Sourcebook, Third Edition

University. It utilizes magnetic nanoparticles (MMPs), which are functionalized with monoclonal antibodies specific to the target protein of interest and then mixed with the sample to promote the capture of target proteins. The MMP-protein hybrid structures are then combined with gold nanoparticle (Au-NP) probes that carry DNA barcodes. Target protein-specific DNA barcodes are released into the solution and detected using the scanometric assay with sensitivities in the femtomolar and picomolar range.

James Heath's laboratory at Caltech designed sandwich immunoassay devices that rely on DNA-encoded antibody libraries (DEAL). The DEAL technique uses DNA-directed immobilization of antibodies in microfluidic channels allowing the conversion of a prepatterned single-stranded DNA (ssDNA) barcode microarray into an antibody microarray. ssDNA oligomers attached to the sensor surface are robust and can withstand elevated temperatures of channel fabrication. Subsequent flow-through of the DNA-antibody conjugates in channels transforms the DNA microarray into an antibody microarray and allows to perform multiplex surface-bound sandwich immunoassays. These devices allow for on-chip blood separation and measurement of large protein panels directly from blood.

The diagnostic magnetic resonance (DMR) sensor platform was designed in the laboratory of Ralph Weissleder at Massachusetts General Hospital. The DMR mechanism exploits changes in the transverse relaxation signal of water molecules in a magnetic field as a sensing mechanism for magnetic nanoparticle-labeled analytes. Highly integrated systems, including microfluidic processing circuits and nuclear magnetic resonance (NMR) detection heads with high signal-to-noise ratio, were built and are capable of detecting the presence of cells, vesicles, and proteins in clinical samples.

Shan Wang's laboratory at Stanford University designed giant magnetoresistive (GMR) biosensors for protein detection. These nanosensors operate by changing their electrical resistance in response to changes in the local magnetic field. They were adapted to the detection of biological signatures in solution by implementing a traditional sandwich assay directly on GMR nanosensors. Antibodies are immobilized on the GMR sensor surface and are used as capture probes for the sample containing target proteins.

Technology in Cancer Treatment

A magnetic particle is used to label the biomolecule of interest in the sample, and a GMR sensor is used for signal transduction. These sensors were used to measure protein levels in complex sample mixtures and also were employed to assess the kinetics of protein interactions.

The devices described above are capable of analyzing large panels of biological signatures at the same time, providing for a high level of multiplexing. The data analysis can establish correlations among different biomarker levels and map correlations of network signaling and thus provide tools for patient stratification based on their response to different treatments and ultimately improve the therapeutic efficacy of the one selected. New advancements in microfluidic technologies opened opportunities to integrate sample preparation and sample processing with biosensors and to realize fully integrated devices that directly deliver full data for a medical diagnosis from a single sample.

Measuring Response to Therapy and the Liquid Biopsy

Measurement of an individual patient's response to therapeutics during the course of their disease is the basis for precise and prognostic medical care. Accurate and disease-relevant monitoring can allow for optimized treatment regimens (e.g., therapeutic course correction, drug combinations, and dose attenuation), preemptive clinical decision-making (e.g., therapeutic responders versus nonresponders, and more), and patient stratification for clinical trials. Beyond the more traditional gold standards of in vivo imaging, tissue biopsy, and in vitro diagnostics available for this purpose, the "liquid biopsy" offers the ability to measure response to therapy by way of simple and serial blood draws. Traditional biopsies involve the resection of small volumes of the tumor tissue directly and thus remain invasive procedures that cannot offer the sampling necessitated to track disease progression relative to the course of therapy or the dynamics of its evolving biology. Liquid biopsies rely on the fact that tumors shed material (e.g., cells, DNA, other cancer-specific biomolecules) into circulation over time and in response to therapy. However, the amount of materials shed by any given tumor and/or stage is typically at incredibly low concentrations

Health Technology Sourcebook, Third Edition

relative to the rest of the blood's constituents (e.g., erythrocytes, leukocytes, thrombocytes, plasma, etc.). This requires specific and sensitive tools to detect, capture, and purify the circulating tumor material relative to the rest. Nanotechnology is enabling these tools to become a reality.

Technological advances in the coupling of complex microfluidics and nanoscale materials have allowed the high-purity capture and downstream functional characterization of circulating tumor cells (CTCs), cell-free tumor DNA, microemboli, exosomes, proteins, neoantigens, and more. Recent examples include the capture and subsequent release of CTCs within microfluidic systems to maintain viable cells for downstream whole genome sequencing, ex vivo expansion, RNA sequencing, and more. Of these examples, one type of device uses magnetic nanoparticles to enrich whole blood prior to magnetic separation within the microfluidic, and the other device uses thermoresponsive nanopolymers that specifically capture CTCs as they flow through the microfluidic then release upon a change in temperature once blood processing is complete. In both cases, the detection sensitivities are very high (e.g., for enumeration >95%), and capture purity is much higher than other non-nanomaterial-based devices. Furthermore, the processing times are increasing every year as the technology evolves, currently averaging 10 mL blood per 30 minutes.

TREATMENT AND THERAPY

Cancer therapies are currently limited to surgery, radiation, and chemotherapy. All three methods risk damage to normal tissues or incomplete eradication of cancer. Nanotechnology offers the means to target chemotherapies directly and selectively to cancerous cells and neoplasms, guide in surgical resection of tumors, and enhance the therapeutic efficacy of radiation-based and other current treatment modalities. All of this can add up to a decreased risk to the patient and an increased probability of survival.

Research on nanotechnology cancer therapy extends beyond drug delivery into the creation of new therapeutics available only through the use of nanomaterial properties. Although small compared to cells, nanoparticles are large enough to encapsulate many

Technology in Cancer Treatment

small molecule compounds, which can be of multiple types. At the same time, the relatively large surface area of the nanoparticle can be functionalized with ligands, including small molecules, DNA or RNA strands, peptides, aptamers, or antibodies. These ligands can be used for therapeutic effects or to direct nanoparticle fate in vivo. These properties enable combination drug delivery, multimodality treatment, and combined therapeutic and diagnostic, known as "theranostic," action. The physical properties of nanoparticles, such as energy absorption and reradiation, can also be used to disrupt diseased tissue, as in laser ablation and hyperthermia applications.

Integrated development of innovative nanoparticle packages and active pharmaceutical ingredients will also enable the exploration of a wider repertoire of active ingredients, no longer confined to those with acceptable pharmacokinetic or biocompatibility behavior. In addition, immunogenic cargo and surface coatings are being investigated as adjuvants to nanoparticle-mediated and traditional radiotherapy and chemotherapy, as well as stand-alone therapies. Innovative strategies include the design of nanoparticles as artificial antigen-presenting cells and in vivo depots of immunostimulatory factors that exploit nanostructured architecture for sustained anti-tumor activity.

Delivering Chemotherapy

The traditional use of nanotechnology in cancer therapeutics has been to improve the pharmacokinetics and reduce the systemic toxicities of chemotherapies through the selective targeting and delivery of these anticancer drugs to tumor tissues. The advantage of nanosized carriers is that they can increase the delivered drug's overall therapeutic index through nanoformulations in which chemotherapeutics are either encapsulated or conjugated to the surfaces of nanoparticles. This capability is largely due to their tunable size and surface properties. Size is a major factor in the delivery of nanotechnology-based therapeutics to tumor tissues. Selective delivery of nanotherapeutic platforms depends primarily on the passive targeting of tumors through the EPR effect. This phenomenon relies on defects specific to the tumor microenvironment, such as defects in lymphatic drainage, along with increased

Health Technology Sourcebook, Third Edition

tumor vasculature permeability, to allow nanoparticles (<200 nm) to accumulate in the tumor microenvironment. Furthermore, the timing or site of drug release can be controlled by triggered events, such as ultrasound, pH, heat, or by material composition.

Several members of the NCI Alliance for Nanotechnology are working toward developing nanomaterial-based delivery platforms that will reduce the toxicity of chemotherapeutics and increase their overall effectiveness. In the Centers for Cancer Nanotechnology Excellence (CCNEs), the Center for Multiple Myeloma Nanotherapy (CMMN) at Washington University is developing a strategy for photodynamic therapy, which would bypass the toxicity that currently limits the effectiveness of chemotherapy for multiple myeloma patients. This strategy is designed for use in bone marrow, which is normally inaccessible to external radiation sources.

The awardees of the Innovative Research in Cancer Nanotechnology (IRCNs) are focused on understanding the fundamental aspects of nanomaterial interactions with the biological system to improve the development of cancer therapeutics and diagnostics. Several of these awardees are studying nanoparticle-based delivery and have proposed nanosystems that deliver chemotherapeutics by penetrating through physiological barriers for access to more restricted tumors via targeting and/or mechanical deformation of particles (Yang, Karathanasis, Kabanov). One of them is dedicated to using a synergistic approach for the delivery of paclitaxel and gemcitabine chemotherapeutics in mesoporous silica nanoconstructs (Nel).

Nano-Enabled Immunotherapy

Immunotherapy is a promising new front in cancer treatment encompassing a number of approaches, including checkpoint inhibition and cellular therapies. Although results for some patients have been spectacular, only a minority of patients being treated for just a subset of cancers experience durable responses to these therapies. Expanding the benefits of immunotherapy requires a greater understanding of tumor-host immune system interactions. New technologies for molecular and functional analysis of single cells are being used to interrogate tumor and immune cells and

Technology in Cancer Treatment

elucidate molecular indicators and functional immune responses to therapy. To this end, nano-enabled devices and materials are being leveraged to sort, image, and characterize T cells in the Alliance's NanoSystems Biology Cancer Center (NSBCC).

Nanotechnologies are also being investigated to deliver immunotherapy. This includes the use of nanoparticles for the delivery of immunostimulatory or immunomodulatory molecules in combination with chemotherapy or radiotherapy or as adjuvants to other immunotherapies. Stand-alone nanoparticle vaccines are also being designed to raise sufficient T-cell response to eradicate tumors through co-delivery of antigen and adjuvant, the inclusion of multiple antigens to stimulate multiple dendritic cell targets, and continuous release of antigens for prolonged immune stimulation. Molecular blockers of immune-suppressive factors produced can also be co-encapsulated in nanoparticle vaccines to alter the immune context of tumors and improve response, an approach being pursued in the Nano Approaches to Modulate Host Cell Response for Cancer Therapy Center at UNC. Researchers in this center are also investigating the use of nanoparticles to capture antigens from tumors following radiotherapy to create patient-specific treatments similar in principle to a "dendritic-cell-activating scaffold" currently in a phase I clinical trial.

Additional uses of nanotechnology for immunotherapy include immune depots placed in or near tumors for in situ vaccination and artificial antigen-presenting cells. These and other approaches will advance and be refined as our understanding of cancer immunotherapy deepens.

Delivering or Augmenting Radiotherapy

Roughly half of all cancer patients receive some form of radiation therapy over the course of their treatment. Radiation therapy uses high-energy radiation to shrink tumors and kill cancer cells. Radiation therapy kills cancer cells by damaging their DNA, inducing cellular apoptosis. Radiation therapy can either damage DNA directly or create charged particles (atoms with an odd or unpaired number of electrons) within the cells that can, in turn, damage the DNA. Most types of radiation used for cancer treatment utilize x-rays, gamma rays, and charged particles. As such, they are inherently toxic to all cells, not just cancer cells, and are given in doses that are as efficacious as possible while not being too harmful to the body or fatal. Because of this tradeoff between efficacy and safety relative to tumor type, location, and stage, often the efficacy of treatment must remain at reduced levels in order to not be overtly toxic to surrounding tissue or organs near the tumor mass.

Nanotechnology-specific research has been focusing on radiotherapy as a treatment modality that could greatly benefit from nanoscale materials' properties and increased tumor accumulation. The primary mechanisms on which these nanoscale platforms rely are enhancement of the effect of the radiotherapy, augmentation of the therapy, and/or novel externally applied electromagnetic radiation modalities. More specifically, most of these nanotechnology platforms rely on the interaction between x-rays and nanoparticles due to the inherent atomic-level properties of the materials used. These include high-Z atomic number nanoparticles that enhance the Compton and photoelectric effects of conventional radiation therapy, in essence, increasing efficacy while maintaining the current radiotherapy dosage and its subsequent toxicity to the surrounding tissue. Other platforms utilize x-ray-triggered drug-releasing nanoparticles that deliver the drug locally at the tumor site or to sensitize the cancer cells to radiotherapy in combination with the drug.

Another type of therapy that relies upon external electromagnetic radiation is photodynamic therapy (PDT). It is an effective anticancer procedure for a superficial tumor that relies on tumor localization of a photosensitizer followed by light activation to generate cytotoxic reactive oxygen species (ROS). Several nanomaterials platforms are being researched to this end. Often made of a lanthanide- or hafnium-doped high-Z core, once injected, these can be externally irradiated by x-rays allowing the nanoparticle core to emit the visible light photons locally at the tumor site. The emission of photons from the particles subsequently activates a nanoparticle-bound or local photosensitizer to generate singlet oxygen ($^1O_2$) ROS for tumor destruction. Furthermore, these nanoparticles can be used as both PDT that generates ROS and for enhanced radiation therapy via the high-Z core. Although

Technology in Cancer Treatment

many of these platforms are initially being studied in vivo by intratumoral injection for superficial tumor sites, some are being tested for delivery via systemic injection to deep tissue tumors. The primary benefits to the patient would be local delivery of PDT to deep tissue tumor targets, an alternative therapy for cancer cells that have become radiotherapy resistant, and a reduction in toxicity (e.g., light sensitivity) common to traditional PDT. Finally, other platforms utilize a form of Cherenkov radiation to a similar end of local photon emission to utilize as a trigger for local PDT. These can be utilized for deep tissue targets as well.

Delivering Gene Therapy

The value of nanomaterial-based delivery has become apparent for new types of therapeutics, such as those using nucleic acids, which are highly unstable in systemic circulation and sensitive to degradation. These include DNA- and RNA-based genetic therapeutics such as small interfering RNAs (siRNAs) and microRNAs (miRNAs). Gene silencing therapeutics, siRNAs, have been reported to have significantly extended half-lives when delivered either encapsulated or conjugated to the surface of nanoparticles. These therapeutics are used in many cases to target "undruggable" cancer proteins. Additionally, the increased stability of genetic therapies delivered by nanocarriers and often combined with controlled release has been shown to prolong their effects.

Members of the Alliance are exploring nanotechnology-based delivery of nucleic acids as effective treatment strategies for a variety of cancers. In particular, the Nucleic Acid-Based Nanoconstructs for the Treatment of Cancer Center at Northwestern University is focused on the design and characterization of spherical nucleic acids for the delivery of RNA therapeutics to treat brain and prostate cancers. Project 1 of the Nano Approaches to Modulate Host Cell Response for Cancer Therapy Center at UNC-Chapel Hill targets vemurafenib-resistant melanoma for direct suppression of drug resistance through the delivery of siRNA using their polymetformin nanoparticles. Among the Innovative Research in Cancer Nanotechnology awardees, the Ohio State project (Guo) is focused on the systematic characterization of in vitro and in vivo RNA nanoparticle behavior for optimized delivery of siRNA to tumor cells, as well as cancer immunotherapeutics.

CURRENT NANOTECHNOLOGY TREATMENTS

The use of nanotechnology for the diagnosis and treatment of cancer is largely still in the development phase. However, there are already several nanocarrier-based drugs on the market and many more nano-based therapeutics in clinical trials. The application of nanotechnology to medicine includes the use of precisely engineered materials to develop novel therapies and devices that may reduce toxicity as well as enhance the efficacy and delivery of treatments. As a result, the application of nanotechnology to cancer can lead to many advances in the prevention, detection, and treatment of cancer. The first nanotechnology-based cancer drugs have passed regulatory scrutiny and are already on the market, including Doxil® and Abraxane®.

In recent years, the U.S. Food and Drug Administration (FDA) has approved numerous Investigational New Drug (IND) applications for nano-formulations, enabling clinical trials for breast, gynecological, solid tumor, lung, mesenchymal tissue, lymphoma, central nervous system, and genito-urinary cancer treatments. The majority of these trials repurpose the previously approved technologies described above.

The NCI Alliance for Nanotechnology funds the development of new technologies to bring the next generation of cancer treatments and diagnostics to the clinic.

SAFETY OF NANOTECHNOLOGY CANCER TREATMENT

Nanotechnology is a powerful tool for combating cancer and is being put to use in other applications that may reduce pollution, energy consumption, and greenhouse gas emissions and help prevent diseases. The NCI's Alliance for Nanotechnology in Cancer is working to ensure that nanotechnologies for cancer applications are developed responsibly.

There is nothing inherently dangerous about being nanosized. Our ability to manipulate objects at the nanoscale has developed

Technology in Cancer Treatment

relatively recently, but nanoparticles are as old as the earth. Many nanoparticles occur naturally (e.g., in volcanic ash and sea spray) and as by-products of human activities since the Stone Age (nanoparticles are in smoke and soot from fire). There are so many ambient incidental nanoparticles, in fact, that one of the challenges of nanoparticle exposure studies is that background incidental nanoparticles are often at order-of-magnitude higher levels than the engineered particles being evaluated.

As with any new technology, the safety of nanotechnology is continuously being tested. The small size, high reactivity, and unique tensile and magnetic properties of nanomaterials—the same properties that drive interest in their biomedical and industrial applications—have raised concerns about implications for the environment, health, and safety (EHS). There has been some as yet unresolved debate recently about the potential toxicity of a specific type of nanomaterial—carbon nanotubes (CNTs)—which has been associated with tissue damage in animal studies. However, the majority of available data indicate that there is nothing uniquely toxic about nanoparticles as a class of materials.

In fact, most engineered nanoparticles are far less toxic than household cleaning products, insecticides used on family pets, and over-the-counter (OTC) dandruff remedies. Certainly, the nanoparticles used as drug carriers for chemotherapeutics are much less toxic than the drugs they carry and are designed to carry drugs safely to tumors without harming organs and healthy tissue.

To ensure that the potential risks of nanotechnology are thoroughly evaluated, the NCI Alliance for Nanotechnology in Cancer makes the services of its Nanotechnology Characterization Laboratory (NCL) available to the nanotech and cancer research communities. The NCL, an intramural program of the Alliance, performs nanomaterial safety and toxicity testing in vitro (in the laboratory) and using animal models. The NCL tests are designed to characterize nanomaterials that enter the bloodstream, regardless of route. This testing is just one part of the NCL's cascade of tests to evaluate the physicochemical properties, biocompatibility, and efficacy of nanomaterials intended for cancer therapy and diagnosis. To date, the NCL has evaluated more than 125 different nanoparticles intended for medical applications.

Health Technology Sourcebook, Third Edition

The NCL works closely with the FDA and National Institutes of Standards and Technology (NIST) to devise experiments that are relevant to nanomaterials, to validate these tests on a variety of nanomaterial types, and to disseminate its methods to the nanotech and cancer research communities. The NCL also facilitates the development of voluntary-consensus standards for reliably and proactively measuring and monitoring the environment, health, and safety ramifications of nanotech applications.

Whether actual or perceived, the potential health risks associated with the manufacture and use of nanomaterials must be carefully studied in order to advance our understanding of this field of science and to realize the significant benefits that nanotechnology has to offer society, such as for cancer research, diagnostics, and therapy.

Section 25.4 | Biomarker Testing for Cancer Treatment

This section includes text excerpted from "Biomarker Testing for Cancer Treatment," National Cancer Institute (NCI), December 14, 2021.

WHAT IS BIOMARKER TESTING FOR CANCER TREATMENT?

Biomarker testing is a way to look for genes, proteins, and other substances (called "biomarkers" or "tumor markers") that can provide information about cancer. Each person's cancer has a unique pattern of biomarkers. Some biomarkers affect how certain cancer treatments work. Biomarker testing may help you and your doctor choose a cancer treatment for you.

There are also other kinds of biomarkers that can help doctors diagnose and monitor cancer during and after treatment.

Biomarker testing is for people who have cancer. People with solid tumors and people with blood cancer can get biomarker testing.

Biomarker testing for cancer treatment may also be called:

- Tumor testing
- Tumor genetic testing

370

Technology in Cancer Treatment

- Genomic testing or genomic profiling
- Molecular testing or molecular profiling
- Somatic testing
- Tumor subtyping

A biomarker test may be called a "companion diagnostic test" if it is paired with a specific treatment.

Biomarker testing is different from genetic testing that is used to find out if someone has inherited mutations that make them more likely to get cancer. Inherited mutations are those you are born with. They are passed on to you by your parents.

HOW ARE BIOMARKER TESTS USED TO SELECT CANCER TREATMENT?

Biomarker tests can help you and your doctor select a cancer treatment for you. Some cancer treatments, including targeted therapies and immunotherapies, may only work for people whose cancers have certain biomarkers.

For example, people with cancer that has certain genetic changes in the *EGFR* gene can get treatments that target those changes, called "EGFR inhibitors." In this case, biomarker testing can find out whether someone's cancer has an *EGFR* gene change that can be treated with an EGFR inhibitor.

Biomarker testing could also help you find a study of a new cancer treatment (a clinical trial) that you may be able to join. Some studies enroll people based on the biomarkers in their cancer instead of where in the body the cancer started growing. These are sometimes called "basket trials."

For some other clinical trials, biomarker testing is part of the study. For example, studies such as NCI-MATCH and NCI-COG Pediatric MATCH use biomarker tests to match people to treatments based on the genetic changes in their cancers.

IS BIOMARKER TESTING PART OF PRECISION MEDICINE?

Yes, biomarker testing is an important part of precision medicine, also called "personalized medicine." Precision medicine is an

Health Technology Sourcebook, Third Edition

approach to medical care in which disease prevention, diagnosis, and treatment are tailored to the genes, proteins, and other substances in your body.

For cancer treatment, precision medicine means using biomarkers and other tests to select treatments that are most likely to help you while at the same time sparing you from getting treatments that are not likely to help.

The idea of precision medicine is not new, but recent advances in science and technology have helped speed up the pace of this area of research. Scientists now understand that cancer cells can have many different changes in genes, proteins, and other substances that make the cells grow and spread. They have also learned that even two people with the same type of cancer may not have the same changes in their cancer. Some of these changes affect how certain cancer treatments work.

Even though researchers are making progress every day, the precision medicine approach to cancer treatment is not yet part of routine care for most patients. But it is important to note that even the "standard" approach to cancer treatment (selecting treatments based on the type of cancer you have, its size, and whether it has spread) is effective and is personalized to each patient.

SHOULD YOU GET BIOMARKER TESTING TO SELECT CANCER TREATMENT?

Talk with your health-care provider to discuss whether biomarker testing for cancer treatment should be part of your care. Doctors usually suggest genomic biomarker testing (also called "genomic profiling") for people with cancer that has spread or come back after treatment (what is called "advanced cancer").

Biomarker testing is also done routinely to select treatment for people who are diagnosed with certain types of cancer—including nonsmall cell lung cancer, breast cancer, and colorectal cancer.

It is also a good idea to check with your health insurance provider to see if they will cover biomarker testing for your cancer. Biomarker testing is not available at every hospital. Check with your health-care provider to see if biomarker testing is offered at the hospital or place where you get your cancer care.

Technology in Cancer Treatment

HOW IS BIOMARKER TESTING DONE?

If you and your health-care providers decide to make biomarker testing part of your care, they will take a sample of your cancer cells. If you have a solid tumor, they may take a sample during surgery. If you are not having surgery, you may need to have a biopsy of your tumor.

If you have blood cancer or are getting a biomarker test known as a "liquid biopsy," you will need to have a blood draw. You might get a liquid biopsy test if you cannot safely get a tumor biopsy, for example, because your tumor is hard to reach with a needle.

Your samples will be sent to a special lab where they will be tested for certain biomarkers. The lab will create a report that lists the biomarkers in your cancer cells and if there are any treatments that might work for you. Your health-care team will discuss the results with you to decide on a treatment.

For some biomarker tests that analyze genes, you will also need to give a sample of your healthy cells. This is usually done by collecting your blood, saliva, or a small piece of your skin. These tests compare your cancer cells with your healthy cells to find genetic changes (called "somatic mutations") that arose during your lifetime. Somatic mutations cause most cancers and cannot be passed on to family members.

ARE THERE DIFFERENT TYPES OF BIOMARKER TESTS?

Yes, there are many types of biomarker tests that can help select cancer treatment. Most biomarker tests used to select cancer treatment look for genetic markers. But some look for proteins or other kinds of markers.

Some tests check for a single biomarker. Others check for many biomarkers at the same time and may be called "multigene tests" or "panel tests." One example is the Oncotype DX test, which looks at the activity of 21 different genes to predict whether chemotherapy is likely to work for someone with breast cancer.

Some tests are for people with a certain type of cancer, such as melanoma. Other tests look for biomarkers that are found in many cancer types, and such tests can be used by people with different kinds of cancer.

373

Health Technology Sourcebook, Third Edition

Some tests, called "whole-exome sequencing," look at all the genes in your cancer. Others, called "whole-genome sequencing," look at all the DNA (both genes and outside of genes) in your cancer.

Still, other biomarker tests look at the number of genetic changes in your cancer (what is known as "tumor mutational burden"). This information can help figure out if a type of immunotherapy known as "immune checkpoint inhibitors" may work for you.

Biomarker tests, known as "liquid biopsies," look in blood or other fluids for biomarkers from cancer cells. There are two liquid biopsy tests approved by the U.S. Food and Drug Administration (FDA), called "Guardant360 CDx" and "FoundationOne Liquid CDx."

WHAT DO THE RESULTS OF A BIOMARKER TEST MEAN?

The results of a biomarker test could show that your cancer has a certain biomarker that is targeted by a known therapy. It means that the therapy may work to treat your cancer. The matching therapy may be available as an FDA-approved treatment, as an off-label treatment, or through participation in a clinical trial.

The results could also show that your cancer has a biomarker that may prevent a certain therapy from working. This information could spare you from getting a treatment that would not help you.

In many cases, biomarker testing may find changes in your cancer that would not help your doctor make treatment decisions. For example, genetic changes that are thought to be harmless (benign) or whose effects are not known (a variant of unknown significance) are not used to make treatment decisions.

Based on your test results, your health-care provider may recommend a treatment that is not FDA-approved for your cancer type but is approved for the treatment of a different type of cancer that has the same biomarker as your cancer. This means the treatment would be used off-label, but it may work for you because your cancer has the biomarker that the treatment targets.

Some biomarker tests can find genetic changes that you may have been born with (inherited) that increase your risk of cancer or other diseases. These genetic changes are also called "germline mutations." If such a change is found, you may need to get another

Technology in Cancer Treatment

genetic test to confirm whether you truly have an inherited mutation that increases cancer risk.

Finding out that you have an inherited mutation that increases cancer risk may affect you and your family. For that reason, your health-care provider may recommend that you speak with a genetic health-care provider (such as a genetic counselor, clinical geneticist, or certified genetic nurse) to help you understand what the test results mean for you and your family.

WILL BIOMARKER TESTING FOR CANCER TREATMENT HELP YOU?

Biomarker tests do not help everyone who gets them. There are several different reasons why they may not help you. Biomarker testing may not help you if:

- You are unable to safely get a biopsy needed for testing.
- There is not enough tumor tissue in your biopsy sample to have biomarker testing done.
- The test does not find any biomarkers in your cancer that match with available therapies.
- The test identifies a matching therapy that would be used off-label, and your insurance does not cover the cost.
- The test identifies a matching therapy that is being tested in a clinical trial, and you are not able to participate in the trial.

Even if your test finds a biomarker that matches an available treatment, the therapy may not work for you. Sometimes, other features of your cancer or your body affect how well a treatment works, such as how the medicine is broken down in your body.

Another reason the treatment might not work is that not all of your cancer cells have the same biomarkers. It means that a biomarker test may find a treatment that will kill some, but not all, of your cancer cells. Cancer cells that are not killed by the treatment could keep growing, preventing the treatment from working or causing the cancer to quickly come back.

One other reason biomarker tests might not help is because the biomarkers in your cancer can change over time. But a test only

Health Technology Sourcebook, Third Edition

captures a "snapshot" of the changes at one point in time. So the results of a biomarker test done in the past may not reflect the biomarkers in your cancer now. Your health-care provider may want to test your cancer again, for example, if it comes back after treatment.

HOW MUCH DOES BIOMARKER TESTING FOR CANCER TREATMENT COST?

The cost of biomarker testing varies widely depending on the type of test you get, the type of cancer you have, and your insurance plan.

For people with advanced cancer, some biomarker tests are covered by Medicare and Medicaid. Private insurance providers often cover the cost of a biomarker test if there is enough proof that the test is required to guide treatment decisions. Tests without enough proof to support their value may be considered experimental and are likely not covered by insurance.

Many clinical trials involve biomarker testing. If you join one of these clinical trials, the cost of biomarker testing might be covered. The study coordinator can give you more information about related costs.

Chapter 26 | What Is Precision Medicine?

Most medical treatments are designed for the "average patient" as a one-size-fits-all approach, which may be successful for some patients but not for others. Precision medicine, sometimes known as "personalized medicine," is an innovative approach to tailoring disease prevention and treatment that takes into account differences in people's genes, environments, and lifestyles. The goal of precision medicine is to target the right treatments to the right patients at the right time.

Advances in precision medicine have already led to powerful new discoveries and treatments approved by the U.S. Food and Drug Administration (FDA) that are tailored to specific characteristics of individuals, such as a person's genetic makeup or the genetic profile of an individual's tumor. Patients with a variety of cancers routinely undergo molecular testing as part of patient care, enabling physicians to select treatments that improve chances of survival and reduce exposure to adverse effects.

NEXT-GENERATION SEQUENCING TESTS

Precision care will only be as good as the tests that guide diagnosis and treatment. Next-generation sequencing (NGS) tests are capable of rapidly identifying or "sequencing" large sections of a person's genome and are important advances in the clinical applications of precision medicine.

This chapter includes text excerpted from "Precision Medicine," U.S. Food and Drug Administration (FDA), September 27, 2018. Reviewed November 2022.

Health Technology Sourcebook, Third Edition

Patients, physicians, and researchers can use these tests to find genetic variants that help them diagnose, treat, and understand more about human disease.

THE U.S. FOOD AND DRUG ADMINISTRATION'S ROLE IN ADVANCING PRECISION MEDICINE

The FDA is working to ensure the accuracy of NGS tests so that patients and clinicians can receive accurate and clinically meaningful test results.

The vast amount of information generated through NGS poses novel regulatory issues for the FDA. While current regulatory approaches are appropriate for conventional diagnostics that detect a single disease or condition (such as blood glucose or cholesterol levels), these new sequencing techniques contain the equivalent of millions of tests in one. Because of this, the FDA has worked with stakeholders in the industry, laboratories, academia, and patient and professional societies to develop a flexible regulatory approach to accommodate this rapidly evolving technology that leverages consensus standards, crowd-sourced data, and state-of-the-art open-source computing technology to support NGS test development. This approach will enable innovation in testing and research and will speed access to accurate, reliable genetic tests.

STREAMLINING THE U.S. FOOD AND DRUG ADMINISTRATION'S REGULATORY OVERSIGHT OF NGS TESTS

In April 2018, the FDA issued two final guidances that recommend approaches to streamline the submission and review of data supporting the clinical and analytical validity of NGS-based tests. Figure 26.1 provides recommendations that are intended to provide an efficient and flexible regulatory oversight approach: as technology advances, standards can rapidly evolve and be used to set appropriate metrics for fast-growing fields such as NGS. Similarly, as clinical evidence improves, new assertions could be supported. This adaptive approach would ultimately foster innovation among test developers and improve patients' access to these new technologies.

378

What Is Precision Medicine?

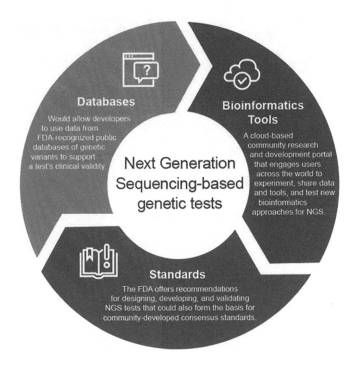

Figure 26.1. Next-Generation Sequencing Tests Flowchart

Chapter 27 | **Human Genome Project**

WHAT WAS THE HUMAN GENOME PROJECT?

The Human Genome Project was a large, well-organized, and highly collaborative international effort that generated the first sequence of the human genome and that of several additional well-studied organisms. Carried out from 1990 to 2003, it was one of the most ambitious and important scientific endeavors in human history.

WHAT WERE THE GOALS OF THE HUMAN GENOME PROJECT?

A special committee of the U.S. National Academy of Sciences (NAS) outlined the original goals for the Human Genome Project in 1988, which included sequencing the entire human genome in addition to the genomes of several carefully selected nonhuman organisms.

Eventually, the list of organisms came to include the bacterium *Escherichia coli* (*E. coli*), baker's yeast, fruit fly, nematode, and mouse. The project's architects and participants hoped the resulting information would usher in a new era for biomedical research, and its goals and related strategic plans were updated periodically throughout the project.

In part due to a deliberate focus on technology development, the Human Genome Project ultimately exceeded its initial set of goals, doing so by 2003, two years ahead of its originally projected

This chapter contains text excerpted from the following sources: Text beginning with the heading "What Was the Human Genome Project?" is excerpted from "Human Genome Project," National Human Genome Research Institute (NHGRI), August 24, 2022.

381

Health Technology Sourcebook, Third Edition

2005 completion. Many of the project's achievements were beyond what scientists thought possible in 1988.

WHAT IS DNA SEQUENCING? HOW WAS IT PERFORMED DURING THE HUMAN GENOME PROJECT?

Deoxyribonucleic acid (DNA) sequencing involves determining the exact order of the bases in DNA—the As, Cs, Gs, and Ts that make up segments of DNA. Because the Human Genome Project aimed to sequence all of the DNA (i.e., the genome) of a set of organisms, significant effort was made to improve the methods for DNA sequencing.

Ultimately, the project used one particular method for DNA sequencing, called "Sanger DNA sequencing," but first greatly advanced this basic method through a series of major technical innovations.

WHOSE DNA WAS SEQUENCED BY THE HUMAN GENOME PROJECT? HOW WAS IT COLLECTED?

The sequence of the human genome generated by the Human Genome Project was not from a single person. Rather, it reflects a patchwork from multiple people whose identities were intentionally made anonymous to protect their privacy.

The project researchers used a thoughtful process to recruit volunteers, acquire their informed consent, and collect their blood samples. Most of the human genome sequence generated by the Human Genome Project came from blood donors in Buffalo, New York: specifically, 93 percent from 11 donors and 70 percent from one donor.

WHO CARRIED OUT THE HUMAN GENOME PROJECT?

The Human Genome Project could not have been completed as quickly and effectively without the dedicated participation of an international consortium of thousands of researchers. In the United States, the researchers were funded by the Department of Energy (DOE) and the National Institutes of Health (NIH), which created the Office for Human Genome Research in 1988 (later renamed the

Human Genome Project

National Center for Human Genome Research in 1990 and then the National Human Genome Research Institute (NHGRI) in 1997).

The sequencing of the human genome involved researchers from 20 separate universities and research centers across the United States, United Kingdom, France, Germany, Japan, and China. The groups in these countries became known as "the International Human Genome Sequencing Consortium."

HOW MUCH DID THE HUMAN GENOME PROJECT COST?

The initially projected cost for the Human Genome Project was $3 billion, based on its envisioned length of 15 years. While precise cost accounting was difficult to carry out, especially across the set of international funders, most agree that this rough amount is close to the accurate number.

The cost of the Human Genome Project, while in the billions of dollars, has been greatly offset by the positive economic benefits that genomics has yielded in the ensuing decades. Such economic gains reflect direct links between resulting products and advances in the pharmaceutical and biotechnology industries, among others.

DID THE HUMAN GENOME PROJECT PRODUCE A PERFECTLY COMPLETE GENOME SEQUENCE?

No. Throughout the Human Genome Project, researchers continually improved the methods for DNA sequencing. However, they were limited in their abilities to determine the sequence of some stretches of human DNA (e.g., particularly complex or highly repetitive DNA).

In June 2000, the International Human Genome Sequencing Consortium announced that it had produced a draft human genome sequence that accounted for 90 percent of the human genome. The draft sequence contained more than 150,000 areas where the DNA sequence was unknown because it could not be determined accurately (known as "gaps").

In April 2003, the consortium announced that it had generated an essentially complete human genome sequence, which was significantly improved from the draft sequence. Specifically, it

Health Technology Sourcebook, Third Edition

accounted for 92 percent of the human genome and less than 400 gaps; it was also more accurate.

On March 31, 2022, the Telomere-to-Telomere (T2T) consortium announced that it had filled in the remaining gaps and produced the first truly complete human genome sequence.

HOW DID THE HUMAN GENOME PROJECT CHANGE PRACTICES AROUND DATA SHARING IN THE SCIENTIFIC RESEARCH COMMUNITY?

Human Genome Project scientists made every part of the draft human genome sequence publicly available shortly after production.

This routine came from two meetings in Bermuda in which project researchers agreed to the "Bermuda Principles," which set out the rules for the rapid release of sequence data. This landmark agreement has been credited with establishing a greater awareness and openness to the sharing of data in biomedical research, making it one of the most important legacies of the Human Genome Project.

HOW DID THE HUMAN GENOME PROJECT FOSTER ETHICS IN BIOLOGICAL RESEARCH?

The leaders of the Human Genome Project recognized the need to be proactive in addressing a wide range of ethical and social issues related to the acquisition and use of genomic information. They were especially aware of the potential risks and benefits of incorporating new genomic knowledge into research and medicine. Similarly, they were aware of the potential misuse of genomic information when it came to insurance and employment, among others.

To help understand and address these issues, NHGRI established the Ethical, Legal, and Social Implications (ELSI) Research Program in 1990.

The early appreciation of the value of this program later led the U.S. Congress to mandate that NHGRI dedicates at least five percent of its research budget to studying the ethical, legal, and social implications of genomic advances. The NHGRI ELSI Research Program has become a model for bioethics research worldwide.

Human Genome Project

HOW DID THE HUMAN GENOME PROJECT AFFECT BIOLOGICAL RESEARCH IN GENERAL?

The Human Genome Project demonstrated that production-oriented, discovery-driven scientific inquiry—which did not involve the investigation of a specific hypothesis or the direct answering of preformed questions—could be remarkably valuable and beneficial to the broader scientific community.

The project was also a successful example of "big science" in biomedical research. The magnitude of the technological challenges prompted the Human Genome Project to assemble interdisciplinary groups from across the world, involving experts in engineering, biology, and computer science, among other areas. It also required the work to be concentrated in a modest number of major centers to maximize economies of scale.

Before the Human Genome Project, the biomedical research community viewed projects of such scale with deep skepticism. These kinds of massive scientific undertakings have become more commonplace and well-accepted based in part on the success of the Human Genome Project.

Chapter 28 | Robots and Their Use in Health Care

Chapter Contents
Section 28.1—Image-Guided Robotic Interventions 389
Section 28.2—Robot-Assisted Surgery 392
Section 28.3—Fiber-Optic-Enabled Sensitive
                 Surgery Tools 395

Section 28.1 | Image-Guided Robotic Interventions

This section includes text excerpted from "Image-Guided Robotic Interventions Fact Sheet," National Institute of Biomedical Imaging and Bioengineering (NIBIB), December 2019.

WHAT ARE IMAGE-GUIDED ROBOTIC INTERVENTIONS?

Image-guided robotic interventions are medical procedures that integrate sophisticated robotic and imaging technologies, primarily to perform minimally invasive surgery. This integrated technology approach offers distinct advantages for both patients and physicians.

Imaging. In image-guided procedures, the surgeon is guided by images from various techniques, including magnetic resonance (MR) and ultrasound. Images can also be obtained using tiny cameras attached to probes that are small enough to fit into a minimal incision. The camera allows the surgery to be performed using a much smaller incision than in traditional surgery.

Robotics. The surgeon's hands and traditional surgical tools are too large for small incisions. Instead, thin, finger-like robotic tools are used to perform the surgery. As the surgeon watches the image on the screen, she or he uses a telemanipulator to transmit and direct hand and finger movements to a robot, which can be controlled by hydraulic, electronic, or mechanical means.

Robotic tools can also be controlled by computers. One advantage of a computerized system is that a surgeon could potentially perform the surgery from anywhere in the world. This type of long-distance surgery is currently in the experimental phase. The experiments illustrate the life-saving potential for such surgeries when a delicate operation requires a specially trained surgeon who is in a distant location.

WHAT ARE THE ADVANTAGES OF MINIMALLY INVASIVE PROCEDURES?

Minimally invasive surgery can reduce the damage to surrounding healthy tissues, thus decreasing the need for pain medication and reducing patients' recovery time. For surgeons, image-guided interventions using robots also have the advantage of reducing

Health Technology Sourcebook, Third Edition

fatigue during long operations, allowing the surgeon to perform the procedure while seated.

WHAT ARE SOME EXAMPLES OF IMAGE-GUIDED ROBOTIC INTERVENTIONS, AND HOW ARE THEY USED?

Robotic prostatectomy. Complete prostate removal is performed through a series of small incisions, compared with a single large incision of 4–5 inches in traditional surgery. The small incisions result in a shorter postoperative recovery, less scarring, and a faster return to normal activities.

Ablation techniques for early cancers. Patients with early kidney cancer can be treated with minimally invasive procedures to destroy small tumors. Cryoablation uses cold energy to destroy tumors. Doctors use computed tomography (CT) and ultrasound imaging to position a needle-like probe within each kidney tumor. Once in position, the tip of the probe is supercooled to encase the tumor in a ball of ice. Alternate freeze/thaw cycles kill the tumor cells. Other minimally invasive methods of destroying early kidney cancers include heating the tumor cells and surgical removal using a robotic device. Many patients can go home the same day and are able to perform regular activities for several days.

Orthopedics. Image-guided robotic procedures are improving the precision and outcome of a number of orthopedic procedures. For example, partial knee resurfacing surgeries aim to target only the damaged sections of the knee joint. Orthopedic surgeons are combining the use of a robotic surgical arm and fiber optic cameras in such procedures, which results in patients retaining more of their normal healthy tissue. Image-guided robotic procedures also improve total knee replacements, allowing precise alignment and positioning of knee implants. The result is more natural knee function, better range of motion, and improved balance for patients.

WHAT ARE NIBIB-FUNDED RESEARCHERS DEVELOPING IN THE AREA OF IMAGE-GUIDED ROBOTIC INTERVENTIONS TO IMPROVE MEDICAL CARE?

- **Portable robot uses three-dimensional (3D) near-infrared imaging to guide needle insertion into veins.**

Robots and Their Use in Health Care

Drawing blood and inserting IV lines are the most commonly performed medical procedures in hospitals and clinics. However, for many patients, it can be difficult to find veins and accurately insert the needle, resulting in patient injury. The scientists funded by the National Institute of Biomedical Imaging and Bioengineering (NIBIB) are developing a portable, lightweight medical robot to help perform these procedures. The device uses 3D near-infrared imaging to identify an appropriate vein for the robot to insert the needle. The current goal is to integrate the imaging system and software into a miniaturized version of the prototype robot. The outcome will be a compact, low-cost system that will greatly improve the safety and accuracy of accessing veins.

- **Robot-assisted needle guidance aids in the removal of liver tumors.** Radio frequency ablation (RFA) is a minimally invasive treatment that kills tumors with heat and can be a life-saving option for patients who are not eligible for surgery. However, the broad use of RFA has been limited because the straight paths taken by the needles that carry tumor-killing electrodes may damage the lung or other sensitive organs. Also, large tumors require multiple needle insertions, which increases the bleeding risk. To address the problem of tissue damage using straight needles, NIBIB-funded scientists are developing highly flexible needles that can be guided along controlled, curved paths through tissue, allowing the removal of tumors that are not accessible by a straight-line path. The technology combines needle flexibility with a 3D ultrasound guidance system that allows the doctor to correct the path of the needle to avoid unexpected obstacles as the needle advances toward the tumor. The device will ultimately increase the accuracy and reduce the damage to healthy tissue during tumor removal resulting in wider use of the technology for better patient outcomes.
- **Swallowable capsule identifies and biopsies abnormal tissue in the esophagus.** Barrett esophagus is a precancerous condition that requires repeated biopsies to

Health Technology Sourcebook, Third Edition

monitor abnormal tissue. NIBIB-funded researchers are developing a swallowable, pill-sized device to improve the management and treatment of this condition. The unsedated patient can easily swallow the pill, which is attached to a thin tether made of cable and optic fiber. The device detects microscopic areas of the esophagus that may show evidence of disease and uses a laser to collect samples from the suspicious tissue—a technology known as "laser capture microdissection." The physician then retrieves the device from the patient without discomfort, and the collected microsamples are examined for visual evidence of disease, as well as genetic analysis. This minimally invasive device improves patient comfort and provides a precise molecular profile of the biopsied regions, which helps the physician better monitor and treat the disorder.

Section 28.2 | Robot-Assisted Surgery

This section includes text excerpted from "Computer-Assisted Surgical Systems," U.S. Food and Drug Administration (FDA), June 21, 2022.

WHAT ARE COMPUTER-ASSISTED SURGICAL SYSTEMS?

Different types of computer-assisted surgical systems can be used for preoperative planning and surgical navigation and to assist in performing surgical procedures. Robotically assisted surgical (RAS) devices are one type of computer-assisted surgical system. Sometimes referred to as "robotic surgery," RAS devices enable the surgeon to use computer and software technology to control and move surgical instruments through one or more tiny incisions in the patient's body (minimally invasive) for a variety of surgical procedures.

The benefits of a RAS device may include its ability to facilitate minimally invasive surgery and assist with complex tasks in confined areas of the body. The device is not actually a robot because it cannot perform surgery without direct human control.

Robots and Their Use in Health Care

The RAS devices generally have several components, which may include the following:

- **Console.** Where the surgeon sits during surgery. The console is the control center of the device and allows the surgeon to view the surgical field through a three-dimensional (3D) endoscope and control the movement of the surgical instruments;
- **Bedside cart.** Includes three or four hinged mechanical arms, camera (endoscope), and surgical instruments that the surgeon controls during surgical procedures;
- **Separate cart.** Contains supporting hardware and software components, such as an electrosurgical unit (ESU), suction/irrigation pumps, and a light source for the endoscope.

Most surgeons use multiple surgical instruments and accessories with the RAS device, such as scalpels, forceps, graspers, dissectors, cautery, scissors, retractors, and suction irrigators.

COMMON USES OF ROBOTICALLY ASSISTED SURGICAL DEVICES

The FDA has cleared RAS devices for use by trained physicians in an operating room environment for laparoscopic surgical procedures in general surgery, cardiac, colorectal, gynecologic, head and neck, and thoracic and urologic surgical procedures. Some common procedures that may involve RAS devices are gallbladder removal, hysterectomy, and prostatectomy (removal of the prostate).

While robotically assisted surgery is safe and effective for performing certain procedures when used appropriately and with proper training, the U.S. Food and Drug Administration (FDA) has not granted marketing authorization for any robotically assisted surgical device system for use in the United States specifically for the prevention or treatment of cancer.

RECOMMENDATIONS FOR PATIENTS AND HEALTH-CARE PROVIDERS ABOUT ROBOTICALLY ASSISTED SURGERY
Patients

Robotically assisted surgery is an important treatment option but may not be appropriate in all situations. Talk to your physician

Health Technology Sourcebook, Third Edition

about the risks and benefits of robotically assisted surgeries, as well as the risks and benefits of other treatment options.

Patients who are considering treatment with robotically assisted surgeries should discuss the options for these devices with their health-care provider and feel free to inquire about their surgeon's training and experience with these devices.

Health-Care Providers

Robotically assisted surgery is safe and effective for performing certain procedures when used appropriately and with proper training. The FDA regulates devices to provide reasonable assurance of their safety and effectiveness for their intended uses. For RAS devices, this includes assuring manufacturers implement adequate training programs for both new and experienced users. The FDA does not supervise or provide accreditation for physician training, nor does it oversee training and education related to legally marketed medical devices. Instead, the development and implementation of training is the responsibility of the manufacturer, physicians, and health-care facilities. In some cases, professional societies and specialty board certification organizations may also develop and support training for their specialty physicians. Specialty boards also maintain the certification status of their specialty physicians.

Physicians, hospitals, and facilities that use RAS devices should ensure surgeons are trained properly and have appropriate credentials to perform surgical procedures with these devices. Device users should ensure they maintain their credentialing. Hospitals and facilities should also ensure that other surgical staff who use these devices complete proper training.

Users of the device should realize there are several different models of RAS devices. Each model may operate differently and may not have the same functions. Users should know the differences between the models and make sure to get appropriate training on each model.

If you suspect a problem or complications associated with the use of RAS devices, the FDA encourages you to file a voluntary report through MedWatch, the FDA Safety Information

Robots and Their Use in Health Care

and Adverse Event Reporting program. Health-care personnel employed by facilities that are subject to the FDA's user facility reporting requirements should follow the reporting procedures established by their facilities. Prompt reporting of adverse events can help the FDA identify and better understand the risks associated with medical devices.

Section 28.3 | Fiber-Optic-Enabled Sensitive Surgery Tools

This section includes text excerpted from "Fiber-Optic "Nerves" Enable Sensitive Surgery Tools," National Aeronautics and Space Administration (NASA), 2020.

NATIONAL AERONAUTICS AND SPACE ADMINISTRATION TECHNOLOGY

Can you make a robot feel? This was the question posed to Johnson Space Center engineer Toby Martin.

It was not a heart that NASA wanted to give its Robonaut, though—it was tactile sensing for the robot's hands.

"It didn't have an autonomous grasping capability," Martin says of the first version of NASA's robot astronaut. A control systems specialist, he was tasked in 2004 with looking for a way to give it that ability. "First we had to figure out how to sense when it's grasping something," he says. "We wanted the hand to be able to grab an object and adjust finger forces and positions and tensions to pick up irregular objects."

At least one company that responded to Martin's request for proposals, Intelligent Fiber Optic Systems (IFOS) Corporation, was no stranger to NASA. Much of the Silicon Valley, California-based company's funding to develop its initial technology had come from two Small Business Innovation Research (SBIR) contracts with Langley Research Center a decade earlier.

The NASA's SBIR and Small Business Technology Transfer (STTR) programs make relatively small investments in promising technologies that could prove useful to the Space Agency's missions and also show commercial potential.

395

For the Langley project, the company had proposed developing "smart surfaces" for aerospace materials and other applications by creating what IFOS calls "optical nerves." These are optical fibers with reflective microstructures called "fiber Bragg gratings" imprinted within their cores at intervals. A device known as an "optical interrogator" sends light along the fiber, and each grating reflects back a particular wavelength signature, which changes slightly if there are changes to strain or temperature.

"If you stretch a grating, the wavelength that comes back becomes longer, proportional to the strain," a phenomenon known as "redshift," explains Dr. Richard Black, chief scientist at IFOS. "If the grating is compressed, there's a proportional blue shift." Similarly, a rise in temperature causes a redshift, while a drop leads to a blueshift. The IFOS interrogator can detect changes in wavelength on the order of picometers to femtometers, the infinitesimal unit used to measure atoms, which it uses to determine strain or temperature change.

With a series of fibers attached to or embedded in a surface, each with several fiber Bragg grating sensors along its length, the interrogator can monitor strain and temperature across the entire surface, a capability that has a multitude of possible applications across many fields.

For Robonaut's hand, the company proposed that its technology could determine the position of each finger in real time by measuring the strain that comes with bending, and if it took readings fast enough, it could even detect vibrations and textures.

TECHNOLOGY TRANSFER

"I was kind of dubious that it would work for our application, but I was intrigued," says Martin. "It provided many of the benefits of strain gauges without some of the negatives, like external electrical noise and interference. With several gratings per fiber, the density of sensors that could fit into a small space was also a plus." Johnson granted the company an SBIR contract to explore the concept's feasibility. To avoid rebuilding the hands, NASA asked for a glove that fit over the existing hands.

Robots and Their Use in Health Care

At the time, IFOS was still using much the same interrogator it had developed for Langley, supporting no more than 10 sensors. To outfit an entire hand requiring many more sensors, though, the company made a fundamental change by developing a scalable architecture that produced an enduring improvement in its sensing capabilities, says Black.

With Johnson funding, the company took an optical chip concept made for telecommunications applications, modified it for its massively parallel sensing architecture, and worked with a foundry to customize a photonic spectral processor—a single chip with many waveguides stamped into it. The processor acts like a prism, sending different parts of the spectrum to different photodetectors in an array. The interrogator monitors changes in the ratios of various spectral components simultaneously to allow precise determination of the sensor wavelengths.

The ability to monitor multiple sensors simultaneously allows for much faster readings, which is important for detecting, for example, the tiny, rapid vibrations caused by friction with a textured surface.

The glove did not work well due to misfires caused by wrinkles and other issues, says Martin. Under a Phase II SBIR contract, however, IFOS and the Mechanical Engineering Department at Stanford University developed their own finger prototype. "We tested it and verified the experiments the company had run showing it worked," Martin says. At the time, both the finger prototype and the interrogator were too large to incorporate into a human-sized hand.

That was as far as the project went, but someone from the Johnson team pushed Behzad Moslehi, the company's chief executive and chief technology officer, to pursue funding for possible medical applications through the National Institutes of Health (NIH), he says. "I looked into it, and I found it was the right home."

BENEFITS

The IFOS has since found a multitude of possible medical applications for its fiber-sensing technology.

Health Technology Sourcebook, Third Edition

Shortly after the Robonaut project, as the company was exploring medical applications, Intuitive Surgical Inc. acquired one of IFOS' fiber-optic sensor systems to investigate its use on dexterous surgical robots. A few years later, IFOS produced several instrumented grasper assemblies with haptic sensing for a medical application Samsung was evaluating. Moslehi says he sees the medical robot market as an opportunity for the company's future through strategic partnerships with other companies.

Closer to commercialization are instrumented biopsy needles that surgeons can use in conjunction with both magnetic resonance imaging (MRI) and ultrasound machines. Stanford has been collaborating with IFOS through its engineering and medical schools to evaluate and test the technology on animals in the MRI environment.

Tools used in real-time MRI-guided surgery—where the surgeon is either reaching into the MRI machine or working remotely from a control room—must not react to magnets or use electricity, Black says. "Optical-fiber sensors are ideal for the sort of sensing we're doing." But such a needle is almost invisible in the MRI image.

"We came up with a way to measure the shape of a biopsy needle in real time, down to the tip of the needle, and superimpose the precise shape over the blurry artifacts from an MRI," he says. This lets surgeons see what they are doing.

The tool can also measure forces on the tip, which relate to tissue hardness. This provides another clue for surgeons, as tumors are typically harder than the surrounding tissue. The team is working on providing haptic feedback, such as a joystick for remote surgery that vibrates according to strain on the needle.

A catheter for sucking up fluids during surgery would work much the same way.

The company has successfully tested the technology on pigs but has yet to go through clinical trials and approval of the U.S. Food and Drug Administration (FDA), so the operating room is still a ways off. IFOS is also working with Civco Medical Solutions to develop needles with optical fiber sensing.

Meanwhile, at the University of Calgary, another team is working on a similar device for MRI-guided neurosurgery, known as

Robots and Their Use in Health Care

NeuroArm. IFOS sold the team an interrogator and outfitted a pair of surgical forceps with its fiber-optic sensors.

Sleep centers at Stanford and at the University of California, Los Angeles, are collaborating with IFOS on a device to monitor sleep apnea with a real-time pressure profile of the airway, and the company has a proposal pending with the NIH for similar technology to monitor male incontinence.

In all these applications, fiber-optic sensing allows for a thinner probe or surgical tool and uniquely high-resolution, multidimensional mapping.

In another project, the company is building on its robotic-hand experience to work with the NIH and George Mason University to develop a robotic prosthetic hand that combines IFOS' fiber-optic sensors with ultrasonic imaging technology that senses the activation of finger-specific muscles in the forearm. This lets the user control the fingers with high precision.

More recent NASA work will also likely lead to commercial applications in medicine and beyond. Under recent Small Business Technology Transfer (STTR) funding from Goddard Space Flight Center and Johnson, IFOS and Stanford are collaboratively developing specialized photonic integrated circuits (PICs), in this case for a "lab-on-a-chip" device to monitor concentrations of biochemicals such as protein and creatinine in animals and humans, including astronauts. The technology is similar to electronic integrated circuits, with a light source and various optical tools densely interconnected within a chip smaller than a fingernail.

"It's like a miniaturized, specialized photonic computing device or signal processor," says Moslehi. "And it works at the speed of light."

IFOS is already working with several PIC foundries to fabricate the optical chips, which could find a multitude of uses.

Black notes that while the interrogator used in the Robonaut work was desktop-sized, the one now being used for surgical devices is half the size of a shoebox. The company is working to reduce that to the size of a smartphone.

In the early days, says William Price, IFOS' strategic programs manager, "the cost to build a high-performance interrogator was

Health Technology Sourcebook, Third Edition

a significant limiting factor, but IFOS is continually working to reduce costs." IFOS recently completed beta testing and will soon launch a family of interrogators priced under $10,000, a fraction of the price of its first interrogators, he says, noting that he expects these new products to open up new applications for fiber-optic sensing beyond the medical industries. They will complement IFOS' other high-performance interrogators for acoustic and vibration measurements.

Moslehi says NASA in particular, as well as other federal agencies, has been instrumental in providing the funding needed to develop the company's technology innovations into products since the beginning. "Certainly, in the early days when IFOS was still run out of a garage in Silicon Valley, NASA funding was what helped us take off and develop this technology," he says.

Many of the projects since then, intended for use in spaceflight, rocket testing, atmospheric reentry, and other extreme environments, have kept that technology robust, reliable, and cutting-edge.

Chapter 29 | Advanced Therapies

Chapter Contents
Section 29.1—Tissue Engineering and Regenerative
Medicine...403
Section 29.2—NIST and the National Biotechnology
and Biomanufacturing Initiative.......................410
Section 29.3—Cartilage Engineering...412
Section 29.4—Light Therapy and Brain Function....................413
Section 29.5—Radiofrequency Thermal Ablation
as Tumor Therapy 416

Section 29.1 | Tissue Engineering and Regenerative Medicine

This section contains text excerpted from the following sources: Text beginning with the heading "What Are Tissue Engineering and Regenerative Medicine?" is excerpted from "NIBIB Tissue Engineering and Regenerative Medicine," National Institute of Biomedical Imaging and Bioengineering (NIBIB), November 2019; Text beginning with heading "Tissue Engineering and Regenerative Medicine Research Program" is excerpted from "Tissue Engineering and Regenerative Medicine Research Program," National Institute of Dental and Craniofacial Research (NIDCR), July 2018. Reviewed November 2022.

WHAT ARE TISSUE ENGINEERING AND REGENERATIVE MEDICINE?

Tissue engineering evolved from the field of biomaterials development and refers to combining scaffolds, cells, and biologically active molecules into functional tissues. The goal of tissue engineering is to assemble such fully functional constructs that restore, maintain, or improve damaged tissue or a whole organ. Skin and cartilage are examples of engineered tissue that have already been approved by the U.S. Department of Food and Drug Administration (FDA); however, currently, they have limited use in human patients.

Regenerative medicine is a broad field that includes tissue engineering but also incorporates the idea of self-healing—where the body uses its own systems, sometimes with help from added biological material from outside the body, to recreate cells or rebuild organs. The terms "tissue engineering" and "regenerative medicine" have become largely interchangeable, as the field hopes to focus on the cure instead of treatment for complex, often chronic diseases.

The field continues to evolve. In addition to medical applications, nontherapeutic applications include using tissues as biosensors to detect biological or chemical threat agents and tissue chips that can be used to test the toxicity of an experimental medication.

HOW DO TISSUE ENGINEERING AND REGENERATIVE MEDICINE WORK?

Cells are the building blocks of tissue, but tissues are the basic unit of function in the body. Generally, groups of cells make and secrete their own support structures, called the "extracellular matrix." This matrix, or scaffold, does more than just support the cells; it also

403

Health Technology Sourcebook, Third Edition

acts as a relay station for various signaling molecules. Thus, cells receive messages from many sources that become available from the local environment. Each signal can start a chain of responses that determine what happens to the cell. By understanding how individual cells respond to signals, interact with their environment, and organize into tissues and organisms, researchers have been able to manipulate these processes to mend damaged tissues or even create new ones.

The process often begins with building a scaffold from a wide set of possible sources, from proteins to plastics. Once scaffolds are created, cells with or without a "cocktail" of growth factors can be introduced. If the environment is fertile, a tissue develops. In some cases, the cells, scaffolds, and growth factors are all mixed together at once, allowing the tissue to "self-assemble."

Another method to create new tissue uses an existing scaffold. The cells of a donor organ are stripped, and the remaining collagen scaffold is used to grow new tissue. This process has been used to bioengineer heart, liver, lung, and kidney tissue. This approach holds great promise for using scaffolding from human tissue discarded during surgery, combined with a patient's own cells, to make customized organs that would not be rejected by the immune system.

HOW DO TISSUE ENGINEERING AND REGENERATIVE MEDICINE FIT IN WITH CURRENT MEDICAL PRACTICES?

Currently, tissue engineering plays a relatively small role in patient treatment. Supplemental bladders, small arteries, skin grafts, cartilage, and even a full trachea have been implanted in patients, but the procedures are still experimental and very costly. While more complex organ tissues, such as heart, lung, and liver tissue, have been successfully recreated in the lab, they are a long way from being fully reproducible and ready to implant in a patient. These tissues, however, can be quite useful in research, especially in drug development. Using functioning human tissue to help screen medication candidates could speed up development, saving money and animals, and provide key tools for facilitating personalized medicine.

Advanced Therapies

WHAT ARE NIBIB-FUNDED RESEARCHERS DEVELOPING IN THE AREAS OF TISSUE ENGINEERING AND REGENERATIVE MEDICINE?

Research supported by the National Institute of Biomedical Imaging and Bioengineering (NIBIB) includes the development of new scaffold materials and new tools to fabricate, image, monitor, and preserve engineered tissues. Some examples of research in this area are described below:

- **Controlling stem cells through their environment.** For many years, scientists have searched for ways to control how stem cells develop into other cell types in the hopes of creating new therapies. Two NIBIB researchers have grown pluripotent cells—stem cells that have the ability to turn into any kind of cell—in different types of defined spaces and found that this confinement triggered very specific gene networks that determined the ultimate fate of the cells. Most other medical research on pluripotent stem cells have focused on modifying the combination of growth solutions in which the cells are placed. The discovery that there is a biomechanical element to controlling how stem cells transform into other cell types is an important piece of the puzzle as scientists try to harness stem cells for medical uses.
- **Implanting human livers in mice.** The NIBIB-funded researchers have engineered human liver tissue that can be implanted in a mouse. The mouse retains its own liver as well and therefore its normal function, but the added engineered human liver can metabolize drugs in the same way humans do. This allows researchers to test susceptibility to toxicity and to demonstrate species-specific responses that typically do not show up until clinical trials. Using engineered human tissue in this way could cut down on the time and cost of producing new drugs, as well as allow critical examinations of drug–drug interactions within a humanlike system.
- **New hope for the bum knee.** An NIBIB-funded tissue engineer has developed a biological gel that can be

Health Technology Sourcebook, Third Edition

injected into a cartilage defect following microfracture surgery to create an environment that facilitates regeneration. However, in order for this gel to stay in place within the knee, researchers also developed a new biological adhesive that is able to bond to both the gel as well as the damaged cartilage in the knee, keeping the newly regrown cartilage in place. The gel/adhesive combo was successful in regenerating cartilage tissue following surgery in a clinical trial of 15 patients, all of whom reported decreased pain at six months post-surgery. In contrast, the majority of microfracture patients, after an initial decrease in pain, returned to their original pain level within six months. This researcher worked in collaboration with another NIBIB grantee to image the patients who had undergone surgery, enabling scientists to combine new, noninvasive methods to see the evolving results in real time.

- **Engineering mature bone stem cells.** Researchers funded by NIBIB completed the first published study that has been able to take stem cells all the way from their pluripotent—state to mature bone grafts that could potentially be transplanted in a patient. Previously, investigators could only differentiate the cells into a primitive version of the tissue, which was not fully functional. Additionally, the study found that when the bone was implanted in immunodeficient mice, there was no abnormal growth afterward—a problem that often occurs after implanting stem cells or bone scaffolds alone.

TISSUE ENGINEERING AND REGENERATIVE MEDICINE RESEARCH PROGRAM

The National Institute of Dental and Craniofacial Research (NIDCR) encourages basic and translational research that takes advantage of advances in biology, chemistry, material science, nanotechnology, computer science, and engineering to develop tissue

Advanced Therapies

constructs that mimic the structure and function of native oral and craniofacial tissues including bone, cartilage, skeletal muscle, vascular and neural components of the craniofacial skeleton and temporomandibular joint, teeth, periodontal ligament, oral mucosa, and salivary glands. Areas of interest include but are not limited to:

- Cell-instructive and structural scaffolds, including biomimetic and nanotechnology-based scaffolds, capable of delivering bioactive molecules at specific concentrations in a temporally and spatially defined fashion and conferring external geometry, internal architecture, and mechanical properties to engineered constructs
- Scaffolds fabricated from smart materials able to respond to environmental cues
- Three-dimensional in vitro bioreactors, including nanotechnology and microfluidics-based bioreactors that recapitulate normal and pathological tissue development, structure, and function
- Medium- and high-throughput assay systems, including nanotechnology and microfluidics-based microphysiological systems (also called "tissue chips") for drug screening, studying mechanisms of disease, and other applications
- Tissue and organ biofabrication or "printing" technologies that use layered manufacturing processes, such as rapid prototyping
- Functional dynamic imaging of the dental and craniofacial tissues
- Application of mechanical forces and electrical stimulation in shaping functional characteristics of engineered tissues
- Isolation, characterization, expansion, and differentiation of stem and progenitor cells for the engineering of dental, oral, and craniofacial (DOC) tissues
- Optimization, standardization, and side-by-side comparison and quality control of stem and progenitor

cell sources for use in DOC tissue engineering and regeneration

- Engineering of composite multi-tissue constructs, such as vascularized and innervated bone and skeletal muscle

FUNCTIONAL INTEGRATION OF ENGINEERED CONSTRUCTS INTO NATIVE HOST TISSUE

The NIDCR encourages research concerning functional and structural integration between the engineered tissue constructs and host DOC tissues. Areas of interest include but are not limited to:

- Optimization of grafting strategies of engineered tissue constructs
- Biocompatibility, immunogenicity, biotoxicity, and biodegradability of tissue engineering biomaterials and scaffolds in animal models, including preclinical large animal models
- Vascularization and innervation of grafted engineered constructs
- Augmentation of hierarchical intertissue interfaces in the tooth, craniofacial skeleton, and temporomandibular joint
- Cell tracing approaches to monitor in vivo cell proliferation, differentiation, reprogramming, survival, and migration
- Small and large animal models to assess short- and long-term structural and functional integrity of engineered tissue constructs in vivo

MECHANISTIC STUDIES OF DOC TISSUE DAMAGE AND REGENERATION

The NIDCR encourages research on cellular and molecular mechanisms of DOC tissue damage, degeneration, aging, and regeneration. Areas of interest include but are not limited to:

- Destruction and regeneration of the periodontium and inflammatory bone erosion associated with periodontal disease

Advanced Therapies

- Distinct molecular and cellular mechanisms of intramembranous and endochondral bone regeneration
- Osteogenesis, angiogenesis, and matrix remodeling during bone regeneration
- Augmentation of craniofacial bone regeneration
- Characterization of in situ stem and progenitor populations and stem cell niches that contribute to tissue regeneration of DOC tissues
- Responses of fibrocartilage to injury and trauma
- Dentin-pulp complex homeostasis, injury, regeneration, and other types of therapy
- Inflammation resolution, wound healing, connective tissue remodeling, and scarless wound healing
- Impact of biophysical forces on tissue damage and regeneration

PROMOTING ENDOGENOUS HOST TISSUE HEALING AND REGENERATION

The NIDCR encourages research that takes advantage of advances in biology, chemistry, material science, nanotechnology, computer science, and engineering to facilitate the regeneration of endogenous DOC tissues. This part of the program welcomes basic and translational research directed at the patterning of the host tissue microenvironment to resolve acute and chronic inflammation, reduce tissue fibrosis, and promote vascularization, innervation, and scarless wound healing. Areas of interest include but are not limited to:

- Targeted and controlled delivery, including temporal, spatial, and combinatorial delivery to tissues of therapeutic molecules, genes, and gene products that modify endogenous tissue microenvironment
- Scaffolds and biomolecules that guide the self-organization of endogenous or exogenous cells into tissues in vivo
- Recapitulation of structure and function of native stem cell niches in vivo
- Directed cell homing and migration and reprogramming in vivo

Health Technology Sourcebook, Third Edition

Section 29.2 | **NIST and the National Biotechnology and Biomanufacturing Initiative**

This section includes text excerpted from "NIST and the National Biotechnology and Biomanufacturing Initiative," National Institute of Standards and Technology (NIST), September 14, 2022.

President Biden's Executive Order 14028 on Advancing Biotechnology and Biomanufacturing Innovation for a Sustainable, Safe, and Secure American Economy was issued on September 12, 2022. This Executive Order (EO) launches a National Biotechnology and Biomanufacturing Initiative to focus federal investments that transform biotechnology discoveries into solutions for critical problems.

The EO directs the National Institute of Standards and Technology (NIST), in partnership with federal and other stakeholders, to:

- Create and make publicly available a lexicon to assist in the development of measurements and measurement methods of the bioeconomy. The lexicon will support important needs in economic measurement, risk assessments, and the application of machine learning and other artificial intelligence tools.
- Take steps to improve the nation's cybersecurity for biological data and bio-related software, consistent with President Biden's Executive Order 14028. The NIST will coordinate with relevant interagency partners to identify and recommend relevant cybersecurity best practices for biological data stored on federal government information systems and consider bio-related software, including software for laboratory equipment, instrumentation, and data management, in establishing baseline security standards for the development of software sold to the government.

The NIST will also play a role, along with other Department of Commerce (DOC) bureaus, in contributing to a report assessing how biotechnology and biomanufacturing can be used to strengthen the resilience of U.S. supply chains and help address

Advanced Therapies

challenges in biomanufacturing supply chains and related biotechnology development infrastructure in creating a vibrant, domestic biomanufacturing ecosystem.

Under Secretary of Commerce for Standards and Technology and NIST, Director Laurie E. Locascio lauded the administration's actions to support biomanufacturing and biotechnology, stating, "The National Institute of Standards and Technology is a leader in advancing measurement science, standards, data, and tools for emerging biotechnologies. This Executive Order emphasizes the importance of federal engagement with industry to achieve a strong and resilient domestic bioeconomy, and NIST's critical role for the nation."

The NIST provides innovative solutions aligned with the goals of the National Biotechnology and Biomanufacturing Initiative through:

- Advancing research and development in engineering biology, biomanufacturing measurements and technologies, standards, and data for impacts in health care, climate change and environmental sustainability, food and agriculture, and supply chain resilience
- Public–private partnerships within the Manufacturing USA network, including the DOC-sponsored National Institute for Innovation in Manufacturing Biopharmaceuticals (NIIMBL), and connections through the Bioindustrial Manufacturing and Design Ecosystem (BioMADE) and BioFabUSA
- Convening industrial, government, and academic stakeholders through NIST-led consortia
- Efforts to strengthen the biomanufacturing and biotechnology supply chains within the Manufacturing Extension Partnership (MEP)

The NIST will work with the DOC bureaus and other federal agencies to support the EO's principles of focusing federal investments to transform biotechnology discoveries into tangible benefits, expand domestic biomanufacturing capacity, and maintain America's competitive edge in biotechnology and biomanufacturing.

Health Technology Sourcebook, Third Edition

Section 29.3 | **Cartilage Engineering**

This section includes text excerpted from "Engineered Cartilage Produces Anti-Inflammatory Drug," National Institute on Aging (NIA), National Institutes of Health (NIH), February 24, 2021.

Joints such as those in the knees and hands rely on cartilage tissue to keep the bones from rubbing together. Wear and tear over a lifetime can cause the cartilage to break down. This leads to a condition called "osteoarthritis."

The symptoms of osteoarthritis can include joint pain, stiffness, and swelling. More than 30 million adults nationwide are living with the condition. Currently, no treatments exist to prevent or reverse its progression.

Researchers have been interested in growing new cartilage in the lab that could be implanted into joints. However, joints with arthritis contain many molecules that promote chronic inflammation. This inflammation, plus the physical stress produced by normal movement, can destroy replacement cartilage quickly.

A research team led by Dr. Farshid Guilak from Washington University in St. Louis has been testing whether cartilage cells could be engineered to protect themselves from inflammation. In a proof-of-concept study, the team altered cartilage cells from pigs to produce an anti-inflammatory molecule when stressed.

The study was funded in part by NIH's National Institute of Arthritis and Musculoskeletal and Skin Diseases (NIAMS), National Institute on Aging (NIA), and National Center for Advancing Translational Sciences (NCATS). Results were published on January 27, 2021, in *Science Advances*.

The researchers first identified a protein called "TRPV4" in the membrane of cartilage cells that senses alterations within cells under compression. They found that TRPV4 becomes activated by a change to the fluid in cells called "osmotic loading." The protein can also be triggered by mechanical forces.

The team showed that in response, TRPV4 activates specific genetic pathways in cartilage cells associated with inflammation and metabolism. The researchers modified these genetic circuits to produce an anti-inflammatory molecule called "interleukin-1

Advanced Therapies

receptor antagonist" (IL-1Ra). Cells with these circuits were then grown to form cartilage.

When exposed to either mechanical forces or osmotic loading, the engineered cells produced IL-1Ra. The timing and duration of production depended on which genetic circuit was used. This suggests that production could be customized by harnessing different cellular pathways that turn on and off at different times.

Finally, the researchers tested whether the production of IL-1Ra could protect cartilage cells in an inflammatory environment, similar to that seen in osteoarthritis. They exposed the engineered cartilage to both an inflammatory molecule and osmotic loading for three days.

By the end of that period, the cartilage that did not produce IL-1Ra was breaking down. In contrast, the cartilage that produced the molecule maintained its structure and strength.

These findings demonstrate the ability to engineer living tissue to produce its own therapeutic drugs. "We think this strategy could be a framework for doing what we might need to do to program cells to deliver therapies in response to a variety of medical problems," Guilak says.

Section 29.4 | Light Therapy and Brain Function

This section includes text excerpted from "Shining a Healing Light on the Brain," Argonne National Laboratory (ANL), U.S. Department of Energy (DOE), March 24, 2021.

Scientists made the pivotal discovery of a method for wireless modulation of neurons with x-rays that could improve the lives of patients with brain disorders. The x-ray source only requires a machinelike that is found in a dentist's office.

Many people worldwide suffer from movement-related brain disorders. Epilepsy accounts for more than 50 million; essential tremor, 40 million; and Parkinson disease (PD), 10 million.

Relief for some brain disorder sufferers may one day be on the way in the form of a new treatment invented by researchers from the U.S. Department of Energy's (DOE) Argonne National Laboratory and four universities. The treatment is based on breakthroughs in both optics and genetics. It would be applicable to not only movement-related brain disorders but also chronic depression and pain.

This new treatment involves stimulation of neurons deep within the brain by means of injected nanoparticles that light up when exposed to x-rays (nanoscintillators) and would eliminate an invasive brain surgery currently in use.

"Our high-precision noninvasive approach could become routine with the use of a small X-ray machine, the kind commonly found in every dental office," said Dr. Elena Rozhkova, a lead author and a nanoscientist in Argonne's Center for Nanoscale Materials (CNM), a DOE Office of Science User Facility.

Traditional deep brain stimulation requires an invasive neurosurgical procedure for disorders when conventional drug therapy is not an option. In the traditional procedure, approved by the U.S. Food and Drug Administration (FDA), surgeons implant a calibrated pulse generator under the skin (similar to a pacemaker). They then connect it with an insulated extension cord to electrodes inserted into a specific area of the brain to stimulate the surrounding neurons and regulate abnormal impulses.

"The Spanish-American scientist José Manuel Rodríguez Delgado famously demonstrated deep brain stimulation in a bullring in the 1960s," said Vassiliy Tsytsarev, a neurobiologist from the University of Maryland and a coauthor of the study. "He brought a raging bull charging at him to a standstill by sending a radio signal to an implanted electrode."

About 15 years ago, scientists introduced a revolutionary neuromodulation technology, "optogenetics," which relies on genetic modification of specific neurons in the brain. These neurons create a light-sensitive ion channel in the brain and, thereby, fire in response to external laser light. This approach, however, requires very thin fiber-optic wires implanted in the brain and suffers from the limited penetration depth of the laser light through biological tissues.

The team's alternative optogenetics approach uses nanoscintillators injected into the brain, bypassing implantable electrodes or

Advanced Therapies

fiber-optic wires. Instead of lasers, they substitute x-rays because of their greater ability to pass through biological tissue barriers.

"The injected nanoparticles absorb the X-ray energy and convert it into red light, which has significantly greater penetration depth than blue light," said Zhaowei Chen, former CNM postdoctoral fellow.

"Thus, the nanoparticles serve as an internal light source that makes our method work without a wire or electrode," added Rozhkova. Since the team's approach can both stimulate and quell targeted small areas, Rozhkova noted, it has other applications than brain disorders. For example, it could be applicable to heart problems and other damaged muscles.

One of the team's keys to success was the collaboration between two of the world-class facilities at Argonne: CNM and Argonne's Advanced Photon Source (APS), a DOE Office of Science User Facility. The work at these facilities began with the synthesis and multi-tool characterization of the nanoscintillators. In particular, the x-ray-excited optical luminescence of the nanoparticle samples was determined at an APS beamline (20-BM). The results showed that the particles were extremely stable over months and upon repeated exposure to the high-intensity x-rays.

According to Zou Finfrock, a staff scientist at the APS 20-BM beamline and Canadian Light Source, "They kept glowing a beautiful orange-red light."

Next, Argonne sent CNM-prepared nanoscintillators to the University of Maryland for tests in mice. The team at the University of Maryland performed these tests over two months with a small portable x-ray machine. The results proved that the procedure worked as planned. Mice whose brains had been genetically modified to react to red light responded to the x-ray pulses with brain waves recorded on an electroencephalogram.

Finally, the University of Maryland team sent the animal brains for characterization using x-ray fluorescence microscopy performed by Argonne scientists. This analysis was performed by Olga Antipova on the Microprobe beamline (2-ID-E) at APS and by Zhonghou Cai on the Hard X-ray Nanoprobe (26-ID) jointly operated by CNM and APS.

Health Technology Sourcebook, Third Edition

This multi-instrument arrangement made it possible to see tiny particles residing in the complex environment of the brain tissue with a super-resolution of dozens of nanometers. It also allowed visualizing neurons near and far from the injection site on a microscale. The results proved that the nanoscintillators are chemically and biologically stable. They do not wander from the injection site or degrade.

"Sample preparation is extremely important in these types of biological analysis," said Antipova, a physicist in the x-ray Science Division (XSD) at the APS. Antipova was assisted by Qiaoling Jin and Xueli Liu, who prepared brain sections only a few micrometers thick with jeweler-like accuracy.

"There is an intense level of commercial interest in optogenetics for medical applications," said Rozhkova. "Although still at the proof-of-concept stage, we predict our patent-pending wireless approach with small X-ray machines should have a bright future."

Section 29.5 | Radiofrequency Thermal Ablation as Tumor Therapy

This section includes text excerpted from "Radiofrequency Thermal Ablation as Tumor Therapy," Clinical Center (CC), National Institutes of Health (NIH), May 19, 2022.

Recent developments in radiofrequency thermal ablation (RFA) have expanded the treatment options for certain oncology patients. Minimally invasive, image-guided therapy may now provide effective local treatment of isolated or localized neoplastic disease and can also be used as an adjunct to conventional surgery, systemic chemotherapy, or radiation. RFA expands the medical application of heat, which for decades has been used as a cautery device to cut tissue. In the procedure, the tumors are located with ultrasound, computed tomography (CT), or magnetic resonance (MR) imaging devices. Then, essentially, the patient is turned into an electrical circuit by placing grounding pads on the thighs. A small needle electrode with an insulated shaft and an uninsulated distal tip is

Advanced Therapies

inserted through the skin and directly into the tumor. Ionic vibration at the needle tip leads to frictional heat. After 10–30 minutes of contact with the tumor, the radio frequency energy kills a 2.5–5 cm sphere. The dead cells are not removed but become scar tissue and eventually shrink. RFA continues to play a time-tested, major role in the treatment of patients with painful osteoid osteomas in the bone and heart arrhythmias. In addition, RFA has been used to treat painful trigeminal neuralgia for 25 years. Today, the mainstream applications of RFA are increasing. In particular, this minimally invasive, percutaneous technique is showing promise as a treatment option for patients with primary or metastatic liver cancer.

Worldwide, primary liver cancer is the most common solid cancer, causing an estimated one million deaths annually. In the United States, 15,300 people were expected to be diagnosed with the disease in 2000, and 13,800 were expected to die. Hepatocellular carcinoma accounts for about 84 percent of primary liver cancers in the United States. The number of people expected to die from colorectal carcinoma metastases to the liver is even greater than that of people expected to die from primary liver cancer. Twenty to 25 percent of patients with colorectal carcinoma liver metastases are eligible for surgery, and of those, the five-year survival rate is approximately 30–40 percent. RFA may provide a safe and effective option for patients with inoperable or recurrent liver cancer who have failed to respond to conventional methods. Given the lack of effective treatment options for the majority of patients with primary liver cancer and metastases to the liver, the oncology team should be aware of this relatively new treatment.

In addition to the treatment of patients with liver cancers, clinical applications of RFA include treatment of kidney, adrenal, and prostate tumors; benign prostatic hyperplasia; painful or abnormal neural tissue; and painful soft tissue or bone masses that are unresponsive to conventional therapy.

Many times RFA can be an alternative to risky surgery, and sometimes, it can change a patient from having an inoperable tumor to being a candidate for surgery. The procedure is proving useful as an adjunct to conventional treatments and as a palliative treatment. What is more, the cauterizing effect of the heated needle

Health Technology Sourcebook, Third Edition

prevents excessive bleeding, leading to low complication rates. Although RFA may not be a magic bullet, it clearly can be a cure in some cases.

Multiple techniques have been studied and used to kill tumor cells. These techniques include laser, focused ultrasound, and microwave, as well as RFA, cryotherapy, and percutaneous ethanol injection (PEI). PEI has proven especially useful in treating primary liver tumors. In PEI, ethanol is injected directly into the tumor in multiple treatment sessions. Prospective, randomized clinical trials comparing PEI and RFA for the treatment of liver tumors are currently in progress. Cryotherapy is an ablation method that has been used primarily during open surgery after mobilizing the liver. It has limited applications due to the size of the treatment probe, expense, and excessive complications, such as liver capsule fracture. Cryotherapy may be less effective and more prone to complications than RFA for liver tumors although this is controversial. While these multiple technologies can destroy tissue, RFA has emerged as safe, cheap, and predictable and is becoming the treatment of choice for small but inoperable tumors of the liver.

Radiofrequency thermal ablation can usually be performed as an outpatient procedure under general anesthesia or conscious sedation. Alternatively, RFA may be performed laparoscopically or during open surgery.

Under light sedation, lidocaine or bupivacaine is administered subcutaneously at the needle entry site and down to the liver capsule. A needle is placed through the skin and into the tumor with imaging guidance. Treatment sessions of percutaneous RFA are easily monitored using real-time ultrasound imaging, computed tomography, or magnetic resonance imaging. Most patients feel little pain during the procedure and go home the same day or the day after the procedure, usually with minimal to no pain or soreness although there is a spectrum, and some patients will experience severe pain the day of the procedure.

During a 10–30 minute treatment session, nitrogen microbubbles gradually create a hyperechoic area on ultrasound that provides a rough estimation of the treated tissue, which is 2.5–5 cm per 10–30 minute treatment sphere. CT, MR imaging, or positron

Advanced Therapies

emission tomography (PET) imaging may provide more exquisite detail for follow-up verification of the treatment zone and for finding residual or recurrent neoplastic tissue. Although real-time MR imaging and CT are available, they are not in widespread use. Ultrasound is a safe, common, and easy guidance method although it is somewhat operator dependent.

Once the needle has been properly positioned within the tumor, the tissue is heated. At temperatures exceeding 50 °C, cells are destroyed. To treat tumors of different sizes and shapes, the needle is available in different lengths and shapes of exposed tips.

Energy is transferred from the uninsulated distal tip of the needle to the tissue as current rather than as direct heat. The circuit is completed with grounding pads placed on the patient's thighs. As the alternating current flows to the grounding pads, it agitates ions in the surrounding tissue, resulting in frictional heat. The tissue surrounding the needle is desiccated, creating an oval or spherical lesion of coagulation necrosis, typically 2.5–5 cm in diameter for each 10–30 minute treatment. These spheres are added together in three dimensions to overlap and completely envelop the tumor. Ideally, the treated tissue will contain the entire tumor plus a variable rim of healthy tissue as a safety margin.

Failure to ablate the entire tumor with clean edges results in the regrowth of the tumor. Depending on the size and configuration of the new growth, the patient may or may not be suited for another treatment session. Over months to years, as the dead necrotic cells are reabsorbed and replaced by scar tissue and fibrosis, the size of the thermal lesion shrinks although the remaining cells are ideally dead. The possibility of successful surgical resection may be augmented by decreasing the number of tumors. Treatment of a tumor in one lobe may broaden the surgical indications of a tumor in the other lobe. Due to the natural course of the disease, new or recurrent tumors may be suited for additional treatment sessions as well.

Various methods of increasing the volume of treated tissue have been explored. One type of ablation needle-electrode consists of a coaxial system or an expandable needle within a needle. The inner hooks are deployed once properly situated within the tumor. Different configurations allow for the treatment of various shapes and locations of tumors. Another ablation system utilizes a triple parallel needle array, which synergistically increases the treated volume.

At temperatures exceeding 100–110 °C, the tissue surrounding the needle vaporizes. The gas from the vaporization insulates the area immediately around the needle, limiting energy deposition in the target zone and decreasing the volume of tissue treated. Overcooking or charring around the outside of the needle also insulates and causes incomplete destruction of target tissue remote from the needle, much like a hamburger cooked too fast on a grill, charred on the outside, and raw in the middle.

The deleterious effects of charring and vaporization may be decreased by monitoring temperature and/or impedance during treatment and adjusting the current accordingly. The generators have computer chips or treatment algorithms to assist in optimizing this process. One system perfuses chilled saline within a closed-tip needle in order to deposit more energy without increasing the temperature. This system allows an increase in the lesion diameter while keeping the temperatures below the vaporization point.

At the end of a treatment session, the active needle is slowly retracted to heat and cauterize the needle pathway. This action prevents bleeding and tumor seeding of the needle track by destroying any cell that becomes attached to the needle or dislodged in the needle tract.

LIVER CANCER AND RADIOFREQUENCY THERMAL ABLATION

Radiofrequency thermal ablation may be most effective in primary liver cancer (hepatocellular carcinoma or hepatoma). Primary tumors are often soft and encapsulated and usually occur in a cirrhotic liver, allowing for effective disbursement and retention of the heat. Although surgery and liver transplant are considered the only curative treatment for hepatocellular carcinoma, few patients are eligible. Eligibility criteria tend to vary by institution and physician. Contraindications include multiple tumors, decreased liver function, or multiple medical problems. While controlled, long-term studies of RFA have not been done, survival rates are likely to be similar to that of patients undergoing surgery or PEI treatment.

Advanced Therapies

With a median follow-up of only 15 months, Curley and colleagues reported a 1.8 percent short-term recurrence rate following RFA of 169 tumors (median diameter 3.4 cm) in 123 patients with primary or metastatic liver cancer. RFA clearly can provide short-term local control of small, early, or focal liver cancer. The question remains if this finding of a low short-term recurrence rate will translate into prolonged survival. Extrapolation of data from the surgical literature for resection of solitary liver tumors suggests that successful local control may lead to prolonged survival. Combination therapies need to be further studied for impact on survival as well.

Current studies are underway to evaluate the long-term efficacy of RFA for liver tumors. As yet, there have been no long-term, randomized studies, and the long-term benefits are thus somewhat speculative. Still, preliminary, short-term results are promising and suggest that this therapy can impact certain patients' survival.

KIDNEY CANCER AND RADIO FREQUENCY THERMAL ABLATION

Radio frequency thermal ablation is being studied as a minimally invasive treatment for patients with kidney cancer. An effective, minimally invasive therapy could postpone kidney failure and prolong kidney function in patients with multiple or hereditary kidney cancer, such as von Hippel-Lindau disease, which causes multiple, recurrent, and diffuse tumors. RFA may also provide a useful option for patients who are not operative candidates or have solitary kidneys, multiple medical problems, or unresectable tumors.

Surgery for benign prostate hyperplasia and prostate cancer is not without morbidity. RFA may provide a safer option for removing abnormal prostate tissue, as well as predictably destroying the entire gland with a low complication rate to the adjacent rectum, sphincter, bladder base, and urethra.

RFA may also provide a method for alleviating pain that is unresponsive to conventional treatment or to complement treatments that have a delayed response. For example, radiation therapy for painful bone metastases can average four weeks to show effect. Studies are underway to investigate the efficacy of RFA in the

Health Technology Sourcebook, Third Edition

palliation of painful bone tumors and painful peripheral soft tissue tumors that are unresponsive or poorly responsive to conventional treatment. Preliminary data suggest that RFA may provide rapid pain relief for many tumors in the days following treatment and thus may decrease dependence on sedating painkillers.

Ablation of nerve and nerve ganglia continues to be used safely and effectively in the treatment of multiple pain syndromes, including trigeminal neuralgia, cluster headaches, chronic segmental thoracic pain, cervicobrachialgia, and plantar fasciitis.

Patients with functional or tumorous disorders of the brain, such as Parkinson disease (PD), and benign or malignant lesions may also be candidates for RFA although it is experimental for brain tumors. One feasibility series on RFA for breast cancer in five patients suggests that it might play a role in select patient populations; however, this is also experimental.

WHAT ARE THE COMPLICATIONS OF RADIO FREQUENCY ABLATION?

Although RFA is relatively safe and minimally invasive, the benefits do not come without slight risks. The reported complication rate has been estimated at nearly two percent and may include bleeding, effusion, fever, and infection. The proximity to vital structures may influence the risk of collateral damage. The risks are kept to a minimum by attention to detail as well as continuous monitoring of vital signs and oxygenation and preprocedural blood tests. Complications are usually managed nonoperatively.

The heating treatment inherent to RFA actually stops bleeding. The 14–17.5 gauge needles are very small; they are the same size needles used for biopsy, with the added benefits of cauterization and coagulation. The low rate of bleeding seen with RFA is likely the result of this cauterization effect, which is similar to electrocautery used to stop bleeding during surgery. This same treatment of the needle track should minimize the risk of needle-track seeding in the systems that are capable of cauterizing the track. The predictable nature of RFA allows for little collateral damage during treatments situated near vital structures. In fact, the "heat sink effect" actually preserves the vessels near a treatment area. However, with

Advanced Therapies

this effect, the inflow of "cool" blood at body temperature (cool relative to the cooked tissue) may impair the heating of the tumor cells closest to the vessels. The protected vessel often harbors an adjacent tumor that may regrow adjacent to large vessels.

Combining RFA therapy with chemoembolization can selectively block blood flow to a tumor and thus may provide more effective treatment for larger tumors. Combining local radiation or local chemotherapy infusion with RFA could also be more effective than any one treatment alone. Doxorubicin has been shown in mice to enhance the effects of RFA by increasing the volume of the tumor treated. Early reports of combining RFA with chemotherapy infusion and chemoembolization should lead to larger studies of such combination therapies.

A wide variety of clinical applications for RFA are being developed. If a target can be seen with CT, MR, or ultrasound, then a needle can be placed into it. If a needle can be placed, then the target tissue or tumor can be ablated and destroyed. If a clean margin is created, then the tumor will not recur at that site. Recent developments in RFA allow this treatment process to be done in a safe, predictable, and cheap fashion with low complication rates and minimal discomfort on an outpatient basis. Further study is required to assess which patients will benefit from this new treatment, and most cancer patients will not be candidates due to the size or location of the tumor. Although long-term data have yet to be reported, early results suggest that RFA may prove to be an effective treatment option or adjunct for many oncology patients.

Part 7 | Rehabilitation and Assistive Technologies

Chapter 30 | **Rehabilitation Engineering**

WHAT IS REHABILITATION ENGINEERING?

Rehabilitation engineering is the use of engineering science and principles to:

- Develop technological solutions and devices to assist individuals with disabilities.
- Aid the recovery of physical and cognitive functions lost because of disease or injury.

Rehabilitation engineers design and build devices and systems to meet a wide range of needs that can assist individuals with mobility, communication, hearing, vision, and cognition. These tools help people with day-to-day activities and tasks related to employment, independent living, and education.

Rehabilitation engineering may involve relatively simple observations of how workers perform tasks and then making accommodations to eliminate further injuries and discomfort. On the other end of the spectrum, more complex rehabilitation engineering is the design of sophisticated brain–computer interfaces that allow a severely disabled individual to operate computers and other assistive devices simply by thinking about the task they want to perform.

This chapter contains text excerpted from the following sources: Text beginning with the heading "What Is Rehabilitation Engineering?" is excerpted from "Rehabilitation Engineering Fact Sheet," National Institute of Biomedical Imaging and Bioengineering (NIBIB), June 2013. Reviewed November 2022; Text under the heading "Disability and Rehabilitation Engineering" is excerpted from "Disability and Rehabilitation Engineering (DARE)," National Science Foundation (NSF), September 10, 2019.

427

Health Technology Sourcebook, Third Edition

Rehabilitation engineers also develop and improve rehabilitation methods used by individuals to regain functions lost due to disease or injury, such as limb (arm and or leg) mobility following a stroke or a joint replacement.

WHAT TYPES OF ASSISTIVE DEVICES HAVE BEEN DEVELOPED THROUGH REHABILITATION ENGINEERING?

The following are examples of the many types of assistive devices:

- Wheelchairs, scooters, and prosthetic devices, such as artificial limbs that provide mobility for people with physical disabilities that affect movement
- Kitchen implements with large, cushioned grips to help people with weakness or arthritis in their hands with everyday living tasks
- Automatic page-turners, book holders, and adapted pencil grips that allow participation in educational activities in school and at home
- Medication dispensers with alarms that can help people remember to take their medicine on time
- Specially engineered computer programs that provide voice recognition to help people with sensory impairments use computer technology

HOW CAN FUTURE REHABILITATION ENGINEERING RESEARCH IMPROVE THE QUALITY OF LIFE FOR INDIVIDUALS?

Ongoing research in rehabilitation engineering involves the design and development of new, innovative assistive devices. An important research area focuses on the development of new technologies and techniques for improved therapies that help people regain physical or cognitive functions lost because of disease or injury. For example:

- **Rehabilitation robotics**. Involves the use of robots as therapy aids instead of solely as assistive devices. Intelligent rehabilitation robotics aids mobility training in individuals suffering from impaired movement, such as following a stroke.

Rehabilitation Engineering

- **Virtual rehabilitation**. Uses virtual reality simulation exercises for physical and cognitive rehabilitation. Compared to conventional therapies, virtual rehabilitation can offer several advantages. It is entertaining and motivates patients. It provides objective measures such as range of motion or game scores that can be stored on the computer operating the simulation. The virtual exercises can be performed at home by a patient and monitored by a therapist over the Internet (known as "telerehabilitation"), which offers convenience as well as reduced costs.
- **Improved prosthetics**. Includes smarter artificial legs. This is an area where researchers continue to make advances in design and function to better mimic natural limb movement and user intent.
- **Increased use of computers**. Involves increasingly sophisticated use of computers as the interface between the user and various devices to enable severely impaired individuals to increase independence and integration into the community. For example, brain–computer interfaces use the brain's electrical impulses to allow individuals to learn to move a computer cursor or a robotic arm that can reach and grab items.
- **Development of new technologies**. Helps analyze human motion, better understand the electrophysiology of muscle and brain activity, and more accurately monitor human functions. These technologies will continue to drive innovation in assistive devices and rehabilitation strategies.

WHAT ARE NIBIB-FUNDED RESEARCHERS DEVELOPING IN THE AREA OF REHABILITATION ENGINEERING?

Promising research currently supported by the National Institute of Biomedical Imaging and Bioengineering (NIBIB) includes a wide range of approaches and technological development. Several examples are described below:

- **Wireless tongue drive system for paralyzed patients**. The NIBIB-funded researchers are developing an assistive technology called the "Tongue Drive System" (TDS). The core TDS technology exploits the fact that even individuals with severe paralysis that impairs limb movement, breathing, and speech can still move their tongue. Simple tongue movements send commands to the computer allowing users to steer their wheelchairs, operate their computers, and generally control their environment in an independent fashion.

- **Neurostimulation in individuals with spinal cord injury (SCI) for recovery of voluntary control of standing and movement and involuntary control of blood pressure, bladder, and sexual function**. Through the NIBIB Rehabilitation Engineering program, researchers are developing the next generation of high-density electrode arrays for stimulation of the spinal cord. The first patient received a current-generation electrical stimulator implant in his lower back. The electrical stimulation and locomotor training resulted in the ability to stand independently for several minutes, some voluntary leg control, and regained blood pressure control, bladder, bowel, and sexual function. Three more patients have received this treatment and had similar results.

- **Smart environment technologies**. As the population ages, increasing numbers of Americans are unable to live independently. The NIBIB-funded researchers are working on creating smart environments that aid with home health monitoring and intervention, allowing individuals with health issues to remain safely at home. For example, researchers are analyzing the needs and limitations of Alzheimer disease patients to develop automated and reminder-based technologies that can be integrated into the home to help with everyday tasks.

- **Artificial hands capable of complex movements and sensations**. Persons with hand amputations expect modern hand prostheses to function like intact hands. Current state-of-the-art prosthetic hands

Rehabilitation Engineering

simply control two movements: "open" and "close." As a result, the NIBIB researchers are developing new artificial hand systems that would perform complex hand motions based on measurements of the residual electrical signals from the remaining muscles of an amputee's forearm. Signals from the muscles (in one project) and nerves (from another project) have the potential to result in much finer control of the fingers in the artificial hand.

In addition, one of the teams is working on capturing the sense of touch, so in the future, the users will be able to also "feel" what they are holding with their artificial hand.

DISABILITY AND REHABILITATION ENGINEERING

Disability and Rehabilitation Engineering (DARE) supports fundamental engineering research that improves the quality of life of persons with disabilities through the development of new technologies. Projects advance knowledge regarding a specific disability, pathological motion, or injury mechanism.

The DARE program is part of the Engineering Biology and Health cluster, which also includes:

- The Biophotonics program
- The Biosensing program
- The Cellular and Biochemical Engineering program
- The Engineering of Biomedical Systems program

The Disability and Rehabilitation Engineering program supports fundamental engineering research that will improve the quality of life of persons with disabilities through the development of new technologies, devices, or software combined with the advancement of knowledge regarding healthy or pathological human motion or advancement in the understanding of injury mechanisms.

Research may be supported that is directed toward the characterization, restoration, rehabilitation, and/or substitution of human functional ability or cognition or to the interaction between persons with disabilities and their environment. Areas of particular

Health Technology Sourcebook, Third Edition

interest are neuroengineering and rehabilitation robotics. The program will also consider research in the areas of new engineering approaches to understand healthy or pathological motion, both as a target for rehabilitation and as a means to characterize motion related to disability or injury; understanding injury at the tissue or system level such that interventions may be developed to reduce the impact of trauma and subsequent disability; or understanding the role of gut microbiota in modulating disability in the context of rehabilitation.

Chapter 31 | Vision and Hearing Loss

Chapter Contents
Section 31.1—Low Vision and Blindness Rehabilitation..........435
Section 31.2—Artificial Retina..446
Section 31.3—Cochlear Implants: Different Kinds
of Hearing 449

Section 31.1 | Low Vision and Blindness Rehabilitation

This section includes text excerpted from "Vision Research: Needs, Gaps, and Opportunities," National Eye Institute (NEI), August 2012. Reviewed November 2022.

Low vision is an impairment to vision that hampers one's ability to function in daily life. Low vision is not correctable with medical or surgical therapies, spectacles, or contact lenses. Although low vision most often includes loss of sharpness or acuity, there may also be reduced field of vision, abnormal light sensitivity, distorted vision, or loss of contrast.

Visual impairment can range from mild to severe, including total blindness or functional blindness, where no useful vision remains. Although important advances have been made in treating and preventing eye diseases and disorders that cause visual impairment, many remain incurable. According to the World Health Organization (WHO), about 314 million people have visual impairment worldwide, of which 45 million are blind. Conservative estimates suggest that there are at least 3.6 million Americans who have visual impairment, of which more than one million are legally blind.

Low vision may occur as a result of birth defects, injury, or aging or as a complication of the disease. More than two-thirds of people with visual impairment are older than 65 years of age, and the leading causes are age-related macular degeneration, glaucoma, diabetic retinopathy, cataract, and optic nerve atrophy. Visual impairment in the elderly decreases independence, increases the risk of falls and fractures, and often leads to isolation and depression. Visual impairment also affects infants and children due to conditions such as retinopathy of prematurity, deficits in the visual centers of the brain, juvenile cataract, and retinal abnormalities. These conditions can severely impair a child's quality of life and can have major consequences on educational advancement and future opportunities for employment. Visual impairment treatment and rehabilitation is an important component of visual health care in the United States. Ophthalmologists and optometrists who specialize in low vision may choose from an assortment of specialized eyewear, filters,

Health Technology Sourcebook, Third Edition

magnifiers, adaptive equipment, closed-circuit television systems, and independent living aids and may offer training and counseling to patients. Although assistive devices and services do not cure visual disorders, research in this field leads to improved devices and new approaches designed to enhance the quality of life for millions of individuals with visual impairment.

RECENT PROGRESS IN LOW VISION AND BLINDNESS REHABILITATION
Assistive Technology

Because most content on the Internet is displayed visually, several new applications are geared to interpret this content for users with visual impairment, such as dynamic pin displays for online Braille and tactile graphics. Recent advances in computing power and image processing have revolutionized applications for individuals with visual impairment. Screen-magnifying and screen-reading software are widely deployed so that computers and smartphones are now accessible to users who have low vision and are blind without the need for costly third-party software accessories. The latest generation of smartphones has stimulated the development of innovative products to aid individuals with visual impairment. These include flexible image magnifiers, mobile optical character recognition, barcode readers, and indoor wayfinding aids. In the past few years, research and development of global positioning system-based navigation aids for people with visual impairment have refined commercially available products.

Behavioral and Neuroscience Basic Research

When we move around our environment, in our mind's eye, we construct a picture of the world around us. This picture, or cognitive map, is attributed to a neural network thought to be located in the medial temporal brain area. The parietal area of the brain is closely tied to the accrual of perceptual information. The interaction between the parietal and temporal regions may explain how ongoing perceptual input leads to the formation of cognitive maps and has implications for understanding how

Vision and Hearing Loss

individuals with visual impairment learn different strategies for orienting and navigating.

Following pathological insult to the retina or brain, perceptual training techniques have been examined using video games. Behavioral studies have demonstrated that extensive practice can improve visual sensitivity. Infants with congenital cataracts or other treatable eye conditions experience visual deprivation during a period of robust visual development. Studies of these children are finding that once vision is restored, substantial functional and organizational changes in the visual cortex occur; whether the same holds true later in life is an actively debated topic. This neuroplasticity can now be studied noninvasively with functional magnetic resonance imaging. These findings regarding plasticity hold promise for informing vision rehabilitation efforts.

Different areas of the brain respond to different types of perceptual stimuli (vision, touch, and sound). Perception depends on integrating this multisensory information. Research shows that normally sighted as well as individuals with visual impairment recruit the visual cortex when interpreting tactile or auditory information. The functional roles of such cross-modal activations are not well understood but are hot topics of current research and may provide the neural basis for sensory substitution, where perceptual processing for one sensory modality is largely replaced for another.

Implications of Vision Loss

With an increased understanding of the interdependence of physical and mental health, vision loss has been shown to be an independent predictor of depression. Depression (both major depressive disorders and subthreshold depression) affects roughly one-third of older adults with vision loss, which is similar to rates found among medically ill populations and those with other chronic conditions. In the visually impaired, depression further exacerbates functional disability in everyday activities. Thus, visual impairment has been found to have widespread negative effects on quality of life and psychological and social well-being.

Quality of Life

Quality-of-life (QOL) issues are gaining increased attention in vision impairment and rehabilitation research. With the development of standardized metrics (e.g., the National Eye Institute (NEI) Visual Functioning Questionnaire), quality-of-life measurements complement objective measures of visual function. Furthermore, there is a growing recognition that QOL is a multidimensional concept that includes financial status, employment, physical and mental health, social relationships, and recreation and leisure time activities.

Activities of Daily Living

Research on activities of daily living includes reading, mobility, and orientation in lab settings and real-world environments. Recent research has focused on the complicated visual environment encountered in the real world to appreciate how normally sighted and individuals with visual impairment process a visually rich environment. Extensive work relating reading to basic processes in visual perception (e.g., eye movement behavior during visual search) in sighted and visually impaired subjects has provided a solid theoretical foundation for developing improved rehabilitation regimens.

There has been significant progress in understanding visually guided behavior in natural settings. Using wavelet-based sensors to capture basic sensory information akin to a crude visual system, researchers are able to model which visual cues are needed to help individuals orient themselves in a complicated environment. In addition, real-world studies that elucidate the challenges that the visually impaired experience in complex public transportation environments and evaluate technologies that enhance safe and efficient street crossings in demanding urban environments have provided important data.

The development of objective measures of abilities to function in daily life has added to our understanding of the capacity for function and adds dimensions to research beyond self-reporting of difficulties with function.

Vision and Hearing Loss

Sight-Recovery Procedures

An impressive array of sight-recovery procedures are being studied in clinical trials, including retinal prostheses, gene therapy, and stem cell transplants. There are also global health initiatives increasing access to established therapies, such as cataract surgery or corrective lenses, to communities in developing countries that would otherwise remain visually impaired. There is an opportunity to study the behavioral and psychosocial impact of site recovery as well as implications for rehabilitation and neurodevelopment.

NEW MOBILE ASSISTIVE TECHNOLOGIES

For individuals with visual impairment, smartphone applications, commonly known as "apps," are emerging as important tools for everyday functioning and independence. The NEI-funded researchers are developing apps to assist individuals in maneuvering around obstacles and reading and recognizing faces and objects. For example, researchers are developing products that will allow the visually impaired to use smartphone cameras to identify packaged food content and prices at the grocery store by scanning the barcodes on the package labels. Another app scans money to determine bill denominations, which provides confidence to the user for transactions at the cash register. Several assistive devices are also under development for the home or the workplace. For example, researchers are developing an app that immediately converts an image of the clock on a microwave oven or the temperature setting on a thermostat into an audio report on the phone's speaker. Indoor wayfinding systems use scannable signs or other locators so that the visually impaired can navigate unfamiliar locations.

For outdoor navigation, researchers are developing apps to capture images of intersections and analyze them to identify crosswalks, curbs, and the status of "Walk/Don't Walk" signs in real time. Others are creating services that provide subscribers with on-demand assistance, where a caller describes a situation or snaps a picture of an item, and an offsite assistant immediately calls back and describes the scene or item to the subscriber. The latest mobile technologies have opened up seemingly unlimited possibilities for

Health Technology Sourcebook, Third Edition

assisting the visually impaired, and the NEI remains committed to supporting the development of these and other cutting-edge technologies.

NEEDS AND OPPORTUNITIES IN LOW VISION AND BLINDNESS REHABILITATION
Understanding Visual Impairment

- Investigate multisensory processes and cross-modal plasticity. Determine whether cross-modal plasticity associated with visual deprivation differs from normal multisensory interactions. Determine the organizing principles and limits that exist for cross-modal plasticity. Determine the informational requirements of a task that affect whether a remaining sensory modality (e.g., touch) can substitute for the absence of sight. Further research using neural network approaches, behavioral, and neuropsychological methods are necessary to inform effective sensory substitution and improve rehabilitation efforts.
- Characterize variation in spatial cognition, which is important for many tasks such as navigation. Spatial cognitive abilities vary widely. Normally sighted individuals with poor spatial cognition may be able to compensate through parallel processing using visual areas of the brain as well as perspective-free cognitive maps. In severe visual impairment, such compensation is limited or impossible, so the consequences of poor spatial cognition (whether innate or through lack of spatial cognitive experience) could be much more profound for the visually impaired than for the normally sighted.
- Determine spatial cognitive abilities of individuals with visual impairment to determine the extent to which nonvisual cues contribute to spatial cognition and how the contribution of nonvisual cues can be enhanced to improve spatial cognition under conditions of visual impairment.
- Understand the use of multisensory spatial representations, or cognitive maps, in learning strategies

Vision and Hearing Loss

and whether learning strategies change with cross-modal plasticity. Does visual impairment result in fundamentally different learning strategies, and does this differ by age?

Screening and Testing

- Design and validate tests of visual perception. Early detection of visual deficits will improve outcomes, but such tests can be used to benchmark outcomes of rehabilitative treatments. Sensitive, efficient testing is important to refine rehabilitation therapies and reduce the burden on patients and clinicians.
- Create and validate vision tests relevant to the tasks of daily living. Eye charts that test letter acuity are not sufficient to characterize functional vision for people with visual impairment. Eye charts of high-contrast patterns are not useful or predictive for a majority of the visual tasks of daily living, which involve dynamic inputs of objects and scenes with varying color and contrast.
- Develop and standardize tests for evaluating more complex visually intensive behavior, such as reading, face recognition, mobility, and driving. Such tests will be useful in determining disability and progress toward rehabilitative goals.
- Develop testing specific to various patient populations. Nonverbal methods for testing vision (e.g., visual fields, retinal function) in special populations (children, neurological patients) are an important, yet unaddressed, area. In addition, developmental testing of visually impaired children, particularly preverbal or nonverbal children, is limited, as current tests require vision to accomplish some or many of the tasks (e.g., stack blocks, match figures). Even motor milestones are affected by vision impairment, but details of how this occurs are unknown, and standards for normal development for visually impaired children are unknown.

Health Technology Sourcebook, Third Edition

Assistive Device Technology

- Develop new technology to improve access to the Internet, print, graphic display, and navigation resources. Some areas require specialized technology innovation (such as online Braille and tactile graphics, specialized embossers, and Braille software), but there are also opportunities for developing new assistive devices and products by modifying devices such as mobile phones, global positioning system, accelerometers, and speech engines. Success in the visually impaired community depends on optimizing format and delivery methods, particularly for elderly, cognitively impaired, or technologically naïve individuals.

- Use models of eccentric vision (using the peripheral retina when the central field is dysfunctional) to translate technology developed for sighted users to visually impaired users. Additionally, basic science on navigation, limited vision use, and multimodal perception can inform new assistive device development. For instance, a fundamental question concerns the limits of sensory substitution: Conveying visual information via auditory and tactile means has proven difficult. Normally, visual recognition of an embossed line drawing is trivial, but using either auditory or tactile means is challenging. Even when sensory substitution succeeds, only fairly simple visual information can be conveyed via these other modalities. A better understanding of the key aspects of visual information that are difficult to convey via other modalities could clearly inform the development of assistive technologies. Furthermore, studies of the effectiveness of these technologies are needed.

Visual Prostheses

- Determine critical parameters for continued improvement of prostheses. Visual prostheses are now being tested on patients. Different approaches include obtaining

Vision and Hearing Loss

visual information (detected by a camera) to electrically stimulate the visual system (retina or the visual cortex). Another relies on sensory substitution (e.g., encoding visual information into sensations on the tongue). In using a prosthesis, certain questions need to be resolved, for example, given a person's state of vision and what tasks can be done. If synchrony between modalities is required, how is one modality affected when the other input is degraded?

- Understand the level of acceptable visual enhancement using prosthetics. This can be determined using models of low vision, such as low-quality images, to determine how much information is necessary for particular visual tasks. "Low-quality" indicates low resolution, reduced fields, poor color contrast, and, more generally, any other image quality decrement that can be associated with low vision. Although normally-sighted humans use high visual acuity to perform tasks such as face recognition, experiments with highly degraded images suggest that many of these skills are exceptionally robust in spite of acuity reductions. Such results could inform prosthesis design engineering and serve as feasibility criteria—if a planned neural prosthesis can only offer a low-resolution image, is it worth implantation? What kinds of visual abilities will it be able to support?

Rehabilitation and Improving Public Health

- Define heterogeneity of visually impaired populations. Within the legally blind/low vision population, there is heterogeneity with respect to visual function, even within a particular disease group. Advanced age is an important variable, ultimately affecting vision in almost all adults. Visual disorders are also associated with concussion and neurocognitive disorders that are not well understood. Studying how behavior and neural processing are altered and differ across the spectrum of visual impairment will improve our understanding

Health Technology Sourcebook, Third Edition

of the sources of the heterogeneity and personalizing rehabilitative efforts.

- Understand the causes and consequences of cortical reorganization in the blind. Several studies have demonstrated that blindness causes visual areas to respond to auditory and tactile stimuli. However, the behavioral consequences of plasticity are not yet clear. Determine if rehabilitative processes can improve functional plasticity. Determine whether such reorganization affects visual learning if sight is restored. Recent studies on establishing sight in previously blind individuals provide opportunities to investigate neuroplasticity and how the brain adapts to new visual input (anatomically and functionally). Determining which visual skills can be acquired, as well as how these changes correlate with age and the extent of visual deprivation, will inform the prospects for recovery.
- Develop and test rehabilitation models and training paradigms. Low vision and blindness rehabilitation models continue to evolve. Interventions that are multimodal and multidisciplinary and address functional and emotional aspects uniquely related to low vision, blindness, loss of vision, and vision restoration hold particular promise. These include findings from basic psychophysical research (e.g., training visual skills to develop a preferred retinal locus in central vision loss or for the use of a visual prosthetic), research on psychosocial implications of vision impairment (e.g., the mechanisms by which visual impairment leads to reduced quality of life), and developing training for prevention and adaptation strategies (e.g., lifestyle changes).
- Create and standardize performance-based outcome assessments as well as the quality of life or other self-reported measures for low-vision interventions, whether they are prosthetic devices, assistive devices, or multidisciplinary rehabilitative strategies.

Vision and Hearing Loss

- Compare the effectiveness of rehabilitation approaches using randomized, controlled clinical trials. Rehabilitation currently lacks standardized methods and outcome assessments. Agreement on protocol and instrumentation will enable large-scale, multisite clinical trials.
- Identify comorbidities that interact with vision impairment and their influence on rehabilitation outcomes and integrate visual rehabilitation models into subacute rehabilitation inpatient units. Poor vision hampers rehabilitation in a variety of age-related conditions (e.g., stroke, falls, hip fracture). Specialized rehabilitation needs for the visually impaired as they age (e.g., arthritis for life-long cane users), as well as for individuals with age-related vision loss, are not understood. Needs can vary depending on the environment (e.g., nursing home residents) and comorbidities (e.g., wheelchair users, hearing-impaired individuals).

Retinal Implants for Vision Restoration

While working to prevent blindness and restore natural vision, the NEI also supports the development of retinal prostheses, also known as "retinal implants." Second Sight Medical Products, Inc. (Second Sight), supported in part by the NEI and by the U.S. Department of Energy (DOE), has engineered the Argus II Retinal Prosthesis System, which provides limited sight to people blinded by retinitis pigmentosa (RP), a genetic eye disease that causes gradual loss of the retina's light-sensing photoreceptor cells. Argus II consists of a video camera mounted on a pair of glasses, which captures and wirelessly transmits electrical signals through a 60-electrode grid surgically attached to the retina. The array bypasses the diseased photoreceptor machinery and directly activates the retinal ganglion cells that bring visual information to the brain.

A clinical trial that included 30 RP patients equipped with the Argus II system showed that not only did the device not hinder the performance of participants with residual vision, but it also improved participants' ability to identify shapes, detect motion,

445

Health Technology Sourcebook, Third Edition

locate objects, walk along a white line, and, in the best cases, read large letters. Although tested in RP patients, Argus II may be suitable for other conditions that damage the photoreceptors but leave the eye's neural networks intact, including AMD. Second Sight is currently developing a newer version of the device that uses a 256-electrode array that promises greater visual resolution. In 2011, Argus II became the eight-millionth patent issued by the U.S. Patent Office, and it is now on the market in Europe.

Other NEI-funded projects use complementary technologies. The Boston Retinal Implant Project is developing a device with external parts small enough to fit on the sclera—the outer wall of the eye. Another prosthetic device captures images with a video camera and then converts them into pulsed near-infrared light. Special glasses worn by the user project the near-infrared light through the eye and onto photodiodes implanted beneath the retina, which then convert the light into electrical signals that stimulate optic neurons. NEI-funded researchers are working to overcome technical barriers to retinal prostheses. They are adapting new nanotechnology to visual prostheses, expanding knowledge of how devices interact with neurons, and developing neurotransmitter-based prostheses.

Section 31.2 | Artificial Retina

This section includes text excerpted from "An Artificial Retina Engineered from Ancient Protein Heads to Space," National Eye Institute (NEI), April 12, 2021.

AN ARTIFICIAL RETINA ENGINEERED FROM ANCIENT PROTEIN HEADS TO SPACE

LambdaVision, the biotech firm that developed the artificial retina based in Farmington, Connecticut, is exploring optimizing the production of the artificial retina in space. In a series of missions to the International Space Station (ISS), the company tested whether microgravity on the station provides just the right conditions for constructing the multilayered protein-based artificial retina.

Vision and Hearing Loss

To get off the ground, LambdaVision received a $5 million commercialization award from the National Aeronautics and Space Administration (NASA), along with its partner, Space Tango, a firm based in Lexington, Kentucky, that provides the logistical support for space-based research.

"When gravity is nearly eliminated, so too are forces such as surface tension, sedimentation, convection driven buoyancy, all of which can interfere with the orientation and alignment important in the creation of crystalline structures, nanoparticles, or improved uniformity in layering processes," said Jana Stoudemire, a commercial innovation officer at Space Tango.

"We're building out not only the feasibility of manufacturing in orbit, but also the good manufacturing practices (GMP) capabilities that enable us to produce products in space for use in people. As in, therapies manufactured in space and returned to Earth for commercial distribution to patients," said Stoudemire.

"The hope is that surgically placing the artificial retina in the eye will restore vision among people with advanced-stage forms of diseases for which there is no treatment such as retinitis pigmentosa and age-related macular degeneration (AMD), a leading cause of vision loss among people age 50 and older," said Dr. Jordan Greco, Ph.D., chief scientific officer at LambdaVision.

In a healthy eye, light from a visual scene reaches the retina, where it is converted into electrical signals by neurons called "photoreceptors." Those signals are communicated to other retinal cells called "bipolar" and "retinal ganglion cells" until they reach the optic nerve, where they travel to the brain. The brain puts the signals together to produce vision.

The aim is for the LambdaVision artificial retina to replace the function of photoreceptors in people who have lost neurons from disease-related damage.

In 2014, the company received funding from the National Eye Institute (NEI) to test a prototype of the artificial retina in animal models. "The Small Business Technology Transfer grant is designed to support biotech companies, such as LambdaVision, as they take steps toward commercializing their innovative products," said Dr. Paek Lee, Ph.D., program manager for small business grants at NEI.

Health Technology Sourcebook, Third Edition

Recipients must be for-profit U.S. businesses that are at least 51 percent owned by individuals and independently operated, with no more than 500 employees. Each year, approximately 40–50 small business grants are awarded for a total of about $25 million.

A LOOK AT THE ARTIFICIAL RETINA

LambdaVision's artificial retina relies on bacteriorhodopsin, a light-activated protein that acts as a proton pump. Bacteriorhodopsin is synthesized by halobacterium salinarum, a microorganism found in extremely salty marshes. Halobacteria are of the Archaea domain, which are among the oldest forms of life on Earth.

As its name implies, bacteriorhodopsin shares some similarities with rhodopsin, the light-activated visual pigment protein within photoreceptors. Both proteins contain retinal, a chromophore that is key to absorbing light energy. In the case of bacteriorhodopsin, light energy is converted into metabolic energy. When light activates bacteriorhodopsin, hydrogen ions get pumped across a membrane, creating a proton gradient.

LambdaVision's founder Dr. Robert Birge, Ph.D., distinguished chair in chemistry at the University of Connecticut, has been studying bacteriorhodopsin for over 40 years and has made a career of incorporating light-activated proteins into biomolecular electronic and therapeutic applications, including the protein-based artificial retina.

In the 1980s, Birge and many other innovators looked to biological systems to see how their structures could inform the development of nano-sized technologies. After all, compared to relatively bulky mechanical electrical circuits, the natural world is full of nano-sized electrical circuits that have evolved over millions of years.

In addition to being light-activated, bacteriorhodopsin's molecular structure is highly ordered and thermally stable, adding to its potential for nanotechnology innovations from light-driven batteries to information processors and the artificial retina.

Within LambdaVision's artificial retina, purified bacteriorhodopsin is layered onto an ion-permeable membrane. The layers are repeated multiple times with the aim of absorbing enough

Vision and Hearing Loss

light to generate an ion gradient that can stimulate the neural circuitry of the bipolar and retinal ganglion cells within the retina, said Greco.

"In patients who've lost their vision from advanced-stage retinal diseases, the artificial retina would mimic the function of photoreceptors. Activated by light entering the eye, the artificial retina pumps protons toward the bipolar and ganglion cells. Receptors on those cells detect the protons, which triggers them to send signals to the optic nerve, where they travel to the brain," said Dr. Nicole Wagner, Ph.D., LambdaVision's president and chief executive officer.

For the artificial retina to function, the bacteriorhodopsin molecular structures must be precisely oriented within each layer to create a unidirectional gradient. That exacting degree of orientation may be more easily established in microgravity, and once achieved, Greco anticipates it should persist even after the implants are exposed to gravity on Earth.

LambdaVision plans to seek Food and Drug Administration approval of the artificial retina for the indication of retinitis pigmentosa. The collection of the preclinical data required to launch a clinical trial is still underway and has yet to be published.

Section 31.3 | Cochlear Implants: Different Kinds of Hearing

This section includes text excerpted from "What Is a Cochlear Implant?" U.S. Food and Drug Administration (FDA), February 4, 2018. Reviewed November 2022.

WHAT IS A COCHLEAR IMPLANT?

A cochlear implant is an implanted electronic hearing device designed to produce useful hearing sensations for a person with severe-to-profound nerve deafness by electrically stimulating nerves inside the inner ear.

These implants usually consist of the following two main components:

- The externally worn microphone, sound processor, and transmitter system
- The implanted receiver and electrode system, which contains the electronic circuits that receive signals from the external system and send electrical currents to the inner ear

Currently made devices have a magnet that holds the external system in place next to the implanted internal system. The external system may be worn entirely behind the ear, or its parts may be worn in a pocket, belt pouch, or harness.

WHO USES COCHLEAR IMPLANTS?

Cochlear implants are designed to help severely to profoundly deaf adults and children who get little or no benefit from hearing aids. Even individuals with severe or profound "nerve deafness" may be able to benefit from cochlear implants.

WHAT DETERMINES THE SUCCESS OF COCHLEAR IMPLANTS?

Many things determine the success of implantation. Some of them are:

- How long the patient has been deaf—as a group, patients who have been deaf for a short time do better than those who have been deaf for a long time
- How old they were when they became deaf—whether they were deaf before they could speak
- How old they were when they got the cochlear implant—younger patients, as a group, do better than older patients who have been deaf for a long time
- How long they have used the implant
- How quickly they learn
- How good and dedicated their learning support structure is

Vision and Hearing Loss

- The health and structure of their cochlea—the number of nerve (spiral ganglion) cells that they have
- Implanting variables, such as the depth and type of implanted electrode and signal processing technique
- Intelligence and communicativeness of patient

HOW DOES A COCHLEAR IMPLANT WORK?

A cochlear implant receives sound from the outside environment, processes it, and sends small electric currents near the auditory nerve. These electric currents activate the nerve, which then sends a signal to the brain. The brain learns to recognize this signal, and the person experiences this as "hearing."

The cochlear implant somewhat simulates natural hearing, where sound creates an electric current that stimulates the auditory nerve. However, the result is not the same as normal hearing.

WHY ARE THERE DIFFERENT KINDS OF IMPLANTS?

Current thinking is that the inner ear responds to sound in at least two separate ways.

One theory, the place theory, says the cochlea responds greater to a simple tone at one place along its length. Another theory is that the ear responds to the timing of the sound.

Researchers, following the place theory, devised implants that separated the sound into groups. For example, they sent the lower pitches to the area of the cochlea, where it seemed more responsive to lower pitches. And they sent higher pitches to the area more responsive to high pitches. Thus, they used several channels and electrodes spaced out inside the cochlea. Since there were also timing theories, researchers devised implants that made the sound signals into pulses to see if the cochlea would respond better to various kinds of pulses.

Most modern cochlear implants are versatile in that they are somewhat capable of being adjusted to respond to sound in various ways. Audiologists try a variety of adjustments to see what works best with a particular patient.

HOW LONG HAVE COCHLEAR IMPLANTS BEEN AVAILABLE?

The first commercial devices were approved by the U.S. Food and Drug Administration (FDA) in the mid-1980s. However, research with this device began in the 1950s.

WHAT ARE THE BENEFITS OF COCHLEAR IMPLANTS?

For people with implants:

- **Hearing ranges from near-normal ability to understand speech to no hearing benefit at all.**
- **Adults often benefit immediately and continue to improve for about three months after the initial tuning sessions.** Then, although performance continues to improve, improvements are slower. Cochlear implant users' performances may continue to improve for several years.
- **Children may improve at a slower pace.** A lot of training is needed after implantation to help the child use the new "hearing" she or he now experiences.
- **Most perceive loud, medium, and soft sounds.** People report that they can perceive different types of sounds, such as footsteps, slamming of doors, sounds of engines, ringing of the telephone, barking of dogs, whistling of the tea kettle, the rustling of leaves, the sound of a light switch being switched on and off, and so on.
- **Many understand speech without lipreading.** However, even if this is not possible, using the implant helps with lipreading.
- **Many can make telephone calls and understand familiar voices over the telephone.** Some good performers can make normal telephone calls and even understand an unfamiliar speaker. However, not all people who have implants are able to use the phone.
- **Many can watch TV more easily,** especially when they can also see the speaker's face. However, listening to the radio is often more difficult as there are no visual cues available.

Vision and Hearing Loss

- **Some can enjoy music.** Some enjoy the sound of certain instruments (e.g., piano or guitar) and certain voices. Others do not hear well enough to enjoy music.

WHAT ARE THE RISKS OF COCHLEAR IMPLANTS?
General Anesthesia Risks

- General anesthesia is drug-induced sleep. The drugs, such as anesthetic gases and injected drugs, may affect people differently. For most people, the risk of general anesthesia is very low. However, for some people with certain medical conditions, it is riskier.

Risks from the Surgical Implant Procedure

- **Injury to the facial nerve.** This nerve goes through the middle ear to give movement to the muscles of the face. It lies close to where the surgeon needs to place the implant, and thus, it can be injured during the surgery. An injury can cause a temporary or permanent weakening or full paralysis on the same side of the face as the implant.
- **Meningitis.** This is an infection of the lining of the surface of the brain. People who have abnormally formed inner ear structures appear to be at greater risk of this rare but serious complication.
- **Cerebrospinal fluid leakage.** The brain is surrounded by cerebrospinal fluid that may leak from a hole created in the inner ear or elsewhere from a hole in the covering of the brain as a result of the surgical procedure.
- **Perilymph fluid leak.** The inner ear or cochlea contains perilymph fluid. This fluid can leak through the hole that was created to place the implant.
- **Infection of the skin wound.**
- **Blood or fluid collection at the site of surgery.**
- **Attacks of dizziness or vertigo.**
- **Tinnitus.** This is a ringing or buzzing sound in the ear

Health Technology Sourcebook, Third Edition

- **Taste disturbances**. The nerve that gives taste sensation to the tongue also goes through the middle ear and might be injured during the surgery.
- **Numbness around the ear**.
- **Reparative granuloma**. The localized inflammation results in reparative granuloma if the body rejects the implant.
- **Other complications**. There may be other unforeseen complications that could occur with long-term implantation that we cannot now predict.

Other Risks Associated with the Use of Cochlear Implants

People with a cochlear implant:

- **May hear sounds differently**. Sound impressions from an implant differ from normal hearing, according to people who could hear before they became deaf. At first, users describe the sound as "mechanical," "technical," or "synthetic." This perception changes over time, and most users do not notice this artificial sound quality after a few weeks of cochlear implant use.
- **May lose residual hearing**. The implant may destroy any remaining hearing in the implanted ear.
- **May have unknown and uncertain effects**. The cochlear implant stimulates the nerves directly with electrical currents. Although this stimulation appears to be safe, the long-term effect of these electrical currents on the nerves is unknown.
- **May not hear as well as others** who have had successful outcomes with their implants.
- **May not be able to understand the language well**. There is no test a person can take before surgery that will predict how well she or he will understand language after surgery.
- **May have to have it removed** temporarily or permanently if an infection develops after the implant surgery. However, this is a rare complication.

Vision and Hearing Loss

- **May have their implant fail**. In this situation, a person with an implant would need to have additional surgery to resolve this problem and would be exposed to the risks of surgery again.
- **May not be able to upgrade their implant**. This may be the case when new external components become available. Implanted parts are usually compatible with improved external parts. That way, as advances in technology develop, one can upgrade his or her implant by changing only its external parts. In some cases, though, this would not work, and the implant will need changing.
- **May not be able to have some medical examinations and treatments**. These treatments include:
  - Magnetic resonance imaging (MRI). MRI is becoming a more routine diagnostic method for the early detection of medical problems. Even being close to an MRI imaging unit will be dangerous because it may dislodge the implant or demagnetize its internal magnet. The FDA has approved some implants, however, for some types of MRI studies done under controlled conditions.
  - Neurostimulation
  - Electrical surgery
  - Electroconvulsive therapy
  - Ionic radiation therapy
- **Will depend on batteries for hearing**. For some devices, new or recharged batteries are needed every day.
- **May damage their implant**. Contact sports, automobile accidents, slips, falls, or other impacts near the ear can damage the implant. This may mean needing a new implant and more surgery. It is unknown whether a new implant would work as well as the old one.
- **May find them expensive**. Replacing damaged or lost parts may be expensive.

Health Technology Sourcebook, Third Edition

- **Will have to use it for the rest of life**. During a person's lifetime, the manufacturer of the cochlear implant could go out of business. Whether a person will be able to get replacement parts or other customer services in the future is uncertain.
- **May have lifestyle changes**. This is because their implant will interact with the electronic environment. An implant may:
  - Set off theft detection systems.
  - Set off metal detectors or other security systems.
  - Be affected by cellular phone users or other radio transmitters.
  - Have to be turned off during takeoffs and landings in aircraft.
  - Interact in unpredictable ways with other computer systems.
- **Will have to be careful of static electricity**. Static electricity may temporarily or permanently damage a cochlear implant. It may be good practice to remove the processor and headset before contact with static-generating materials such as children's plastic play equipment, TV screens, computer monitors, or synthetic fabric. For more details regarding how to deal with static electricity, contact the manufacturer or implant center.
- **Have less ability to hear** both soft sounds and loud sounds without changing the sensitivity of the implant. The sensitivity of normal hearing is adjusted continuously by the brain, but the design of cochlear implants requires that a person manually change the sensitivity setting of the device as the sound environment changes.
- **May develop irritation** where the external part rubs on the skin and have to remove it for a while.
- **Cannot let the external parts get wet**. Damage from water may be expensive to repair, and the person may be without hearing until the implant is repaired. Thus,

Vision and Hearing Loss

the person will need to remove the external parts of the device when bathing, showering, swimming, or participating in water sports.

- **May hear strange sounds** caused by its interaction with magnetic fields, like those near airport passenger screening machines.

Chapter 32 | **Prosthetic Engineering**

Our aim is to improve prosthetic prescription by investigating the efficacy of prosthetic components used in current clinical practice and by developing novel approaches to improve the current standard of care. Our amputee-centric research encompasses improving patient mobility and comfort and preventing injury. Support for this research (2000 to present) includes funding from the Department of Veterans Affairs (VA) Rehabilitation Research and Development (RRD) Service and the National Institutes of Health (NIH).

MOBILITY RESEARCH
Disturbance Response in Amputee Gait
Errors in foot placement while avoiding obstacles and maneuvering in the household and community environments may lead to falls and injuries. This research aims to develop an ankle that can invert and evert and thereby control the center of pressure under the prosthetic foot, enhancing the balance and stability of lower limb amputees.

Foot–Ankle Stiffness
Many ambulatory lower limb amputees exhibit fatigue, asymmetrical gait, and the inability to walk at varying speeds. A rapid prototyping

This chapter includes text excerpted from "Prosthetic Engineering—Overview," Center for Limb Loss and Mobility (CLiMB), U.S. Department of Veterans Affairs (VA), March 30, 2017. Reviewed November 2022.

Health Technology Sourcebook, Third Edition

approach is used to fabricate feet of varying stiffness for exploring the effects of foot stiffness on amputee gait.

Turning Gait

Turning corners and maneuvering around obstacles are essential abilities for a successful community and household ambulation. The aim of this research is to test the efficacy of a compliant torque adapter in the pylons of transtibial amputees.

Energy Storage and Release

Many ambulatory lower limb amputees exhibit fatigue, asymmetrical gait, and the inability to walk at varying speeds. Several approaches aimed at providing the propulsive forces necessary to alleviate these problems.

Stochastic Resonance

Stochastic resonance (subthreshold vibration) may enhance peripheral sensation sufficiently to result in improved postural stability and locomotor function. This research explores the application of this phenomenon to the residual limb and intact plantar surface of diabetic lower limb amputees.

Research in Robotics and Biomechanics

Dr. Aubin's research spans robotics and biomechanics with applications in health and mobility. He motivates his research by engaging with patients and stakeholders to understand shortcomings in the areas of rehabilitation, prosthetics, orthotics, and physical therapy. Dr. Aubin strives to address these unmet patient and caregiver needs by establishing multidisciplinary research teams that leverage state-of-the-art technologies in robotics, neuroscience, and computational intelligence. Dr. Aubin's research goal is to develop and utilizes novel sensors, algorithms, assistive-powered devices, and robotic tools that can augment human performance and/or improve mobility and function for those affected by the disease, age, or trauma.

Prosthetic Engineering

Smart Cane System
People with pain or arthritis in their knee often walk with a cane to reduce knee pain and to improve or maintain their mobility. Increased pressure on the knee joint likely causes knee arthritis, and reducing the pressure on the knee joint may slow the progression of arthritis. Walking with a cane reduces the pressure inside the knee joint but only if the cane supports 10–20 percent of a person's weight. Many people may not be using their cane in the best way they can because they do not know how much force (percent of their body weight) they are putting on the cane when they walk. In this study, we are looking at how using a computerized cane that beeps or vibrates (like a cell phone) when a certain amount of force is applied to it might help people learn to more effectively use a cane. We are also examining how walking with a cane changes the pressure in the knee joint. We hypothesize that giving the user biofeedback, a sound or vibration signal from the cane will help them apply the optimal amount of force on the cane. Our secondary hypothesis is that increased cane loading will result in a decrease in knee joint pressure.

Sensory Feedback for Prosthetic Limbs
It has long been recognized that restoring movement function after amputation is a priority. We are now entering an era in which restoration of sensation may be possible as well through the use of smart sensorized prosthetic devices and haptic feedback. We are working on understanding how feedback of forces and events on foot—for example, the placement of the prosthetic foot as the user is walking down stairs—can lead to improved function.

INJURY PREVENTION RESEARCH
Vacuum Suspension Systems
Many amputees live with an ill-fitting socket and can experience limb pistoning within the socket, which in turn may result in skin irritation, tissue breakdown, discomfort, and a reduction in activity. The aims of this research are to characterize the response of the

Health Technology Sourcebook, Third Edition

lower residual limb to a vacuum suspension system and to measure changes in limb volume with a structured light scanning system.

Socket Systems and Tissue O_2

Limb health and wound healing capacity is closely related to the amount of oxygen present in limb tissues. Using our fiber-optic video-oximetry imaging system, we aim to discover if the prosthetic prescription can influence residual limb tissue oxygenation during both rest and gait.

Distributed Sensing

The goal of the proposed project is to develop enabling sensing technology based on a flexible array and to build a prototype of a prosthetic liner with distributed, unimodal field sensing capability. The specific aims include: (1) the design of the flexible sensing array for measurement of moisture, temperature, pressure, and shear stress; (2) integration of this array into a prosthetic liner/socket; and (3) testing of the device performance.

Torsional Prosthesis

This research seeks to develop a prosthetic limb whose torsional characteristics can adapt depending on activity. Our goal is to reduce torsional stresses and the incidence of residual limb injuries.

PATIENT COMFORT RESEARCH
Thermal Comfort

Lower limb amputations often experience discomfort related in part to higher skin temperatures within their prosthetic socket. Our research has found prosthetic liners and sockets are excellent insulators that can retain heat. Activity can cause a dramatic increase in skin temperature within the prosthesis requiring substantially long periods of inactivity to restore resting state temperatures. Our current work involves developing active cooling systems and embedded sensor networks to monitor skin temperature.

Prosthetic Engineering

Evaporative Cooling and Perspiration Removal

Amputees often complain about uncomfortably warm residual limb skin temperatures and the accumulation of perspiration within their prosthesis. This research will discover if a novel evaporative cooling system can ameliorate these problems.

Chapter 33 | Brain–Computer Interface

Scientists have developed a brain–computer interface (BCI) designed to restore the ability to communicate in people with spinal cord injuries (SCIs) and neurological disorders, such as amyotrophic lateral sclerosis (ALS). This system has the potential to work more quickly than previous BCIs, and it does so by tapping into one of the oldest means of communication we have—handwriting.

The study, published in *Nature*, was funded by the Brain Research Through Advancing Innovative Neurotechnologies® (BRAIN) Initiative of the National Institutes of Health (NIH) as well as the National Institute of Neurological Disorders and Stroke (NINDS) and the National Institute on Deafness and Other Communication Disorders (NIDCD), both part of the NIH.

Researchers focused on the part of the brain that is responsible for fine movement and recorded the signals generated when the participant attempted to write individual letters by hand. In doing so, the participant, who is paralyzed from the neck down following an SCI, trained a machine learning computer algorithm to identify neural patterns representing individual letters. While demonstrated as a proof of concept in one patient so far, this system appears to be more accurate and more efficient than existing communication BCIs and could help people with paralysis rapidly type without needing to use their hands.

"This study represents an important milestone in the development of BCIs and machine learning technologies that are

This chapter includes text excerpted from "Composing Thoughts: Mental Handwriting Produces Brain Activity That Can Be Turned into Text," National Institutes of Health (NIH), May 12, 2021.

Health Technology Sourcebook, Third Edition

unraveling how the human brain controls processes as complex as communication," said Dr. John Ngai, Ph.D., director of the NIH BRAIN Initiative. "This knowledge is providing a critical foundation for improving the lives of others with neurological injuries and disorders."

When a person becomes paralyzed due to SCI, the part of the brain that controls movement still works. This means that while the participant could not move her or his hand or arm to write, her or his brain still produced similar signals related to the intended movement. Similar BCI systems have been developed to restore motor function through devices such as robotic arms.

"Just think about how much of your day is spent on a computer or communicating with another person," said study co-author Dr. Krishna Shenoy, Ph.D., a Howard Hughes Medical Institute (HHMI) Investigator and the Hong Seh and Vivian W. M. Lim Professor at Stanford University. "Restoring the ability of people who have lost their independence to interact with computers and others is extremely important, and that is what is bringing projects like this one front and center."

First, the participant was asked to copy letters that were displayed on the screen, which included the 26 lowercase letters along with some punctuation: ">" that was used as a space and "~" that was used as a "full stop." At the same time, implanted electrodes recorded the brain activity from approximately 200 individual neurons that responded differently while he mentally "wrote" each individual character. After a series of training sessions, the BCI's computer algorithms learned how to recognize neural patterns corresponding to individual letters, allowing the participant to "write" new sentences that had not been printed out before, with the computer displaying the letters in real time.

"This method is a marked improvement over existing communication BCIs that rely on using the brain to move a cursor to "type" words on a screen," said Dr. Frank Willett, Ph.D., an HHMI Research Scientist at Stanford University and the study's lead author. "Attempting to write each letter produces a unique pattern of activity in the brain, making it easier for the computer to identify what is being written with much greater accuracy and speed."

Brain–Computer Interface

Using this system, the participant was able to compose sentences and communicate with others at a speed of about 90 characters per minute, comparable to someone of a similar age typing on a smartphone. In contrast, "point-and-click" interfaces have only achieved about 40 characters per minute.

This system also provides a level of flexibility that is crucial to restoring communication. Some studies have gone as far as attempting direct thought-to-speech BCIs that, while promising, are currently limited by what is possible through recordings from the surface of the brain that averages responses across thousands of neurons.

"Right now, other investigators can achieve about a 50-word dictionary using machine learning methods when decoding speech," said Dr. Shenoy. "By using handwriting to record from hundreds of individual neurons, we can write any letter and thus any word which provides a truly 'open vocabulary' that can be used in most any life situation."

For individuals who are paralyzed or living with "locked-in syndrome" due to brainstem stroke or late-stage ALS, the ability to communicate is largely or even completely lost without technological intervention. While preliminary, the technologies being developed here offer the potential to help those who have completely lost the ability to write and speak.

"Communication is central to how we function in society," said Dr. Debara L. Tucci, M.D., M.S., M.B.A, director, NIDCD. "In today's world of internet-based communication, people with severe speech and physical impairments can face significant communication barriers and, potentially, isolation. We hope these findings will encourage commercial development of this latest BCI technology."

In the future, Dr. Shenoy's team intends to test the system on a patient who has lost the ability to speak, such as someone with advanced ALS. In addition, they are looking to increase the number of characters available to the participants (such as capital letters and numbers).

The clinical trial, called "BrainGate2," a collaboration of internationally recognized laboratories, universities, and hospitals working to advance brain–computer interface technologies, is testing the

Health Technology Sourcebook, Third Edition

safety of BCIs that directly connect a person's brain to a computer. The study was a collaboration between the research group of Dr. Shenoy and Dr. Jaimie Henderson, M.D., at Stanford University and Dr. Leigh Hochberg, M.D., Ph.D., from Brown University, Massachusetts General Hospital, and Providence VA and sponsor-investigator of the BrainGate2 trial. Dr. Henderson at Stanford University also performed the surgery to place the necessary electrodes.

Chapter 34 | **Assistive Devices**

Chapter Contents
Section 34.1—Rehabilitative and Assistive Technology:
  An Overview 471
Section 34.2—Assistive Devices for Communication 476
Section 34.3—Hearing Aids 482
Section 34.4—Mobility Aids 483
Section 34.5—GPS and Wayfinding Apps for People
  with Visual Impairment 489

Section 34.1 | Rehabilitative and Assistive Technology: An Overview

This section includes text excerpted from "Rehabilitative and Assistive Technology," *Eunice Kennedy Shriver* National Institute of Child Health and Human Development (NICHD), October 24, 2018. Reviewed November 2022.

Rehabilitative and assistive technology (AT) refers to tools, equipment, or products that can help people with disabilities successfully complete activities at school, home, and work and in the community. Disabilities are disorders, diseases, health conditions, or injuries that affect a person's physical, intellectual, or mental well-being and functioning. Rehabilitative and assistive technologies can help people with disabilities function more easily in their everyday lives and can also make it easier for a caregiver to care for a person with disabilities. The term "rehabilitative technology" refers to aids that help people recover their functioning after injury or illness. "Assistive technologies" may be as simple as a magnifying glass to improve vision or as complex as a digital communication system.

Some of these technologies are made possible through rehabilitative engineering research, which applies engineering and scientific principles to study how people with disabilities function in society. It includes studying barriers and designing solutions so that people with disabilities can interact successfully in their environments.

The Eunice Kennedy Shriver National Institute of Child Health and Human Development (NICHD) houses the National Center for Medical Rehabilitation Research (NCMRR), which is charged with advancing scientific knowledge on disabilities and rehabilitation while also providing vital support and focus for the field of medical rehabilitation to help ensure the health, independence, productivity, and quality of life of all people. Through the NCMRR, NICHD supports the development and testing of rehabilitative and assistive technologies with a focus on physical rehabilitation.

WHAT ARE SOME TYPES OF ASSISTIVE DEVICES, AND HOW ARE THEY USED?

Some examples of assistive technologies are as follows:

- Mobility aids, such as wheelchairs, scooters, walkers, canes, crutches, prosthetic devices, and orthotic devices
- Hearing aids to help people hear or hear more clearly
- Cognitive aids, including computer or electrical assistive devices, to help people with memory, attention, or other challenges in their thinking skills
- Computer software and hardware, such as voice recognition programs, screen readers, and screen enlargement applications, to help people with mobility and sensory impairments use computers and mobile devices
- Tools, such as automatic page-turners, bookholders, and adapted pencil grips to help learners with disabilities participate in educational activities
- Closed captioning to allow people with hearing problems to watch movies, television programs, and other digital media
- Physical modifications in the built environment, including ramps, grab bars, and wider doorways to enable access to buildings, businesses, and workplaces
- Lightweight, high-performance mobility devices that enable persons with disabilities to play sports and be physically active
- Adaptive switches and utensils to allow those with limited motor skills to eat, play games, and accomplish other activities
- Devices and features of devices to help perform tasks, such as cooking, dressing, and grooming; specialized handles and grips; devices that extend reach; and lights on telephones and doorbells are a few examples

Assistive Devices

WHAT ARE SOME TYPES OF REHABILITATIVE TECHNOLOGIES?

Rehabilitative technologies and techniques help people recover or improve function after injury or illness. Examples include the following:

- **Robotics.** Specialized robots help people regain and improve function in their arms or legs after a stroke.
- **Virtual reality.** People who are recovering from injuries can retrain themselves to perform motions within a virtual environment.
- **Musculoskeletal modeling and simulations.** These computer simulations of the human body can pinpoint underlying mechanical problems in a person with a movement-related disability. This technique can help improve assistive aids or physical therapies.
- **Transcranial magnetic stimulation (TMS).** TMS sends magnetic impulses through the skull to stimulate the brain. This system can help people who have had a stroke recover movement and brain function.
- **Transcranial direct current stimulation (tDCS).** In tDCS, a mild electrical current travels through the skull and stimulates the brain. This can help recover movement in patients recovering from stroke or other conditions.
- **Motion analysis.** Motion analysis captures video of human motion with specialized computer software that analyzes the motion in detail. The technique gives health-care providers a detailed picture of a person's specific movement challenges to guide proper therapy.

Some devices incorporate multiple types of technologies and techniques to help users regain or improve function. For example, the BrainGate project, which was partially funded by the NICHD through the NCMRR, relied on tiny sensors being implanted in the brain. The user could then think about moving their arm, and a robotic arm would carry out the thought.

HOW DOES REHABILITATIVE TECHNOLOGY BENEFIT PEOPLE WITH DISABILITIES?

Rehabilitative technology can help restore or improve function in people who have developed a disability due to disease, injury, or aging. Appropriate assistive technology often helps people with disabilities compensate, at least in part, for a limitation.

For example, assistive technology enables students with disabilities to compensate for certain impairments. This specialized technology promotes independence and decreases the need for other support.

Rehabilitative and assistive technology can enable individuals to:

- Care for themselves and their families.
- Work.
- Learn in typical school environments and other educational institutions.
- Access information through computers and reading.
- Enjoy music, sports, travel, and the arts.
- Participate fully in community life.

Assistive technology also benefits employers, teachers, family members, and everyone who interacts with people who use the technology.

As ATs become more commonplace, people without disabilities are benefiting from them. For example, people for whom English is a second language are taking advantage of screen readers. Older individuals are using screen enlargers and magnifiers.

The person with a disability, along with her or his caregivers and a team of professionals and consultants, usually decide which type of rehabilitative or assistive technology would be most helpful. The team is trained to match particular technologies to specific needs to help the person function better or more independently. The team may include family doctors, regular and special education teachers, speech-language pathologists, rehabilitation engineers, occupational therapists, and other specialists, including representatives from companies that manufacture assistive technology.

Assistive Devices

What Conditions May Benefit from Assistive Devices?

Some disabilities are quite visible, while others are "hidden." Most disabilities can be grouped into the following categories:

- **Cognitive disability.** Intellectual and learning disabilities/disorders, distractibility, reading disorders, inability to remember or focus on large amounts of information.
- **Hearing disability.** Hearing loss or impaired hearing.
- **Physical disability.** Paralysis, difficulties with walking or other movements, inability to use a computer mouse, slow response time, or difficulty controlling movement.
- **Visual disability.** Blindness, low vision, or color blindness.
- **Mental conditions.** Posttraumatic stress disorder (PTSD), anxiety disorders, mood disorders, eating disorders, or psychosis.

Hidden disabilities are those that might not be immediately apparent when you look at someone. They can include visual impairments, movement problems, hearing impairments, and mental health conditions.

Some medical conditions may also contribute to disabilities or may be categorized as hidden disabilities under the Americans with Disabilities Act (ADA). For example, epilepsy, diabetes, sickle cell conditions, human immunodeficiency virus (HIV)/acquired immunodeficiency syndrome (AIDS), cystic fibrosis (CF), cancer, and heart, liver, or kidney problems may lead to problems with mobility or daily functions and may be viewed as disabilities under the law. The conditions may be short or long term, stable or progressive, constant or unpredictable, and changing, treatable, or untreatable. Many people with hidden disabilities can benefit from assistive technologies for certain activities or during certain stages of their diseases or conditions.

People who have spinal cord injuries (SCI), traumatic brain injury (TBI), cerebral palsy (CP), muscular dystrophy (MD), spina bifida, osteogenesis imperfecta (OI), multiple sclerosis (MS),

Health Technology Sourcebook, Third Edition

demyelinating diseases, myelopathy, progressive muscular atrophy (PMA), amputations, or paralysis often benefit from complex rehabilitative technology. The assistive devices are individually configured to help each person with her or his own unique disability.

Section 34.2 | Assistive Devices for Communication

This section includes text excerpted from "Assistive Devices for People with Hearing, Voice, Speech, or Language Disorders," *Eunice Kennedy Shriver* National Institute of Child Health and Human Development (NICHD), November 12, 2019.

WHAT ARE ASSISTIVE DEVICES?

The term assistive device or assistive technology (AT) can refer to any device that helps a person with hearing loss or a voice, speech, or language disorder to communicate. These terms often refer to devices that help a person to hear and understand what is being said more clearly or to express thoughts more easily. With the development of digital and wireless technologies, more and more devices are becoming available to help people with hearing, voice, speech, and language disorders communicate more meaningfully and participate more fully in their daily lives.

WHAT TYPES OF ASSISTIVE DEVICES ARE AVAILABLE?

Health professionals use a variety of names to describe assistive devices:

- Assistive listening devices (ALDs) help amplify the sounds you want to hear, especially where there is a lot of background noise. ALDs can be used with a hearing aid or cochlear implant to help a wearer hear certain sounds better.
- Augmentative and alternative communication (AAC) devices help people with communication disorders to express themselves. These devices can range from a simple picture board to a computer program that synthesizes speech from text.

476

Assistive Devices

- Alerting devices connect to a doorbell, telephone, or alarm that emits a loud sound or blinking light to let someone with hearing loss know that an event is taking place.

WHAT TYPES OF ASSISTIVE LISTENING DEVICES ARE AVAILABLE?

Several types of ALDs are available to improve sound transmission for people with hearing loss. Some are designed for large facilities such as classrooms, theaters, places of worship, and airports. Other types are intended for personal use in small settings and for one-on-one conversations. All can be used with or without hearing aids or a cochlear implant. ALD systems for large facilities include hearing loop systems, frequency-modulated (FM) systems, and infrared systems.

Hearing loop (or induction loop) systems use electromagnetic energy to transmit sound. A hearing loop system involves four parts:

- A sound source, such as a public address system, microphone, or home TV or telephone
- An amplifier
- A thin loop of wire that encircles a room or branches out beneath carpeting
- A receiver worn in the ears or as a headset

Amplified sound travels through the loop and creates an electro-magnetic field that is picked up directly by a hearing loop receiver or a telecoil, a miniature wireless receiver that is built into many hearing aids and cochlear implants. To pick up the signal, a listener must be wearing the receiver and be within or near the loop. Because the sound is picked up directly by the receiver, the sound is much clearer, without as much of the competing background noise associated with many listening environments. Some loop systems are portable, making it possible for people with hearing loss to improve their listening environments, as needed, as they proceed with their daily activities. A hearing loop can be connected to a public address system, a television, or any other audio source. For those who do not have hearing aids with embedded telecoils, portable loop receivers are also available.

Health Technology Sourcebook, Third Edition

FM systems use radio signals to transmit amplified sounds. They are often used in classrooms, where the instructor wears a small microphone connected to a transmitter and the student wears the receiver, which is tuned to a specific frequency or channel. People who have a telecoil inside their hearing aid or cochlear implant may also wear a wire around the neck (called a "neck loop") or behind their aid or implant (called a "silhouette inductor") to convert the signal into magnetic signals that can be picked up directly by the telecoil. FM systems can transmit signals up to 300 feet and are able to be used in many public places. However, because radio signals are able to penetrate walls, listeners in one room may need to listen to a different channel than those in another room to avoid receiving mixed signals. Personal FM systems operate in the same way as larger-scale systems and can be used to help people with hearing loss follow one-on-one conversations.

Infrared systems use infrared light to transmit sound. A transmitter converts sound into a light signal and beams it to a receiver that is worn by a listener. The receiver decodes the infrared signal back to sound. As with FM systems, people whose hearing aids or cochlear implants have a telecoil may also wear a neck loop or silhouette inductor to convert the infrared signal into a magnetic signal, which can be picked up through their telecoil. Unlike induction loop or FM systems, the infrared signal cannot pass through walls, making it particularly useful in courtrooms where confidential information is often discussed and in buildings where competing signals can be a problem, such as classrooms or movie theaters. However, infrared systems cannot be used in environments with too many competing light sources, such as outdoors or in strongly lit rooms.

Personal amplifiers are useful in places in which the above systems are unavailable or when watching TV, being outdoors, or traveling in a car. About the size of a cell phone, these devices increase sound levels and reduce background noise for a listener. Some have directional microphones that can be angled toward a speaker or other source of sound. As with other ALDs, the amplified sound can be picked up by a receiver that the listener is wearing, either as a headset or as earbuds.

Assistive Devices

WHAT TYPES OF AUGMENTATIVE AND ALTERNATIVE COMMUNICATION DEVICES ARE AVAILABLE FOR COMMUNICATING FACE-TO-FACE?

The simplest AAC device is a picture board or touch screen that uses pictures or symbols of typical items and activities that make up a person's daily life. For example, a person might touch the image of a glass to ask for a drink. Many picture boards can be customized and expanded based on a person's age, education, occupation, and interests.

Keyboards, touch screens, and sometimes a person's limited speech may be used to communicate desired words. Some devices employ a text display. The display panel typically faces outward so that two people can exchange information while facing each other. Spelling and word prediction software can make it faster and easier to enter information.

Speech-generating devices go one step further by translating words or pictures into speech. Some models allow users to choose from several different voices, such as male or female, child or adult, and even some regional accents. Some devices employ a vocabulary of prerecorded words, while others have an unlimited vocabulary, synthesizing speech as words are typed in. Software programs that convert personal computers into speaking devices are also available.

WHAT AUGMENTATIVE AND ALTERNATIVE COMMUNICATION DEVICES ARE AVAILABLE FOR COMMUNICATING BY TELEPHONE?

For many years, people with hearing loss have used text telephone or telecommunications devices, called "TTY" or "TDD" machines, to communicate by phone. This same technology also benefits people with speech difficulties. A TTY machine consists of a typewriter keyboard that displays typed conversations onto a readout panel or printed on paper. Callers will either type messages to each other over the system or, if a call recipient does not have a TTY machine, use the national toll-free telecommunications relay service at 711 to communicate. Through the relay service, a communications assistant serves as a bridge between two callers, reading typed messages aloud to the person with hearing while transcribing what is spoken into type for the person with hearing loss.

479

Health Technology Sourcebook, Third Edition

With today's new electronic communication devices, however, TTY machines have almost become a thing of the past. People can place phone calls through the telecommunications relay service using almost any device with a keypad, including a laptop, personal digital assistant, and cell phone. Text messaging has also become a popular method of communication, skipping the relay service altogether.

Another system uses voice recognition software and an extensive library of video clips depicting American Sign Language (ASL) to translate a signer's words into text or computer-generated speech in real time. It is also able to translate spoken words back into sign language or text.

Finally, for people with mild-to-moderate hearing loss, captioned telephones allow you to carry on a spoken conversation while providing a transcript of the other person's words on a read-out panel or computer screen as a backup.

WHAT TYPES OF ALERTING DEVICES ARE AVAILABLE?

Alerting or alarm devices use sound, light, vibrations, or a combination of these techniques to let someone know when a particular event is occurring. Clocks and wake-up alarm systems allow a person to choose to wake up to flashing lights, horns, or gentle shaking.

Visual alert signalers monitor a variety of household devices and other sounds, such as doorbells and telephones. When the phone rings, the visual alert signaler will be activated and will vibrate or flash a light to let people know. In addition, remote receivers placed around the house can alert a person from any room. Portable vibrating pagers can let parents and caretakers know when a baby is crying. Some baby monitoring devices analyze a baby's cry and light up a picture to indicate if the baby sounds hungry, bored, or sleepy.

WHAT RESEARCH IS BEING CONDUCTED ON ASSISTIVE TECHNOLOGY?

The National Institute on Deafness and Other Communication Disorders (NIDCD) funds research into several areas of assistive technology, such as those described below:

- **Improved devices for people with hearing loss.**
  NIDCD-funded researchers are developing devices

480

Assistive Devices

that help people with varying degrees of hearing loss communicate with others. One team has developed a portable device in which two or more users type messages to each other that can be displayed simultaneously in real time. Another team is designing an ALD that amplifies and enhances speech for a group of individuals who are conversing in a noisy environment.

- **Improved devices for nonspeaking people.**
- **More natural synthesized speech.** NIDCD-sponsored scientists are also developing a personalized text-to-speech synthesis system that synthesizes speech that is more intelligible and natural sounding to be incorporated into speech-generating devices. Individuals who are at risk of losing their speaking ability can prerecord their own speech, which is then converted into their personal synthetic voice.
- **Brain–computer interface research.** A relatively new and exciting area of study is called brain–computer interface research. NIDCD-funded scientists are studying how neural signals in a person's brain can be translated by a computer to help someone communicate. For example, people with amyotrophic lateral sclerosis (ALS, or Lou Gehrig's disease) or brainstem stroke lose their ability to move their arms, legs, or body. They can also become locked in, where they are not able to express words, even though they are able to think and reason normally. By implanting electrodes in the brain's motor cortex, some researchers are studying how a person who is locked in can control communication software and type out words simply by imagining the movement of his or her hand. Other researchers are attempting to develop a prosthetic device that will be able to translate a person's thoughts into synthesized words and sentences. Another group is developing a wireless device that monitors brain activity that is triggered by visual stimulation. In this way, people who are locked in can call for help during an emergency by staring at a designated spot on the device.

Health Technology Sourcebook, Third Edition

Section 34.3 | **Hearing Aids**

This section includes text excerpted from "Hearing Aids," U.S. Food and Drug Administration (FDA), August 16, 2022.

More than 30 million adults in the United States have some degree of hearing loss. Hearing loss can have a negative effect on communication, relationships, school or work performance, and emotional well-being. However, hearing loss does not have to restrict your daily activities. Properly fitted hearing aids and aural rehabilitation can help in many listening situations. Aural rehabilitation is the use of techniques to identify and diagnose hearing loss and implement therapies for patients who are hard of hearing, which often involves the use of hearing aids. Aural rehabilitation helps a person focus on adjusting to their hearing loss and the use of their hearing aids. It also explores assistive devices to help improve communication. Most people who are hearing-impaired will need two hearing aids because both ears are often affected by hearing loss though some people may only need one hearing aid.

This section includes information on the difference between hearing aids, which are intended for use by people with hearing loss, and sound amplifiers for consumers with no hearing loss who want to make environmental sounds louder for recreational use.

While the U.S. Food and Drug Administration (FDA) regulates hearing aids, which are medical devices, it does not consider sound amplifiers to be medical devices when labeled for recreational or other use by individuals with normal hearing. However, certain safety regulations related to sound output levels still apply to these products.

The President's Council of Advisors on Science and Technology (PCAST) and the National Academies of Sciences (NAS), Engineering, and Medicine issued reports recommending ways to improve the access and affordability of hearing aids. The FDA considered these recommendations along with input from the public and has issued the "Immediately in Effect Guidance Document: Conditions for Sale for Air-Conduction Hearing Aids" guidance document. The FDA issued this guidance to communicate that it

Assistive Devices

does not intend to enforce certain conditions for sale applicable to hearing aids for users 18 years of age or older (shown in Table 34.1).

Table 34.1. Types of Products

	Over-the-Counter Hearing Aids	Prescription Hearing Aids (Any Hearing Aids That Do Not Meet OTC Requirements)	Personal Sound Amplification Products
Type of product	Medical device Electronic product	Medical device Electronic product	Electronic product
Intended users	People 18 years and older For those with perceived mild-to-moderate hearing loss	People of any age, including those younger than 18 years For people with any degree of hearing loss, including severe	People of any age with normal hearing to amplify sounds in certain environments
Conditions for sale	Purchaser 18 years or older No medical exam No prescription No fitting by an audiologist No need for a licensed seller	Prescription needed Must purchase from a licensed seller in some states	Not applicable FDA requirements regarding conditions for sale

Section 34.4 | Mobility Aids

This section includes text excerpted from "Wheelchairs, Mobility Aids, and Other Power-Driven Mobility Devices," ADA.gov, U.S. Department of Justice (DOJ), January 31, 2014. Reviewed November 2022.

People with mobility, circulatory, respiratory, or neurological disabilities use many kinds of devices for mobility. Some use walkers, canes, crutches, or braces. Some use manual or power wheelchairs or electric scooters. In addition, advances in technology have given rise to new devices, such as Segways®, that some people

Health Technology Sourcebook, Third Edition

with disabilities use as mobility devices, including many veterans injured while serving in the military. And more advanced devices will inevitably be invented, providing more mobility options for people with disabilities.

This section is designed to help title II entities (state and local governments) and title III entities (businesses and nonprofit organizations that serve the public; together, "covered entities") understand how the new rules for mobility devices apply to them. These rules went into effect on March 15, 2011.

- Covered entities must allow people with disabilities who use manual or power wheelchairs or scooters and manually powered mobility aids, such as walkers, crutches, and canes, into all areas where members of the public are allowed to go.
- Covered entities must also allow people with disabilities who use other types of power-driven mobility devices into their facilities unless a particular type of device cannot be accommodated because of legitimate safety requirements. Where legitimate safety requirements bar accommodation for a particular type of device, the covered entity must provide the service it offers in alternate ways if possible.
- The rules set out five specific factors to consider in deciding whether or not a particular type of device can be accommodated.

WHEELCHAIRS

Most people are familiar with the manual and power wheelchairs and electric scooters used by people with mobility disabilities. The term "wheelchair" is defined in the new rules as "a manually operated or power-driven device designed primarily for use by an individual with a mobility disability for the main purpose of indoor or of both indoor and outdoor locomotion."

OTHER POWER-DRIVEN MOBILITY DEVICES

In recent years, some people with mobility disabilities have begun using less traditional mobility devices such as golf cars or Segways®.

Assistive Devices

These devices are called "other power-driven mobility devices" (OPDMDs) in the rule. The OPDMD is defined in the new rules as "any mobility device powered by batteries, fuel, or other engines... that is used by individuals with mobility disabilities for the purpose of locomotion, including golf cars, electronic personal assistance mobility devices... such as the Segway® PT, or any mobility device designed to operate in areas without defined pedestrian routes, but that is not a wheelchair." When an OPDMD is being used by a person with a mobility disability, different rules apply under the ADA than when it is being used by a person without a disability.

CHOICE OF DEVICE

People with disabilities have the right to choose whatever mobility device best suits their needs. For example, someone may choose to use a manual wheelchair rather than a power wheelchair because it enables her to maintain her upper body strength. Similarly, someone who is able to stand may choose to use a Segway® rather than a manual wheelchair because of the health benefits gained by standing. A facility may be required to allow a type of device that is generally prohibited when being used by someone without a disability when it is being used by a person who needs it because of a mobility disability. For example, if golf cars are generally prohibited in a park, the park may be required to allow a golf car when it is being used because of a person's mobility disability unless there is a legitimate safety reason that it cannot be accommodated.

REQUIREMENTS REGARDING MOBILITY DEVICES AND AIDS

Under the new rules, covered entities must allow people with disabilities who use wheelchairs (including manual wheelchairs, power wheelchairs, and electric scooters) and manually powered mobility aids, such as walkers, crutches, canes, braces, and other similar devices into all areas of a facility where members of the public are allowed to go.

In addition, covered entities must allow people with disabilities who use any OPDMD to enter the premises unless a particular type of device cannot be accommodated because of legitimate safety requirements. Such safety requirements must be based on actual

Health Technology Sourcebook, Third Edition

risks, not on speculation or stereotypes about a particular type of device or how it might be operated by people with disabilities using them.

- For some facilities—such as a hospital, a shopping mall, a large home improvement store with wide aisles, a public park, or an outdoor amusement park—covered entities will likely determine that certain classes of OPDMDs being used by people with disabilities can be accommodated. These entities must allow people with disabilities using these types of OPDMDs into all areas where members of the public are allowed to go.
- In some cases, even in facilities such as those described above, an OPDMD can be accommodated in some areas of a facility but not in others because of legitimate safety concerns. For example, a cruise ship may decide that people with disabilities using Segways® can generally be accommodated, except in constricted areas, such as passageways to cabins that are very narrow and have low ceilings.
- For other facilities—such as a small convenience store or a small town manager's office—covered entities may determine that certain classes of OPDMDs cannot be accommodated. In that case, they are still required to serve a person with a disability using one of these devices in an alternate manner if possible, such as providing curbside service or meeting the person at an alternate location.

Covered entities are encouraged to develop written policies specifying which kinds of OPDMDs will be permitted and where and when they will be permitted based on the following assessment factors.

ASSESSMENT FACTORS

In deciding whether a particular type of OPDMD can be accommodated in a particular facility, the following factors must be considered:

- The type, size, weight, dimensions, and speed of the device

Assistive Devices

- The facility's volume of pedestrian traffic (which may vary at different times of the day, week, month, or year)
- The facility's design and operational characteristics (e.g., whether its business is conducted indoors or outdoors, its square footage, the density and placement of furniture and other stationary devices, and the availability of storage for the OPDMD if needed and requested by the user)
- Whether legitimate safety requirements (such as limiting speed to the pace of pedestrian traffic or prohibiting the use of escalators) can be established to permit the safe operation of the OPDMD in the specific facility
- Whether the use of the OPDMD creates a substantial risk of serious harm to the immediate environment or natural or cultural resources or poses a conflict with federal land management laws and regulations

It is important to understand that these assessment factors relate to an entire class of device types, not to how a person with a disability might operate the device. All types of devices powered by fuel or combustion engines, for example, may be excluded from indoor settings for health or environmental reasons but may be deemed acceptable in some outdoor settings. Also, for safety reasons, larger electric devices such as golf cars may be excluded from narrow or crowded settings where there is no valid reason to exclude smaller electric devices like Segways®.

Based on these assessment factors, the U.S. Department of Justice (DOJ) expects that devices such as Segways® can be accommodated in most circumstances. The DOJ also expects that in most circumstances, people with disabilities using ATVs and other combustion engine-driven devices may be prohibited indoors and in outdoor areas with heavy pedestrian traffic.

POLICIES ON THE USE OF OPDMDS

In deciding whether a type of OPDMD can be accommodated, covered entities must consider all assessment factors and, where

Health Technology Sourcebook, Third Edition

appropriate, should develop and publicize rules for people with disabilities using these devices. Such rules may include the following:

- Requiring the user to operate the device at the speed of pedestrian traffic.
- Identifying specific locations, terms, or circumstances (if any) where the devices cannot be accommodated.
- Setting out instructions for going through security screening machines if the device contains technology that could be harmed by the machine.
- Specifying whether or not storage is available for the device when it is not being used.

CREDIBLE ASSURANCE

An entity that determines it can accommodate one or more types of OPDMDs in its facility is allowed to ask the person using the device to provide credible assurance that the device is used because of a disability. If the person presents a valid, state-issued disability parking placard or card or a state-issued proof of disability, it must be accepted as credible assurance on its face. If the person does not have this documentation but states verbally that the OPDMD is being used because of a mobility disability, it must also be accepted as credible assurance unless the person is observed doing something that contradicts the assurance. For example, if a person is observed running and jumping, it may be evidence that contradicts the person's assertion of a mobility disability. However, it is very important for covered entities and their staff to understand that the fact that a person with a disability is able to walk for a short distance does not necessarily contradict a verbal assurance—many people with mobility disabilities can walk but need their mobility device for longer distances or uneven terrain. This is particularly true for people who lack stamina, have poor balance, or use mobility devices because of respiratory, cardiac, or neurological disabilities. A covered entity cannot ask people about their disabilities.

STAFF TRAINING

Ongoing staff training is essential to ensure that people with disabilities who use OPDMDs for mobility are not turned away or

Assistive Devices

treated inappropriately. Training should include instruction on the types of OPDMDs that can be accommodated, the rules for obtaining credible assurance that the device is being used because of a disability, and the rules for the operation of the devices within the facility.

Section 34.5 | GPS and Wayfinding Apps for People with Visual Impairment

This section includes text excerpted from "GPS and Wayfinding Apps," U.S. Library of Congress (LOC), February 2020.

People with visual disabilities use a variety of tools to help them navigate their environment. Nontechnological methods include white canes and service animals. This reference guide offers an overview of the technological solutions for people with disabilities when in transit from one location to another. Listed in this resource are mobile applications (apps) for mobile devices that can aid people with visual impairments in finding destinations. The apps listed below are for use in conjunction with white canes and service animals, not to replace them. Prices are subject to change, and listing in this reference guide does not constitute an endorsement.

MOBILE APPS
The following software mobile apps are designed to work with devices such as iPhones, iPads, and phones and tablets working on the Android platforms. Several are designed specifically for people with visual disabilities, while others are designed for the general public but are accessible to users with visual impairments as of this writing.

Access Now
Access Now informs users of the nearest restaurant, bar, café, or other space open to the public and shares its accessibility to people with

disabilities. A map feature gives directional information to users. Users can enter accessibility information about particular locations.

Apple Maps

Apple Maps offers turn-by-turn navigation and allows users to ask Siri for navigation to locations, as well as provides transit timetables and directions to locations using public transportation. Users can store their favorite places on any additional apple devices they have.

Ariadne GPS

Ariadne interfaces with VoiceOver to provide information regarding the data on its map. Users place their fingers on the map shown on the app, and the app provides them with directional guidance. It has the option of alerting the user with periodic information regarding their location.

AroundMe

AroundMe tells users what is near them. If they are looking for a restaurant or library, AroundMe informs them of the closest one. Designed for the general public, it also has a view feature that uses the device's camera so that the images of items of interest appear on the screen.

Autour

Using three-dimensional (3D) sound, Autour lets users with visual disabilities know of the points of interest around them in real time as they walk. Once users discover a point of interest they want to learn more about, they can select it. The app provides them with additional information.

BlindSquare

BlindSquare interfaces with FourSquare to inform the user of points of interest nearest them and dictates the location in a synthesized voice. The app also announces information about intersections near the user. For an additional in-app credit purchase, it can respond to voice commands.

Assistive Devices

BlindSquare Event
BlindSquare Event is available to organizers of meetings, conferences, social gatherings, and other functions that expect blind or visually impaired individuals to attend. Organizers can register their event with BlindSquare, which makes key information about the event available for free.

Clew
When activated, Clew traces the steps of a user with a visual impairment, so they can follow their steps back. It also saves the route so they can revisit the direction they originally chose. Uses of the app include, for example, finding one's way from a hotel ballroom back to the front door of a lobby.

Embark
Designed for the general public, Embark is a public transportation app that works in over 500 cities around the world and contains maps of their transportation systems. It informs users when they are approaching their stop and saves favorite stops for the rider. Users can bookmark destinations so they can receive step-by-step instructions to those locations. Allows users to access entertainment options from within the app itself.

Get There
Get There is a GPS app designed for people with visual impairments. Gives turn-by-turn navigation and alerts users when they approach and arrive at intersections. Informs users when they veer off their route. Users can set alerts for when they reach specific locations. Speech recognition is available.

Google Maps
Google Maps is available in over 220 countries, offering users point-by-point navigation and real-time mass transit information. It contains information on points of interest and suggests points of interest based on visits to similar locations. Allows users to share points of interest with friends and loved ones.

iMove around

iMove around notifies users regarding their locations, tells them of nearby points of interest, and allows for the recordings of speech notes. It allows the user to share their location via text message and visit the website of the point of interest nearest to them.

Intersection Explorer

Intersection Explorer offers speech instructions about the layout of the intersection to walkers with visual impairments as they "touch and drag" their fingers over the screen.

iWalkStraight

iWalkStraight is an orientation aid that informs users when they are no longer following a straight trajectory and gives them speech instructions when they stray.

Lazarillo

Lazarillo gives users information about their locations as they navigate city streets. It informs them of points of interest nearby and allows them to search for locations, such as restaurants, cafes, and libraries.

Lazzus

Lazzus identifies the current location of users and allows them to preprogram information about common obstacles on routes they frequently travel. For instance, they can program in crosswalks, staircases, and other potential hazards so they will be notified the next time they approach them. It also tells users about nearby points of interest, such as cafes, restaurants, and banks.

Loadstone GPS

Previously available on Nokia devices, Loadstone is now available for iOS. Users navigate their surroundings, learn their addresses, and discover points of interest. It also allows users to input data about a specific location and share that information with other Loadstone users.

Assistive Devices

MyWay Classic

MyWay Classic directs travelers with visual impairments to points of interest. It can access data from the contacts in the phone of the users and direct users to the locations of those addresses. It notifies users of nearby points of interest. Users can import files from Open Street Map to discover additional points of interest.

Nearby Explorer

Nearby Explorer guides users as they move toward a destination. Users can either enter an address or select from points of interest, and the app provides them with point-by-point instructions on how to get there, sharing information about intersections and alerting them when they are veering off the entered course.

Nearby Explorer Online

Nearby Explorer Online is a free version of Nearby Explorer. Unlike its fully functional parent, it only works indoors when connected to the internet.

OverTHERE

When users direct their phone to the point of interest—which are referred to as "signs"—the app informs them what it is. It also allows users to access contact information about those points of interest and informs them of street intersections.

Seeing Assistant AlarmGPS

Seeing Assistant AlarmGPS alarms users as they are making their way to their destinations. Users can set alarms and distance notifications. It also has a "where am I" function that informs users of their current location.

Seeing Assistant Move

Using geolocation from OpenStreetMap, this app gives users directions as they navigate. It provides advanced scanning of a region to

Health Technology Sourcebook, Third Edition

provide directions for the user. It is voice-activated, allowing users to speak commands on their phones.

Seeing Eye GPS

Seeing Eye GPS provides point-by-point navigation to users as they make their way to their destinations. It has a simplified menu with only current location, points of interest, and route. It describes the intersections where users are located. It gives a warning when approaching turns. Routes are recalculated when the users stray.

Soundscape

Designed to be used with stereo headphones, Soundscape allows users with visual disabilities to find desired destinations and tag them with virtual beacons. Users hear a bell sound when facing the beacons. When travelers are not directed toward a beacon, they hear a tapping sound from the direction in which the beacon is located. The app also highlights points of interest and allows users to mark locations such as bus stops.

ViaOptaNav

ViaOptaNav offers turn-by-turn navigation for travelers with visual impairments. It informs them of their current location and alerts them when they have reached their destination. It allows users to set up waypoints for ease of navigation and to save destinations.

Where Am I At?

Designed for the general public, Where Am I At? pinpoints locations of users with information including the address and coordinates. It allows users to share their location information with others.

Where To?

Designed for the general public, Where To? announces points of interest nearest to the user. It lists points of interest near the user's location and provides information on locations, such as the menus of restaurants and special offers from businesses.

Assistive Devices

APPS THAT WORK WITH STRATEGICALLY PLACED BEACONS

The apps and devices listed below work with beacons placed strategically in a venue. Proprietors of the location contract with one of the companies listed below to have them place the beacons. The end user has access to a free app that uses those beacons to help them navigate around the setting.

Aware

Aware uses iBeacons to inform users where they are in a specific location and how to navigate a building. For example, it tells users at an airport how to find their gate or a shopper at a mall how to find a department store. The beacons can also have data specific to a location programmed within them to relay back to users. For example, Aware can tell users if an item at a store is on sale. It is capable of being operated by voice commands.

ClickandGo

ClickandGo offers users a library of venues to choose from, such as college campuses, airports, train stations, bus terminals, hospitals, and so on. It interfaces with iBeacons placed in the location to communicate that information to users with a visual impairment.

LowViz Guide Indoor Navigation

Working with strategically placed beacons throughout a building, the app informs users with visual disabilities of their locations. It provides them with guidance on the best locations and routes within an indoor environment.

RightHear

Using a series of beacons strategically placed throughout a location, RightHear informs users of key locations in that area. It can be used in places such as airports, shopping malls, hotels, and so on. Users have the option of receiving specific instructions from a telephone operator for indoor environments.

Part 8 | Future of Health Technology

Chapter 35 | **Internet of Things in Health Care**

The internet of things (IoT) refers to the technologies and devices that sense information and communicate it to the Internet or other networks and, in some cases, act on that information. These "smart" devices are increasingly being used to communicate and process quantities and types of information that have never been captured before and respond automatically to improve industrial processes, public services, and the well-being of individual consumers. For example, a "connected" fitness tracker can monitor a user's vital statistics and store the information on a smartphone. Electronic processors and sensors have become smaller and less costly, which makes it easier to equip devices with IoT capabilities. This is fueling the global proliferation of connected devices, allowing new technologies to be embedded in millions of everyday products.

FEASIBILITY OF INTERNET OF THINGS DEVICES

The recent advances in the technologies that support IoT devices include:

- **Miniaturized, inexpensive electronics**. The cost and size of electronics are decreasing, making it easier for the electronics to be embedded into objects, enabling them as IoT devices. Smartphones are one of the drivers behind these advances in electronics used in the IoT. As the smartphone market has expanded to

This chapter includes text excerpted from "GAO-17-75, Technology Assessment: Internet of Things: Status and Implications of an Increasingly Connected World," U.S. Government Accountability Office (GAO), May 2017. Reviewed November 2022.

Health Technology Sourcebook, Third Edition

encompass billions of products, the electronics within smartphones—sensors, screens, and communication chips—are also manufactured in large quantities. These electronics have become smaller to meet the requirements of smartphone developers and less costly due to the quantities being produced.

- **Ubiquitous connectivity.** The expansion of networks and decreasing costs allow for easier connectivity. Easily accessible, pervasive networking allows IoT devices to be connected almost anywhere. An example of how networks have expanded is Wi-Fi. The adoption of smartphones has also accelerated connectivity, as smartphones can connect to multiple types of networks, such as Wi-Fi, cellular, and Bluetooth.
- **Cloud computing**. It allows for increased computer processing capabilities. Since IoT devices can create a large amount of data, these devices can require large amounts of computing power to analyze the data. Cloud computing is one way to obtain this computing power. This means that the IoT device itself does not need to have the computation or storage capability but can remotely access cloud computing instead. In addition, the cost of data storage has decreased to the point that cloud computing can store more data for longer periods of time, allowing for the accumulation of large amounts of data.
- **Data analytics**. Advances in data analytics have allowed for the efficient analysis of the rapidly increasing amounts of data created by IoT devices. New advanced analytical tools can be used to examine large amounts of data to uncover subtle or hidden patterns, correlations, and other insights. Advanced algorithms in computing systems enable the automation of functions that appear to require the ability to reason. These advances in data analytics allow valuable information to be extracted from the data collected by IoT devices.

Internet of Things in Health Care

USES AND BENEFITS OF INTERNET OF THINGS IN HEALTH CARE

Internet of things devices are used in health care, both for home health monitoring and in hospitals, with benefits to consumers and the industry. Health-care IoT devices collect data to improve patient quality of life and safety by enabling patients to self-manage and monitor their health. Furthermore, IoT devices can be used together for patients with chronic conditions, such as diabetes. For example, a fitness tracker will generate detailed data on the patient's activity levels. A home monitor will collect data on the patient's blood glucose levels. IoT-enabled pill bottles can collect data on when and how often the patient is taking medication. Aggregating data provide a complete picture of the patient's health by identifying trends and problems that may require intervention by patients and health-care providers. Using IoT devices that transmit health data collected at home to a medical facility can be particularly beneficial to individuals living in rural areas. For example, patients with an implanted heart device can transmit data from their heart device to specialized equipment in their home. The equipment then transmits these data to the patient's health-care provider for review to identify any health-related issues.

Some hospitals rely on IoT devices to monitor and track patients and equipment. For example, a sensor mat under a hospital bed can track patient movement as well as heart and respiration rates. These data are analyzed to monitor movement in and out of bed, to adjust the patient's position while in bed to reduce pressure, and to view trends in heart and respiration rates. Wi-Fi-connected badges worn by patients are used in hospitals and long-term care homes to track patients' locations. Health-care providers can view a patient's location on a monitor, as well as receive alerts if the patient enters a restricted area. This type of monitoring increases patient visibility, mitigates injuries from falls, and monitors a patient's activity. Similarly, hospital equipment, from wheelchairs to vital carts, can be tagged with Wi-Fi devices to provide real-time location and availability information. This reduces the time health-care providers spend searching for equipment and prevents theft by creating an alarm if the equipment is taken off the premises.

Chapter 36 | Use of Blockchain Technology in Health-Care Industry

Blockchain can refer to a data structure that represents a series of immutable transaction records; an algorithm; a collection of technologies; a distributed, peer-to-peer network of systems; or a system of recording information in a way that makes it difficult or impossible to change, hack, or cheat the system.

Blockchain maintains a distributed digital ledger via the use of blocks—a chain of blocks.

Each block contains:

- **Data**. The purpose of the blockchain will dictate the type of data.
- **Hash**. Digital fingerprint identifies a block and all its contents uniquely.
- **Previous hash**. Links current block to the previous block and key to security.

SUPPLY CHAIN TRANSPARENCY

The challenges faced in health-care supply chain, especially with regard to pharmaceuticals, are assuring the authenticity, origin, and supply chain of medical products. Supply chain transparency is important in developing markets where counterfeit prescription

This chapter includes text excerpted from "Blockchain for Healthcare," U.S. Department of Health and Human Services (HHS), October 7, 2021.

Health Technology Sourcebook, Third Edition

medicines and medical devices can cause tens of thousands of deaths annually. To solve this, companies and end consumers need to be able to track each package's end-to-end movement from the point of origin, including manufacturers, wholesale, transport, and so on.

Blockchain can enable companies throughout the prescription drug supply chain to verify the authenticity of medicines, expiry dates, and other important information.

ELECTRONIC HEALTH RECORDS

Electronic health records provide immediate and secure access to health records by patients and their health-care providers. But ensuring that patients have access to all their health/medical records across all service providers is one of the key issues in EHR maintenance.

Blockchain-based medical record systems can be linked to existing medical record software and act as an overarching, single view of a patient's record without placing patient data on the blockchain. Each new record can be appended to the blockchain in the form of a unique hash function, which can only be decoded if the person who owns the data—in this case, the patient—gives their consent.

SMART CONTRACTS

Smart contracts provide immediate, secure, and accurate communications with insurance companies and supply chains. Maintaining contracts of various types can cause unnecessary bureaucratic delays, additional costs, and inaccuracies, which can consume time and legal resources to mitigate.

Blockchain can facilitate transactions between health-care stakeholders, authenticating their organizational identities, logging contract details, and tracking transactions and payments for goods and services. This goes beyond traditional supply chain management to enable business partners and insurance providers in the health sector to operate based on fully digital and automated contract terms. Shared smart contracts between manufacturers, distributors, and health-care organizations included on a blockchain ledger, vice

Use of Blockchain Technology in Health-Care Industry

individual types of contracts, can significantly reduce payment disputes, which can be lengthy and consume resources. Shared smart contracts can be used to manage medical insurance contracts for patients, which once this data is digitized and easily accessible, insurance providers can leverage more advanced analytics to optimize health outcomes and costs.

INTERNET OF THINGS SECURITY FOR REMOTE MONITORING

Remote patient monitoring services require reliable access to the Internet of Things (IoT) technologies. IoT and internet of medical things (IoMT) technologies are susceptible to distributed denial of service (DDoS) and other similar disruptive attacks. 5G is increasing the availability and deployment of these technologies, ultimately increasing the attack surface and making them more attractive targets. Many patients rely on remote monitoring solutions, where sensors measure patients' vital signs to provide health-care practitioners visibility into patients' health, enabling more proactive and preventative care. Security can be an issue due to disruptive attacks.

Blockchain limits unauthorized data access. It enables IoT and IoMT devices to communicate directly that decreases the opportunities for network disruption.

Blockchain is expected to provide the health-care industry with the following:

- Improved confidentiality hand in hand with increased access to more comprehensive data
- Better quality and more trustworthy goods and services (both procedures and medicine)
- Less fraud, lower prices, and more innovation

Chapter 37 | **Nanotechnology**

Chapter Contents

Section 37.1—What Is Nanotechnology?....................................509
Section 37.2—Nanomedicine 510

Chapter 31 | Nephrotechnology

Section 37.1 | What Is Nanotechnology?

This section includes text excerpted from "What Is Nanotechnology," National Nanotechnology Initiative (NNI), September 13, 2014. Reviewed November 2022.

Nanotechnology is science, engineering, and technology conducted at the nanoscale, which is about 1–100 nm.

Nanoscience and nanotechnology are the study and application of extremely small things and can be used across all the other science fields, such as chemistry, biology, physics, materials science, and engineering.

HOW NANOTECHNOLOGY STARTED

The ideas and concepts behind nanoscience and nanotechnology started with a talk entitled "There's Plenty of Room at the Bottom" by physicist Richard Feynman at an American Physical Society meeting at the California Institute of Technology (CalTech) on December 29, 1959, long before the term nanotechnology was used. In his talk, Feynman described a process in which scientists would be able to manipulate and control individual atoms and molecules. Over a decade later, in his explorations of ultraprecision machining, Professor Norio Taniguchi coined the term nanotechnology. It was not until 1981, with the development of the scanning tunneling microscope that could "see" individual atoms, that modern nanotechnology began.

FUNDAMENTAL CONCEPTS IN NANOSCIENCE AND NANOTECHNOLOGY

It is hard to imagine just how small nanotechnology is. One nanometer is a billionth of a meter, or 10^{-9} of a meter. Here are a few illustrative examples:

- There are 25,400,000 nm in an inch.
- A sheet of newspaper is about 100,000 nm thick.
- On a comparative scale, if a marble were a nanometer, then one meter would be the size of the Earth.

Health Technology Sourcebook, Third Edition

Nanoscience and nanotechnology involve the ability to see and control individual atoms and molecules. Everything on Earth is made up of atoms—the food we eat, the clothes we wear, the buildings and houses we live in, and our own bodies.

But something as small as an atom is impossible to see with the naked eye. In fact, it is impossible to see with the microscopes typically used in high school science classes. The microscopes needed to see things at the nanoscale were invented in the early 1980s.

Once scientists had the right tools, such as the scanning tunneling microscope (STM) and the atomic force microscope (AFM), the age of nanotechnology was born.

Although modern nanoscience and nanotechnology are quite new, nanoscale materials have been used for centuries. Alternate-sized gold and silver particles created colors in the stained glass windows of medieval churches hundreds of years ago. The artists back then just did not know that the process they used to create these beautiful works of art actually led to changes in the composition of the materials they were working with.

Today's scientists and engineers are finding a wide variety of ways to make materials deliberately at the nanoscale to take advantage of their enhanced properties, such as higher strength, lighter weight, increased control of the light spectrum, and greater chemical reactivity than their larger-scale counterparts.

Section 37.2 | Nanomedicine

This section includes text excerpted from "Nanomedicine," National Institutes of Health (NIH), October 28, 2019.

The Nanomedicine Initiative program began in 2005 with a national network of eight Nanomedicine Development Centers (NDCs). Now, in the second half of this 10-year program, the four centers best positioned to effectively apply their findings to translational studies were selected to continue receiving support.

Nanotechnology

The following are the two major goals of the Nanomedicine Initiative:

- Understand how the biological machinery inside living cells is built and operates at the nanoscale.
- Use this information to re-engineer these structures, develop new technologies that could be applied to treating diseases, and/or leverage the new knowledge to focus work directly on translational studies to treat a disease or repair damaged tissue.

Nanomedicine, an offshoot of nanotechnology, refers to highly specific medical interventions at the molecular scale for curing disease or repairing damaged tissues, such as bone, muscle, or nerve.

The vision of the National Institutes of Health (NIH) for nanomedicine is built upon the strengths of NIH-funded researchers in probing and understanding the biological, biochemical, and biophysical mechanisms of living tissues. Since the cellular machinery operates at the nanoscale, the primary goal of the program—characterizing the molecular components inside cells at a level of precision that leads to re-engineering intracellular complexes—is a monumental challenge.

The teams selected to carry out this initiative consist of researchers with deep knowledge of biology and physiology, physics, chemistry, math and computation, engineering, and clinical medicine. The choice and design of experimental approaches are directed by the need to solve clinical problems (e.g., treatment of sickle cell disease, blindness, cancer, and Huntington disease). These are very challenging problems, and great breakthroughs are needed to achieve the goals within the projected 10-year time frame. The initiative was selected for the NIH Roadmap (now Common Fund) precisely because of the challenging, high-risk goals, and the NIH team is working closely with the funded investigators to use the funds and the intellectual resources of the network of investigators to meet those challenges.

Health Technology Sourcebook, Third Edition

TEN-YEAR PROGRAM DESIGN: HIGH RISK, HIGH REWARD

The NDCs were funded with the expectation that the first half of the initiative would be more heavily focused on basic science with increased emphasis on the application of this knowledge in the second five years. This was a novel, experimental approach to translational medicine that began by funding basic scientists interested in gaining a deep understanding of an intracellular nanoscale system and necessitated collaboration with clinicians from the outset in order to properly position work at the centers so that during the second half of the initiative, studies would be applied directly to medical applications. The program began with eight NDCs, and four centers remain in the second half of the program.

CLINICAL CONSULTING BOARDS

The program has established Clinical Consulting Boards (CCBs) for each of the continuing centers. These boards consist of at least three disease-specific clinician-scientists who are experts in the target disease(s). The intent is for CCBs to provide advice and insight into the needs and barriers regarding resource and personnel allocations as well as scientific advice as needed to help the centers reach their translational goals. Each CCB reports directly to the NIH project team.

TRANSLATIONAL PATH

In 2011, the principal investigators (PIs) of the NDCs worked with their CCBs to precisely define their translational goals and the translational research path needed to reach those goals by the end of the initiative in 2015. To facilitate this, the NIH project team asked them to develop critical decision points along their path. These critical decision points differ from distinct milestones because they may be adjusted based on successes, challenges, barriers, and progress. Similarly, the timing of these decision points may be revised as the centers progress. Research progress and critical decision points are revisited several times a year by the CCB and the NIH team, and when a decision point is reached, the next steps are re-examined for relevance, feasibility, and timing.

Nanotechnology

TRANSITION PLAN

Throughout the program, various projects have been spun off of work at all the centers, and most have received funding from other sources. This was by design, as work at each center has been shifting from basic science to translational studies. Centers will not be supported by the common fund after 10 years. It is expected that work at the centers will be more appropriately funded by other sources. Preclinical targets will likely be developed, and the work at each center will be focused on a specific disease, so the work will need to transition out of the experimental space of the common fund.

Chapter 38 | Stem Cells and Artificial Intelligence: Better Together

One day in the future when you need medical care, someone will examine you, diagnose the problem, remove some of your body's healthy cells, and then use them to grow a cure for your ailment. The therapy will be personalized and especially attuned to you and your body, your genes, and the microbes that live in your gut. This is the dream of modern medical science in the field of "regenerative medicine."

There are many obstacles standing between this dream and its implementation in real life, however. One obstacle is complexity.

Cells often differ so much from one another and differ in so many ways that scientists have a hard time predicting what the cells will do in any given therapeutic scenario. There are literally millions of parameters when it comes to living products. And that means millions of ways that a medical therapy could possibly go wrong.

"It is notoriously difficult to characterize cell products," says Carl Simon, a biologist at the National Institute of Standards and Technology (NIST). "They are not stable, and they are not homogenous, and the test methods for characterizing them have large error bars."

Simon and his colleagues want to change that by narrowing down the possibilities and increasing the chances, the doctor will know that these cells will do exactly what is expected.

This chapter includes text excerpted from "Stem Cells and AI: Better Together," National Institute of Standards and Technology (NIST), November 18, 2019.

Health Technology Sourcebook, Third Edition

One of the keys is good measurement. Scientists need to be able to measure what happens in cells as they are manufactured into medical products, but how do you efficiently measure something that has millions of parameters?

The cell measurement question has been plaguing medical product researchers and developers for years, including eye researchers. As some people age, they begin to lose their eyesight in a process called "age-related macular degeneration" (AMD). Finding an effective therapy based on stem cells could mean an increased quality of life for people around the world. Personalized, regenerative medicine seems like a strong possibility for this ailment, but quality assurance measurements have been slow and halting.

To help improve that quality assurance piece of the puzzle, Simon's team was working with Kapil Bharti, a researcher at the National Eye Institute at the National Institutes of Health, to use a new kind of microscopy to examine lab-grown eye tissues for treating blindness.

One day when Simon and Nicholas Schaub, one of the postdoctoral researchers on Simon's team, were experimenting with computers in the lab, it struck Schaub that the free, open-source artificial intelligence (AI) program he would use to narrow down good investment choices for personal finance projects might be useful for their research.

They took data they had collected from their experiments with Bharti—which is normally very difficult to decipher—and applied a type of AI program called "deep neural networks."

The results came back with an astounding rate of accuracy. They discovered that the AI program made only one incorrect prediction about cell changes out of the 36 predictions it was asked to make.

The AI program they used was based on a well-known model architecture, GoogLeNet. Their program learned how to predict cell function in different scenarios and settings from annotated images of cells. It could soon rapidly analyze images of the lab-grown eye tissues to classify the tissues as good or bad. Once trained, an AI program can classify eye tissues more accurately and faster than any human.

Stem Cells and Artificial Intelligence: Better Together

What was most novel in this case, however, was that the numbers being plugged into the software were the result of one of the oldest pieces of technology in biology: a basic microscope set up to gather what are called "bright-field" images. This team's effort paired one of the most modern ways to do research with one of the oldest.

Chapter 39 | **Deep Learning for Better Medical Images**

Researchers funded by the National Institute of Biomedical Imaging and Bioengineering (NIBIB) are constructing macroscopic medical images of cells and tissues at speeds 7,000 times faster than current methods allow, using a deep learning approach. Producing high-quality, real-time, macroscopic molecular images could enable medical experts to make better, more informed clinical diagnoses. The new technique, by a team at Rensselaer Polytechnic Institute, may produce better images of living organisms in real time.

Molecular imaging allows medical experts to observe a detailed picture of what is happening inside a person's cells and tissues by exploiting various traits of molecules associated with a disease, also known as "biomarkers." In optical imaging, scientists attach fluorescent tags to the biomarkers.

They can simultaneously monitor multiple biomarkers by varying the fluorescent colors bound to each one, so they are easy to differentiate from one another. With this technique, they can measure the length of time a molecule stays glowing or in an excited state, defined as "lifetime." Measuring the lifetime of a molecule can be useful for monitoring drug delivery or the environment immediately surrounding the molecule (microenvironment).

The length of time it takes for data processing "is one of the main barriers in measuring the lifetime of multiple fluorescent biomarkers, especially for clinical applications," said Dr. Behrouz

---

This chapter includes text excerpted from "Deep Learning Builds Better Medical Images at Ultra-Fast Speeds," National Institute of Biomedical Imaging and Bioengineering (NIBIB), July 18, 2019. Reviewed November 2022.

Health Technology Sourcebook, Third Edition

Shabestari, Ph.D., director of the NIBIB program in artificial intelligence, machine learning, and deep learning. "Developments in artificial intelligence in biomedical imaging, especially deep learning, are beginning to significantly improve image quality and speed up processing times."

Deep learning has been applied to biomedical imaging to improve the quality of an existing image for improved clinical diagnosis. "But what our team is working towards is unique; we are using deep learning to execute the physics behind the original construction of the image," explained Dr. Xavier Intes, Ph.D., codirector of the Biomedical Imaging Center at Rensselaer and the corresponding author of the paper published in the Nature journal *Light: Science and Applications.*

Building upon a previous approach developed by the same team, the new technique called "network for fluorescence lifetime imaging with compressed sensing" ("Net-FLICS") uses deep learning to construct an image from a small number of point measurements.

Intes' and Yan's team created an entirely new deep learning network to build molecular images. Often, a network that is exceptional at identifying images in a Google search can be slightly adapted for similar applications such as facial recognition; this process is called "transfer learning." "There wasn't an existing network for our specific application, so we had to take pieces of other networks to build what we needed," said Yan.

The researchers trained the network using simulations and computer models to generate a large amount of data. Using models gave the team an enormous advantage—they had access to an infinite amount of data, which is a common obstacle in training a network.

However, there are challenges to working with a new network. "It's hard to comprehend what occurs inside a brand-new network like ours—it's kind of like a black box. As we continue to learn more, it will become clearer why the network makes certain decisions, and we can improve it," explained Intes.

The significant advantages of Net-FLICS allow images to be acquired in almost real time, opening new doors to researchers and clinicians due to the improved speed and quality of images. Future applications of the Net-FLICS technique will help identify which

Deep Learning for Better Medical Images

individual cells show uptake of drug treatment and which ones do not. Real-time molecular imaging could also aid surgeons while performing complicated procedures, such as removing a tumor or working around delicate nerves.

Chapter 40 | Emerging Artificial Intelligence Applications in Oncology

Research funded by the National Cancer Institute (NCI) has already led to several opportunities for the use of artificial intelligence (AI).

IMPROVING CANCER SCREENING AND DIAGNOSIS

Scientists in the NCI's intramural research program are leveraging the capabilities of AI to improve cancer screening for cervical and prostate cancer. The NCI investigators developed a deep learning (DL) approach for the automated detection of precancerous cervical lesions from digital images.

Another group of NCI intramural investigators and their collaborators trained a computer algorithm to analyze magnetic resonance imaging (MRI) images of the prostate. Historically, standard biopsies of the prostate did not always produce the most accurate information. Starting 15 years ago, clinicians at NCI began performing biopsies guided by findings from MRI, enabling them to focus on regions of the prostate most likely to be cancerous. MRI-guided biopsy improved diagnosis and treatment when utilized by prostate cancer experts, but the method did not transfer well to clinics without prostate cancer expertise. The NCI clinicians used AI to capture their diagnostic expertise and made the algorithm

This chapter includes text excerpted from "Emerging AI Applications in Oncology," National Cancer Institute (NCI), August 31, 2020.

Health Technology Sourcebook, Third Edition

accessible to clinics across the country as a tool to help with diagnosis and clinical decision-making.

The full potential of the MRI-guided biopsy developed by the NCI researchers is being realized in clinics without prostate-cancer-specific expertise because of this AI tool. New AI algorithms under development now aim to surpass the capabilities of well-trained radiologists by enabling the prediction of patient outcomes from MRI.

AIDING THE GENOMIC CHARACTERIZATION OF TUMORS

Artificial intelligence methods can also be used to identify specific gene mutations from tumor pathology images instead of using traditional genomic sequencing. For instance, NCI-funded researchers at New York University used DL to analyze pathology images of lung tumors obtained from The Cancer Genome Atlas. Not only could the DL method accurately distinguish between two of the most common lung cancer subtypes, adenocarcinoma and squamous cell carcinoma, but it could also predict commonly mutated genes from the images.

In the context of brain tumors, identifying mutations using noninvasive techniques is a particularly challenging problem. With the NCI support, an international team, including investigators at Harvard University and the University of Pennsylvania, recently developed a DL method to identify isocitrate dehydrogenase (IDH) mutations noninvasively from MRI images of gliomas. These research findings suggest that in the future, AI could help identify gene mutations in innovative ways.

ACCELERATING DRUG DISCOVERY

The NCI is leveraging the power of AI in multiple ways to discover new treatments for cancer. The Cancer Moonshot is supporting two major efforts in partnership with the U.S. Department of Energy (DOE) to leverage its supercomputing expertise and power for cancer research. In one effort, AI is being used to detect and interpret

Emerging Artificial Intelligence Applications in Oncology

features of target molecules (e.g., proteins or nucleic acids that are important in cancer growth), make predictions for new drugs to target those molecules, and help evaluate the effectiveness of those drugs. Research is also being done to identify novel approaches for creating new drugs more effectively.

A project that is part of the second effort is using computational methods to model the interaction of Kirsten rat sarcoma virus (KRAS) protein with the cell membrane in detailed ways that were not previously possible. A cross-agency research team collaborating with the RAS Initiative developed a model of KRAS–lipid membrane binding to simulate the behavior of KRAS at the membrane. This model could help identify novel ways to inhibit the activity of mutant KRAS protein. This work will help scientists find new avenues to target mutations in the *KRAS* gene, one of the most frequently mutated oncogenes in tumors. In the future, this could be applied to other important oncogenes.

IMPROVING CANCER SURVEILLANCE

The NCI–DOE collaboration is also enabling the application of DL to analyze patient information and cancer statistics collected by the NCI Surveillance, Epidemiology, and End Results (SEER) program. As part of this effort, DL algorithms were developed to extract tumor features automatically from pathology reports, saving thousands of hours of manual processing time. The goal of the project is to transform cancer care by applying AI capabilities to population-based cancer data in real time. This will help better understand how new diagnostic methods, treatments, and other factors affect patient outcomes. Real-time data analysis will also allow for newly diagnosed individuals to be linked with clinical trials that may benefit them. The NCI's long-term investment in the SEER program and its infrastructure, coupled with newer investments in AI, will enable pattern recognition in population data that was impossible before. AI will aid in predicting treatment response, the likelihood of recurrence (local or metastatic), and survival.

REALIZING THE PROMISE OF ARTIFICIAL INTELLIGENCE IN ONCOLOGY AND AVOIDING THE PITFALLS

The potential applications of AI in medicine and cancer research hold great promise. Leveraging these opportunities will require increasing investments and addressing some challenges that will have to be overcome.

Understanding the Method behind the Machine

One challenge of AI, and DL specifically, is the "black box" problem: not fully understanding what features of the data a computer has used in its decision-making process. For example, a DL algorithm that predicts the optimal treatment for a patient does not provide the reasoning it used to make that prediction. Additional efforts are needed to reveal how algorithms arrive at a decision or prediction so that the process becomes transparent to scientists and clinicians. Making these algorithms transparent could help researchers identify new biological features relevant to disease diagnosis or treatment.

Incorporating information about biological processes into the algorithm is likely to improve its accuracy and decrease dependence on large amounts of annotated data, which may not be available. One danger of the "black box" problem is that DL may inadvertently perpetuate existing unconscious biases. Researchers need to carefully consider how potential biases affect the data being used to develop a model, adopt practices to address and monitor those biases, and monitor the performance and applicability of AI models.

With increased investments, the NCI's efforts to realize AI's potential will lead to more accurate and rapid diagnoses, improved clinical decision-making, and, ultimately, better health outcomes for patients with cancer and those at risk.

Chapter 41 | **Drug Delivery Systems**

WHAT ARE DRUG DELIVERY SYSTEMS?

Drug delivery systems describe technologies that carry drugs into or throughout the body. These technologies include the method of delivery, such as a pill that you swallow or a vaccine that is injected. Drug delivery systems can also describe the way that drugs are "packaged"—such as a micelle or a nanoparticle—that protects the drug from degradation and allows it to travel wherever it needs to go in the body. The field of drug delivery has advanced dramatically in the past few decades, and even greater innovations are anticipated in the coming years. Biomedical engineers have contributed substantially to our understanding of the physiological barriers to efficient drug delivery and have also contributed to the development of several new modes of drug delivery that have entered clinical practice.

Yet, with all of this progress, many disease treatments still have unacceptable side effects. Side effects occur because drugs interact with healthy organs or tissues, and this can limit our ability to treat many diseases, such as cancer, neurodegenerative diseases, and infectious diseases. Continuing advances in this space will help facilitate the targeted delivery of drugs while also mitigating their side effects.

This chapter includes text excerpted from "Drug Delivery Systems," National Institute of Biomedical Imaging and Bioengineering (NIBIB), July 2022.

How Are Drug Delivery Systems Used in Current Medical Practice?

Clinicians historically have attempted to administer interventions to areas of the body directly affected by the disease. Instead of delivering drugs systemically, which affects the whole body, some drugs can be administered locally, which can decrease side effects and drug toxicity while maximizing a treatment's impact. A topical (used on the skin) antibacterial ointment for the treatment of localized infection or a cortisone injection to relieve pain in a joint can avoid some of the systemic side effects of these medications. There are other ways to achieve targeted drug delivery, but some medications can only be given systemically.

Another example of a drug delivery system includes the components of a vaccine that helps it travel inside the body. Vaccines work by providing your immune system with instructions to recognize and attack a pathogen. These "instructions"—such as mRNA, in the case of some COVID-19 vaccines—must be packaged so that it is not degraded by the body and can reach its target. The packaging used for COVID-19 mRNA vaccines is lipid nanoparticles, which protects the fragile mRNA cargo and facilitates its delivery into cells.

WHAT TECHNOLOGIES ARE NIBIB-FUNDED RESEARCHERS DEVELOPING FOR DRUG DELIVERY?

Current research on drug delivery systems can be described in two broad categories: routes of delivery and delivery vehicles.

Routes of Delivery

Medications can be taken in a variety of ways—by swallowing, by inhalation, by absorption through the skin, or by injection. Each method has advantages and disadvantages, and not all methods can be used for every medication. Improving current delivery methods or designing new ones can enhance the use of existing medications.

- **Microneedle patch for painless vaccination.**
  Microneedle arrays are one example of a new method of delivering medications through the skin. In these

Drug Delivery Systems

arrays, dozens of microscopic needles, each far thinner than a strand of human hair, can be fabricated to contain a medicine. The needles are so small that although they penetrate the skin, they do not reach the nerves and can deliver medications painlessly. NIBIB-funded scientists are developing such a patch with an array of dissolvable microneedles for vaccine delivery. These patches are easy to use and do not require refrigeration or special disposal methods, so they can be used by patients at home. This technology could be especially helpful in low-resource communities that may not have many health-care providers or adequate storage facilities for traditional, refrigerated medicines.

- **Robotic pill for oral drug delivery of complex drugs.** Self-injections are used to manage some diseases, such as diabetes and Crohn's disease. Medications for these conditions may require an injection because the drugs used are often complex and easily degradable and therefore cannot be taken orally. However, self-injection can represent burdens for patients, including the frequency of the injections and the potential for needle stick injuries.

  NIBIB-funded scientists are developing an alternative method for self-injection: a robotic pill that can be loaded with complex, liquid drugs. Once swallowed, this pill makes its way to the stomach, where the drug is injected into the stomach tissue. The pill is then excreted through the gastrointestinal tract. While these robotic pills have only been evaluated in animal models so far, they could potentially offer an alternative to self-injection across a range of conditions.

Drug Delivery Vehicles

Drug delivery vehicles represent different ways that medications can be packaged so that the drug can safely travel within the body. Some common examples of drug delivery vehicles include micelles,

Health Technology Sourcebook, Third Edition

liposomes, or nanoparticles. Different drug delivery vehicles can improve the targeting of the drug by helping the medication travel exactly where it needs to go. Additionally, research in this space allows for the development of new ways to package hard-to-use drugs for reasons such as size or fragility. These improvements in biotechnology are leading to improved medications that can target diseases more effectively and precisely.

- **Nanoparticle carriers for the treatment of eye disorders**. Gene transfer therapies—where genetic material that codes for therapeutic proteins is introduced into cells—represent a promising way to treat a variety of eye disorders, including macular degeneration. Current delivery methods have limitations, such as the size of the genetic material that they can hold and their tendency to initiate an immune response.

NIBIB-funded scientists are developing a nanoparticle to carry genetic material that overcomes these limitations. These nanoparticles are not readily detected by the immune system and can hold larger genes than current methods. In a mouse model of macular degeneration, the researchers found that injection with their gene-loaded nanoparticles resulted in a 60 percent reduction in abnormal blood vessels (a characteristic of the disease that causes vision impairments) compared with controls. While still in the early stages, this research could lead to better treatments for eye disorders.

- **Mimicking immune cells to combat inflammation**. While inflammation is an essential part of your immune response to harmful substances, excessive inflammation in the vascular system can ultimately cause tissue injury, notably in the lungs. Acute respiratory distress syndrome (ARDS) is a life-threatening condition characterized by sudden and severe damage in the lungs, which can cause low blood oxygen levels. Treatments typically include mechanical ventilation, but there are no recommended

Drug Delivery Systems

pharmacological interventions. Mortality rates for ARDS are high, ranging from 35 to 46 percent.

Part of the vascular inflammation process includes the migration and adhesion of neutrophils, a type of immune cell, into the lungs, where they bind to endothelial cells. Taking advantage of this behavior, NIBIB-funded researchers are designing nanovesicles that mimic neutrophils, which could be loaded with anti-inflammatory drugs that then deposit their therapeutic cargo in the lungs. This new drug delivery system, inspired by biology, is still early in development.

Chapter 42 | Smart Operating Rooms of the Future

SURGERY OF THE FUTURE

In the not-too-distant future, operating rooms will feature devices that will revolutionize surgery for patients and doctors. You can get a sneak peek at these tools in a new mobile app.

The Surgery of the Future app provides a three-dimensional (3D) virtual tour of the operating room of the future. This app is provided by the National Institute of Biomedical Imaging and Bioengineering (NIBIB).

More than a dozen surgical technologies are featured in the app. You can download it on iOS and Android devices. All of the featured technologies are still in development and are funded by the NIBIB.

"NIBIB funds a wide range of advanced technologies, including tools for imaging the body, biomaterials, and robotics," says Margot Kern, who led the development of the app. "One arena where all of these technologies come into play is in the operating room, in surgery."

"When people think about the types of research NIH supports, they don't necessarily think of surgery," she adds. "But surgery is a critical part of our health-care system, and advances in surgical

This chapter contains text excerpted from the following sources: Text under the heading "Surgery of the Future" is excerpted from "Surgery of The Future: A Glimpse of What's to Come in the Operating Room," MedlinePlus, National Institutes of Health (NIH), July 14, 2017. Reviewed November 2022. Text under the heading "NIH-Supported Technologies of the Future" is excerpted from "NIH-Supported Technologies of the Future," MedlinePlus, National Institutes of Health (NIH), July 14, 2017. Reviewed November 2022.

533

Health Technology Sourcebook, Third Edition

technologies have the potential to greatly improve patient care. We thought showcasing some of the technologies NIBIB is funding in a virtual surgical operating room would be an exciting way for the public to learn how their tax dollars are being used to make surgery safer and more effective."

In the app, users can view a number of NIH-funded technologies. These include robots that can stitch tissues by themselves, biomaterials that change shape or dissolve inside the body, and a tool that reduces a surgeon's natural hand tremor.

"This project demonstrates ways that patients and surgeons may benefit from the next generation of technologies conceived, tested, and developed in biomedical engineering and team science laboratories," says Dr. Roderic I. Pettigrew, Ph.D., M.D., director of NIBIB. "This virtual tour provides a sneak peek at what the surgery of the future could entail, all engineered to assist surgical teams and achieve better outcomes for their patients."

NIH-SUPPORTED TECHNOLOGIES OF THE FUTURE

The Surgery of the Future app of the NIBIB lets users see different medical technologies that are coming down the pipeline.

Silk Screws

Silk has been used to stitch up wounds for centuries. Now, researchers have created silk screws and plates to repair fractured bones. Unlike metal, silk can safely break down in the body. This means that patients who receive temporary silk devices to hold their bones in place would not need a second surgery to remove them.

Biopsy Guidance

The Clear Guide ONE is a device that helps target tumors for biopsy. The tool attaches to an ultrasound probe, which produces images of the inside of the body. It helps the physician see the path the needle would take if inserted at that spot.

Smart Operating Rooms of the Future

High-Intensity-Focused Ultrasound
High-intensity-focused ultrasound lets surgeons operate deep within the body without making a cut. In a procedure that uses this technology, multiple beams of ultrasound focus on a target in the body. At the focal point, the energy from the ultrasound beam causes the temperature of the tissue to rise and then destroy it. It does this while leaving surrounding tissue unharmed.

Flexible Endoscope with Fluorescent Capabilities
Researchers have developed a flexible endoscope that can help spot precancerous growths in the colon. The endoscope has a single optical fiber that uses laser light and shows images of fluorescent molecules, which stick to the precancerous growths.

Minimally Invasive Neurosurgical Intracranial Robot
Researchers are creating robots to use inside a magnetic resonance imaging (MRI) machine so surgeons can more easily see tumors. One researcher is developing a worm-like robot that could be directed inside the brain while a patient has an MRI scan.

Fluorescent Tumor Paint
Researchers created fluorescent molecules that cause cancer cells to glow. The molecules can be injected before surgery and are just taken up by cancer cells. Surgeons can see the glowing cancer tissue or tumors using a special camera. Researchers are also developing molecules to light up nerves, which can get wrapped up in tumors.

Self-Stitching Surgical Robot
This robot can stitch soft tissues all by itself. It has 3D and special light cameras to keep track of tissue position.

Tremor-Reducing Instrument

This handheld tool reduces a surgeon's shaking when operating on small structures such as the eye. It estimates the tremor of the surgeon and then adjusts to provide smooth control.

Biodegradable Stent

Each year, approximately half a million Americans receive a stent to hold open an artery in their heart that has been unclogged during a procedure called "angioplasty." A stent is a small wire-mesh tube. It is usually made of stainless steel or another metal. The NIBIB-funded researchers have invented a new material that makes a stent dissolve over time. This new solution could eliminate some of the disadvantages of metal stents.

Chapter 43 | **Telecritical Care**

Shreveport VA has introduced veteran patients to a new form of critical care that expands on the traditional intensive care unit (ICU) model. This new structure is based on telehealth and is known as "telecritical care."

Physicians and nurses from connected parts of the country can join simultaneously, offer discussions, and control a camera. The clarity is remarkable enough to allow critical care specialists to see or identify areas of concern based on the detail needed.

"TeleCritical Care offers 24-hour care at the push of a button," says Kristine Miller, the operations and nurse manager for VA's TeleCritical Care West hub based in Minneapolis, VA.

A Minneapolis team of critical care specialists has spent the last several months in Shreveport helping test the sophisticated equipment, install software, and hard-wire 20 rooms capable of providing telecritical care. The team also offered face-to-face and one-on-one training for Shreveport VA's ICU care teams.

PHYSICIANS IN TWO STATES IMMEDIATELY RESPOND

"TeleCritical Care has transformed the ICU to allow continuity of critical care with licensed intensivists and critical-care nurses using live audio and video," said Matthew Goede, the medical director for the western-based TeleCritical Care hub in Minneapolis.

This chapter includes text excerpted from "TeleCritical Care—ICU of the Future Here Today," U.S. Department of Veterans Affairs (VA), July 13, 2021.

Health Technology Sourcebook, Third Edition

"We have learned, especially over the last many months, that we must embrace technology," said Richard Crockett, Shreveport Medical Center director. "Seeing is believing. When the ICU nurse pushed the call button, it was amazing to see intensive care physicians in two different states immediately respond. Having this Telehealth technology at our medical center is a proud moment in Shreveport VA history."

The arrangement of hi-tech equipment appears as simple as any webcam experience. But there is so much more.

The technology allows staff to monitor blood pressure, heart rate, and lab results. Intensivists can prescribe medications, order tests or procedures, make diagnoses, and discuss health care with patients and family members.

"At the push of a button, any member of the ICU team can receive on-demand critical care from an intensivist or ICU nurse," Miller illustrated. "The hi-resolution camera produces excellent imagery and audio for a one-on-one experience long distance."

ANOTHER SAFETY BARRIER FOR AN ORGANIZATION FOCUSED ON HIGH RELIABILITY

Currently, Minneapolis serves as the central network for VA's TeleCritical Care. Seasoned intensivists and nurses in locations such as Chicago, Las Vegas, Los Angeles, and Iowa City have the knowledge and ability to serve as on-call telecritical care specialists from thousands of miles away.

Goede points out, "VA has taken the TeleCritical lead and we expect to have the largest TeleCritical Care System in the world when all VA hospitals that have opted in and are online. Within moments you can get an intensivist at the bedside."

The inclusion of TeleCritical Care upgrades any ICU and adds another safety barrier for an organization focused on high reliability. The added layer of support improves care and allows the Shreveport VA's ICU to offer the best possible outcome.

Part 9 | Health Technology: Legal and Ethical Concerns

Chapter 44 | **Health Information Privacy Law and Policy**

WHAT TYPE OF PATIENT CHOICE EXISTS UNDER HIPAA?

Most health-care providers must follow the Health Insurance Portability and Accountability Act (HIPAA) Privacy Rule (Privacy Rule), a federal privacy law that sets a baseline of protection for certain individually identifiable health information ("health information").

The Privacy Rule generally permits, but does not require, covered health-care providers to give patients a choice as to whether their health information may be disclosed to others for certain key purposes. These key purposes include treatment, payment, and health-care operations.

HOW CAN PATIENT CHOICE BE IMPLEMENTED IN ELECTRONIC HEALTH INFORMATION EXCHANGE?

While it is not required, health-care providers may decide to offer patients a choice as to whether their health information may be exchanged electronically, either directly or through a health information exchange (HIE) organization.

This chapter includes text excerpted from "Health Information Privacy Law and Policy," HealthIT.gov, Office of the National Coordinator for Health Information Technology (ONC), September 1, 2022.

ARE THERE SPECIFIC LEGAL REQUIREMENTS FOR OPT-IN OR OPT-OUT POLICIES?

The U.S. Department of Health and Human Services (HHS) does not set out specific steps or requirements for obtaining a patient's choice of whether to participate in electronic HIE. However, adequately informing patients of these new models for exchange and giving them a choice of whether to participate is one means of ensuring that patients trust these systems. Health-care providers are therefore encouraged to enable patients to make a "meaningful" consent choice rather than an uninformed one.

ARE THERE PRIVACY LAWS THAT REQUIRE PATIENT CONSENT?

Yes. There are some federal and state privacy laws that require health-care providers to obtain patients' written consent before they disclose their health information to other people and organizations, even for treatment. Many of these privacy laws protect information that is related to health conditions considered "sensitive" by most people.

HOW DOES HIPAA AFFECT THESE OTHER PRIVACY LAWS?

The HIPAA created a baseline of privacy protection. It overrides (or "preempts") other privacy laws that are less protective. But HIPAA leaves in effect other laws that are more privacy-protective. Under this legal framework, health-care providers and other implementers must continue to follow other applicable federal and state laws that require obtaining patients' consent before disclosing their health information.

The resources listed below provide links to some federal, state, and organization resources that may be of interest to those setting up electronic HIE policies in consultation with legal counsel. Implementers may also want to visit their state's law and policy sites for additional information.

Chapter 45 | **Health Information Technology Legislation and Regulations**

21ST CENTURY CURES ACT

There are many provisions of the 21st Century Cures Act (Cures Act) that will improve the flow and exchange of electronic health information. The Office of the National Coordinator for Health Information Technology (ONC) is responsible for implementing those parts of Title IV, delivery, related to advancing interoperability, prohibiting information blocking, and enhancing the usability, accessibility, and privacy and security of health information technology. ONC works to ensure that all individuals, their families, and their health-care providers have appropriate access to electronic health information to help improve the overall health of the nation's population.

In addition to supporting medical research, advancing interoperability, clarifying Health Insurance Portability and Accountability Act (HIPAA) privacy rules, and supporting substance abuse and mental health services, the Cures Act defines interoperability as the ability to exchange and use electronic health information without

This chapter includes text excerpted from "Health IT Legislation," HealthIT.gov, Office of the National Coordinator for Health Information Technology (ONC), August 9, 2022.

Health Technology Sourcebook, Third Edition

special effort on the part of the user and as not constituting information blocking.

The ONC focuses on the following provisions as we implement the Cures Act:

- Section 4001: Health IT Usability
- Section 4002(a): Conditions of Certification
- Section 4003(b): Trusted Exchange Framework and Common Agreement
- Section 4003(e): Health Information Technology Advisory Committee
- Section 4004: identifying reasonable and necessary activities that do not constitute information blocking

The ONC is also supporting and collaborating with our federal partners, such as the Centers for Medicare & Medicaid Services (CMS), the Office of Civil Rights (OCR) of the United States Department of Health and Human Services (HHS), the HHS Inspector General, the U.S. Agency for Healthcare Research and Quality (AHRQ), and the National Institute for Standards and Technology (NIST).

MEDICARE ACCESS AND CHIP REAUTHORIZATION ACT

The Medicare Access and CHIP Reauthorization Act (MACRA) of 2015 ended the Sustainable Growth Rate formula and established the Quality Payment Program (QPP). The QPP rewards high-value, high-quality Medicare clinicians with payment increases while reducing payments to clinicians who do not meet performance standards. The quality, eligible clinicians have two tracks to choose from in the QPP based on their practice size, specialty, location, or patient population.

- Advanced Alternative Payment Models (APMs)
- The Merit-Based Incentive Payment System (MIPS)

Under MACRA, the Medicare EHR Incentive Program, commonly referred to as meaningful use, was transitioned to become one of the four components of the MIPS, which consolidated multiple quality programs into a single program to improve care.

Clinicians participating in MIPS earn a performance-based payment adjustment, while clinicians participating in an advanced APM may earn an incentive payment for participating in an innovative payment model.

HEALTH INFORMATION TECHNOLOGY FOR ECONOMIC AND CLINICAL HEALTH ACT

The Health Information Technology for Economic and Clinical Health (HITECH) Act of 2009 provides HHS with authority to establish programs to improve health-care quality, safety, and efficiency through the promotion of health information technology (IT), including electronic health records and private and secure electronic health information exchange.

U.S. FOOD AND DRUG ADMINISTRATION SAFETY AND INNOVATION ACT

Section 618 of the U.S. Food and Drug Administration Safety and Innovation Act (FDASIA) of 2012 directed the U.S. Secretary of Health and Human Services, acting through the Commissioner of the U.S. Food and Drug Administration (FDA), and in consultation with ONC and the chairman of the Federal Communications Commission (FCC), to develop a report that contains a proposed strategy and recommendations on an appropriate, risk-based regulatory framework for health IT, including medical mobile applications, that promotes innovation, protects patient safety, and avoids regulatory duplication. The Health IT Policy Committee formed an FDASIA workgroup and issued recommendations to ONC, FDA, and FCC as of the September 4, 2013, Health IT Policy Committee meeting.

HEALTH INSURANCE PORTABILITY AND ACCOUNTABILITY ACT

The HIPAA of 1996 protects health insurance coverage for workers and their families when they change or lose their jobs, requires the establishment of national standards for electronic health-care transactions, and requires the establishment of national identifiers for providers, health insurance plans, and employers.

Health Technology Sourcebook, Third Edition

The HHS's OCR administers the HIPAA Privacy and Security Rules. The HIPAA Privacy Rule describes what information is protected and how protected information can be used and disclosed. The HIPAA Security Rule describes who is covered by the HIPAA privacy protections and what safeguards must be in place to ensure appropriate protection of electronic protected health information.

The CMS administers and enforces the HIPAA Administrative Simplification Rules, including the Transactions and Code Set Standards, Employer Identifier Standard, and National Provider Identifier Standard. The HIPAA Enforcement Rule provides standards for the enforcement of all the Administrative Simplification Rules.

AFFORDABLE CARE ACT

The Affordable Care Act (ACA) of 2010 establishes comprehensive health-care insurance reforms that aim to increase access to health care, improve quality and lower health-care costs, and provide new consumer protections.

Chapter 46 | **HIPAA Privacy Rule's Right of Access and Health Information Technology**

The federal Privacy, Security, and Breach Notification Rules implemented under Health Insurance Portability and Accountability Act (HIPAA) and administered and enforced by the Office of Civil Rights (OCR) of the U.S. Department of Health and Human Services (HHS) continue to serve as the national foundation of protections for individually identifiable health information and of individuals' rights with respect to their information, including the right to see and obtain copies of their health information from their health-care providers and health plans. In addition, HIPAA-covered entities and their business associates continue to use the required HIPAA electronic transactions and code set standards to exchange health information for essential administrative purposes, such as submitting insurance claims.

As the Office of the National Coordinator for Health Information Technology (ONC) and OCR work toward achieving the individual access and interoperability promises of the 21st Century Cures Act (Cures Act), they reflect on the fact that the "P" in HIPAA stands for portability. While the portability provision in HIPAA refers to the portability of health insurance coverage for individuals and

This chapter includes text excerpted from "HIPAA & Health Information Portability: A Foundation for Interoperability," HealthIT.gov, Office of the National Coordinator for Health Information Technology (ONC), August 30, 2018. Reviewed November 2022.

Health Technology Sourcebook, Third Edition

their families, they want to talk about the "P" in HIPAA, also signifying the secure portability—or the flow—of health information across the health ecosystem.

HIPAA SUPPORTS DATA PORTABILITY

The HIPAA recognizes the importance of providing individuals with the portability of their data. With limited exceptions, the HIPAA Privacy Rule provides individuals with a right, upon request, to see and receive copies of information in their medical and other health records (a "designated record set") maintained by a HIPAA-covered entity, such as an individual's health-care provider or health plan. At the direction of an individual or personal representative, a covered entity must transmit health information about the individual directly to any person or designated entity within 30 days (with the possibility of one 30-day extension). Covered entities are strongly encouraged to provide individuals with access to their health information much sooner and to take advantage of technologies that enable individuals to have faster or even immediate access to the information.

The ONC and OCR recently began a campaign encouraging individuals to get, check, and use copies of their health information and the two offices offer training for health-care providers about the HIPAA right of access. The OCR and ONC have developed guidance to empower individuals to take more control of decisions regarding their health and well-being through easy access to their health information. These guidelines include access guidance for professionals, HIPAA right of access training for health-care providers, and Get It. Check It. Use It. (https://www.hhs.gov/hipaa/for-individuals/right-to-access/index.html) resources for individuals.

The HIPAA also supports the sharing of health information among health-care providers, health plans, and those operating on their behalf for treatment, payment, and health-care operations (TPO) purposes and provides avenues for transmitting health information to loved ones involved in an individual's care as well as for research, public health, and other important activities.

TECHNOLOGY FACILITATES PORTABILITY: PAST, PRESENT, AND FUTURE

To further promote the portability of health information, the HHS encourages the development, refinement, and use of health information technology (health IT) to provide health-care providers, health plans, and individuals and their personal representatives the ability to more rapidly access, exchange, and use health information electronically.

Now, more health-care providers and health plans are offering individuals electronic access to their health information. In addition, the Cures Act directs the HHS to address information blocking and promote the trusted exchange of health information, which will further promote the portability of this information.

The HHS and its components, such as the Centers for Medicare & Medicaid Services (CMS) and the National Institutes for Health (NIH), along with the White House Office of American Innovation, are working to support the portability of health information and encourage the growth of a health ecosystem that encourages health-care providers, health plans, and individuals to share health information electronically.

- The CMS is calling on health-care providers and health plans (HIPAA-covered entities) to share health information directly with patients upon their request.
- The NIH has established a research program to help improve health care for all individuals that will require the portability of health information.
- The White House Office of American Innovation also has an initiative, MyHealthEData, that aims to break down the barriers preventing patients from having electronic access to their own health records; this initiative also facilitates individuals their HIPAA privacy rule right of access to obtain their health information and direct copies to share with third parties.

Health IT can improve the portability of digital health information and facilitate the HIPAA individual right of access. For example, health-care providers using Certified Electronic Health Record Technology (CEHRT) certified to the 2015 edition of standards, implementation specifications, and certification criteria adopted by HHS for ONC's Health IT Certification Program have view, download, and transmit (VDT) technical capabilities. These capabilities support individuals' ability to use Internet-based technology to transmit their health information to a third party directly from the health-care provider's technology (such as through a patient portal or personal health record) to any e-mail address, as requested by the patient. In the 2015 edition, the "application access" certification criteria require health IT developers to demonstrate that the health IT can provide application access to a common set of patient clinical data via an application programming interface (API). An API is a technology that allows one software application to access programmatically the services another software application provides, including supporting the sharing of electronic health information.

The health app developer portal of the OCR offers resources for health IT developers and others interested in the intersection of health IT and HIPAA privacy and security protections, including those wanting to build privacy and security protections into technology to enable individual choices for secure health information access and sharing.

The Cures Act builds on the capabilities of the 2015 edition by calling for the development of APIs that enable the user to access and use health information "without special effort." As we focus on accelerating individuals' ability to access, share, and use their health information on their smartphones or other mobile devices, APIs should increase data portability and serve as a technology to further implement the health information portability concept. For example, the HHS is currently looking at how developers and users of health IT enable individuals to use an API to make a request to exercise their HIPAA right of access and to request that their health information be transmitted to a designated third party, such as the All of Us Research Program.

LOOKING AHEAD

The guiding principle of the HHS is to make policy choices that will give consumers, health-care professionals, and innovators more options for getting and using health information. Their interoperability efforts focus on improving individuals' ability to access and share their health information to better enable them to shop for and coordinate their own care. They are dedicated to putting patients first, allowing them to be empowered consumers of health care by making the information they need to be engaged and active decision-makers in their care available on their smartphones or other mobile devices.

Chapter 47 | **Telehealth Privacy and Legal Considerations**

Telehealth is a safe and secure way of connecting with your health-care provider online. Just like in-person care, your telehealth appointments, messages, and information are protected by privacy rules.

CONNECTING SECURELY ONLINE

Telehealth connects patients with health care online using a computer, tablet, or smartphone.

Although your appointment will use your regular Internet service or data plan, health-care providers typically use secure patient portals to message, call, and video chat with patients. During the COVID-19 public health emergency, federal policy changes have also allowed health-care providers to sometimes use popular video chat programs for telehealth care.

PRIVACY DURING YOUR APPOINTMENT

Your health-care provider will call you from a private setting, such as their office or an appointment room. You should also be

---

This chapter contains text excerpted from the following sources: Text in this chapter begins with excerpts from "Telehealth Privacy for Patients," U.S. Department of Health and Human Services (HHS), June 29, 2022; Text beginning with the heading "Protecting Patient Health Information" is excerpted from "Legal Considerations," U.S. Department of Health and Human Services (HHS), August 10, 2022.

Health Technology Sourcebook, Third Edition

in a private, safe location where you feel safe to openly discuss your health.

Private locations for your appointment include:

- A private room in your home
- Your car
- A private room in a friend's home
- Outdoors, away from other people

If you cannot find a private place for a video telehealth appointment, let your health-care provider know. You may be able to e-mail, chat, or text through your provider's patient portal instead. They can also help you reschedule or suggest a better location for a visit.

TIPS FOR SAFELY SHARING INFORMATION ONLINE

Telehealth makes it possible to get some health-care services wherever you are. Keeping telehealth private and secure is the responsibility of patients and health-care providers. Take steps to protect yourself when you begin connecting with your health-care provider online.

- Only enter your personal information on secure websites with a lock icon in the address bar.
- Keep your devices protected with updated antivirus software.
- Protect your wireless connection with a password.
- Avoid using public Wi-Fi to access telehealth services.
- Avoid accessing telehealth on devices shared with people outside of your home or family.
- Do not set up a telehealth appointment or share your information with a health-care provider you do not know or with those whose information you do not recognize. Call your regular health-care provider's main phone number to confirm their identity first.

PROTECTING PATIENT HEALTH INFORMATION
The HIPAA Compliance

The Health Insurance Portability and Accountability Act of 1996 (HIPAA) ensures that health-care providers protect patients' personal health information. When we are not in the COVID-19

Telehealth Privacy and Legal Considerations

public health emergency, all of the telehealth services you provide need to be in compliance with HIPAA rules.

The HIPAA Flexibility during the COVID-19 Public Health Emergency

The Office for Civil Rights (OCR) of the U.S. Department of Health and Human Services (HHS) issued a Notification of Enforcement Discretion to empower covered health-care providers to use widely available communications applications without the risk of penalties imposed by the HHS' OCR for violations of HIPAA rules for the good faith provision of telehealth services.

While the HHS' OCR has issued a notice of enforcement discretion to waive HIPAA penalties, the State Attorney Generals have not issued the same notices. Under Section 13410(e) of the Health Information Technology for Economic and Clinical Health (HITECH) Act, State Attorney Generals are permitted to obtain civil money penalties on behalf of state residents for HIPAA violations. You should check with any applicable states to see if they have also waived these penalties.

The HIPAA Flexibility after the COVID-19 Public Health Emergency

The HHS' OCR released guidance to help health-care providers and health plans bound by HIPAA and HIPAA rules understand how they can use remote communication technologies for audio-only telehealth post-COVID-19 public health emergency. Information in the guidance includes the ability to comply with HIPAA when using remote communications to provide audio-only telehealth services, the need to meet HIPAA rules for electronic protected health information transmitted over electronic media, and when a business associate agreement with a telecommunication service provider is not necessary.

PROTECTING YOURSELF FROM LIABILITY AND MALPRACTICE
Before You Offer Telehealth
- Check with your insurance company to make sure they cover telehealth. In some cases, liability insurance will

Health Technology Sourcebook, Third Edition

already cover it, and in others, you may need to purchase supplemental coverage.

- If you plan to offer telehealth in more than one state, you will need to confirm that your insurance policy covers you for all locations.
- You will also want to be aware of any state laws that regulate how you collect and store protected health information.

Chapter 48 | Security and Privacy Risks of Wearable Devices

SECURITY AND PRIVACY RISKS AND CHALLENGES OF WEARABLE HEALTH-CARE DEVICES

When consumers use wearable health-care devices, the technology needs to assure appropriate data protection. Wearable health-care devices should include capabilities that assure security and privacy controls that protect the data that the device collects, stores, and transmits. At the same time, device manufacturers should maximize device use flexibility and convenience to the consumer. A few of the security and privacy considerations inherent in wearable health-care devices are discussed below.

Limiting the Use of User Data

With the rise in the use of wearable health-care devices that track health and wellness activities, there has been a corresponding rise in the use of these devices by employers to incentivize and measure participation in workplace wellness programs. As individuals adopt wearable device usage, sensitive health-related or personal data may be created. Privacy and security controls may not be present in these programs, and data governance programs may be unclear without a clearly established regulatory obligation that

This chapter includes text excerpted from "Securing Consumer Mobile Healthcare Devices," U.S. Department of Homeland Security (DHS), October 1, 2021.

Health Technology Sourcebook, Third Edition

provides guidance on safeguarding the data. For example, programs offered to all employees may not fall under the purview of the Health Insurance Portability and Accountability Act (HIPAA), and therefore, compliance requirements with the HIPAA security and privacy rules may not be defined clearly, or not applicable. Some of these programs link back directly to health insurance companies and employers with the data being used in determining health-care premiums.

Inadvertent Disclosure of Ancillary Information

Users of wearable health-care devices often share information gathered by those devices without realizing how that data could be used to discover information that they do not intend to share. An example of this came to light in 2018 when the global heat map created by Strava, a fitness tracking app used by military personnel in Iraq, was shown to reveal the location of several U.S. military strongholds. Security experts also speculated that the user-generated map could show not only the locations of military bases but also specific routes most heavily traveled as military personnel unintentionally shared their jogging paths and other routes.

Innovation Outpacing Security

The popularity of wearables, such as fitness trackers and smartwatches, is growing at a staggering rate, but the security of these wearables is not keeping up. The increase in the number of native applications available for smartwatches will create new opportunities for fraudsters to compromise wearable health-care devices for access to highly valuable personal information.

Unauthorized Use and Sale of Data by Data Brokers

The ambiguity in terms of use for wearables is used to reserve some actions with "third parties," also known as "data brokers." The U.S. Federal Trade Commission (FTC) released a report to Congress in May 2014 after an in-depth study of nine data brokers. The report revealed that these companies acquired data from various sources,

Security and Privacy Risks of Wearable Devices

including wearables, to be sold in packages to companies with diverse interests, all private and lucrative. In 2012, these businesses invoiced $426 million within the United States. Although regulations are in place in almost all parts of the world that moderately protect the digital consumer from apathy when being made aware of what information is shared, the wearable health-care devices data highway assumes a free hand to an abundance of data for these companies.

Data Is Vulnerable in Transit

Wearable health-care devices are dependent on underlying operating systems and software. Two popular mobile device operating systems are iOS and Android. Smart cellular phones and tablets use these operating systems. Wearable health-care devices may be "tethered" to a smartphone or a tablet, for example, for network communications capabilities or may use these operating systems to support the wearable device's software. Operating systems may include vulnerabilities that are targeted by hackers. Successful vulnerability exploitation may expose private data.

With wearable health-care devices, consumers may be limited in controlling or imposing limits on the wearable device's data collection process. Consumers may not have the option to shut down a wearable device's sensors individually or cancel the device's data collection. Consumers may find it difficult to limit a device manufacturer or other parties from viewing or using collected data. Furthermore, device manufacturers may not implement appropriate data-in-transit protections.

Lack of Industry Standards, Laws, and Regulations

The data transmission formats, encryption and confidentiality, integrated platform interfaces, and data transmission protocols generated by various devices lack uniform industry standards, and a series of problems, such as information silos and privacy protection, have emerged. There is also no uniform industry standard for the data format and content collected by health-care wearable health-care devices, creating difficulties in the storage and management

Health Technology Sourcebook, Third Edition

of data as well as integration and utilization of data. Additionally, there is a lack of cohesive federal policies and regulations on data security and privacy protection for wearable health-care devices, including wearable health-care devices. Certain uses of wearable health-care devices do not fall under HIPAA regulations, allowing wearable device manufacturers to sell user data.

SECURING WEARABLE HEALTH-CARE DEVICES
Consumers

Wearable health-care devices may interoperate with a consumer's smartphone device. Consumers should ensure that they apply appropriate cyber hygiene practices on mobile devices such as their smartphone devices. Consumers may find smartphone security guidance by leveraging tools offered by the Federal Communications Commission (FCC). For example, the FCC implemented FCC Smartphone Security Checker. The FCC (www.fcc.gov/) provides a tool that smartphone users can use to secure their phones. Consumers may navigate the website's interface, select a mobile device operating system, and then click on the "Generate Your Checker" button.

While cursory searching may identify that mobile and wearable devices pose challenges to consumers, device manufacturers may be remiss in proactively providing privacy and security measures. Device safeguarding guidance is available. This paper identifies several links that may serve as starting points for consumers that need information on securing their devices. Some common approaches are as follows:

- Use the passcode lock on smartphones, smartwatches, and other devices. This will make it more difficult for thieves to access information if a device is lost or stolen.
- Protect a smartphone from viruses and malicious software. It is necessary to protect smartphones and other devices from malware, as one would do for a workstation, by installing mobile security software.
- Use caution when downloading apps. Consumers should avoid third-party apps (e.g., apps not purchased through a trusted or managed application distribution

Security and Privacy Risks of Wearable Devices

store). Apps can contain malicious software, worms, and viruses. Consumers should beware of apps that ask for unnecessary "permissions."

- Delete apps that are not needed. Clearing up unwanted apps can boost the performance of your device.
- Check the privacy setting on any apps that collect personal data and limit what gets shared. Consumers should limit sharing between apps.
- Limit location permissions.
- Apply caution when using social network accounts to sign into apps.
- Keep your software/firmware updated on your phone, mobile apps, and wearable health-care devices.
- Avoid storing sensitive information, such as passwords or a Social Security number, on your mobile device.
- Beware of "shoulder surfers" or other social engineering tactics. A common form of information theft is observation. As a consumer, you should beware of your surroundings, especially when you are punching in sensitive information.
- Wipe data off your mobile device before you donate, sell, or trade it using specialized software or using the manufacturer's recommended technique.
- Enable settings that deter theft. Some mobile device features allow the consumer to wipe their device remotely if it is lost or stolen.
- Beware of mobile phishing. Avoid opening links and attachments in e-mails and texts, especially from unknown senders.
- Apply caution when using public Wi-Fi connections. Public Wi-Fi access points may not promote appropriate security measures, and using public Wi-Fi access points may result in exposing sensitive data.
- When available, enable data encryption (data-at-rest protection) and use two-factor authentication or security keys to access network services and applications.

Remanufacturing and Servicing

The U.S. Food and Drug Administration (FDA) has also taken steps to provide guidelines applicable to servicing or remanufacturing medical devices. In the proposed guidelines, the FDA recognizes that medical devices are often reusable and need preventive maintenance and repair during their useful life. Recognizing that remanufacturing has implications for specific regulatory responsibilities and a direct impact on the safety of the ultimate user of the medical device, the FDA issued the draft guidelines to help clarify when remanufacturing is occurring. In the draft, the FDA defines (1) remanufacturing as processing, conditioning, renovating, repackaging, restoring, or other changes to a finished device that significantly changes the devices' performance safety specifications or intended use and (2) servicing as repair or preventive or routine maintenance of one and more parts in a device after distribution. These guidelines can be applied to wearable health-care devices.

Safer Technologies Program

The FDA has also implemented a safer technologies program (STeP) to provide a collaborative opportunity for manufacturers of medical devices that are expected to significantly improve the safety of currently available treatments or diagnostics targeting certain diseases or conditions that are generally nonlife-threatening or reversible. To be eligible, the medical devices must be subject to a premarket approval, De Novo classification request, or premarket notification. The FDA's intent is to allow manufacturers of those devices to interact with FDA experts to address topics as they arise during premarket review phase and improve the efficiencies of those communications. The FDA's goal in the STeP program is to facilitate the delivery of qualified medical devices to end users more quickly by expediting their development, assessment, and review while also preserving statutory standards for their delivery to the market. These guidelines can also be applied to wearable health-care devices.

Chapter 49 | **Tips for Cybersecurity in Health Care**

ESTABLISH A SECURITY CULTURE

Security professionals are unanimous: The weakest link in any computer system is the user. Researchers who study the psychology and sociology of information technology (IT) users have demonstrated time and again how very difficult it is to raise people's awareness about threats and vulnerabilities that can jeopardize the information they work with daily. The tips provided in this chapter describe some ways to reduce the risk, decreasing the likelihood that patients' personal health information will be exposed to unauthorized disclosure, alteration, and destruction or denial of access. But none of these measures can be effective unless the health-care practice is willing and able to implement them, enforce policies that require these safeguards to be used, and effectively and proactively train all users so that they are sensitized to the importance of information security. In short, each health-care practice must instill and support a security-minded organizational culture.

One of the most challenging aspects of instilling a security focus among users is overcoming the perception that "it can't happen to me." People, regardless of their level of education or IT sophistication, are alike in believing that they "will never succumb to sloppy

This chapter includes text excerpted from "Top 10 Tips for Cybersecurity in Health Care," HealthIT.gov, Office of the National Coordinator for Health Information Technology (ONC), January 13, 2015. Reviewed November 2022.

Health Technology Sourcebook, Third Edition

practices or place patient information at risk. That only happens to other people."

The checklists included in this chapter are one proven way to overcome the human blind spot with respect to information security. By following a set of prescribed practices and checking them each time, at least some of the errors due to overconfidence can be avoided. But checklists alone are not enough. It is incumbent on any organization where lives are at stake to support proper information security by establishing a culture of security. Every person in the organization must subscribe to a shared vision of information security so that habits and practices are automatic.

Security Practices Must Be Built In, Not Bolted On

No checklist can adequately describe all that must be done to establish an organization's security culture, but there are some obvious steps that must be taken:

- Education and training must be frequent and ongoing.
- Those who manage and direct the work of others must set a good example and resist the temptation to indulge in exceptionalism.
- Accountability and taking responsibility for information security must be among the organization's core values.

Protecting patients through good information security practices should be as second nature to the health-care organization as sanitary practices.

PROTECT MOBILE DEVICES

Mobile devices—laptop computers, handhelds, smartphones, and portable storage media—have opened a world of opportunities to untether electronic health records (EHRs) from the desktop. But these opportunities also present threats to information privacy and security. Some of these threats overlap those of the desktop world, but others are unique to mobile devices.

Tips for Cybersecurity in Health Care

- Because of their mobility, these devices are easy to lose and vulnerable to theft.
- Mobile devices are more likely than stationary ones to be exposed to electromagnetic interference, especially from other medical devices. This interference can corrupt the information stored on a mobile device.
- Because mobile devices may be used in places where the device can be seen by others, extra care must be taken by the user to prevent unauthorized viewing of the electronic health information displayed on a laptop or handheld device.
- Not all mobile devices are equipped with strong authentication and access controls. Extra steps may be necessary to secure mobile devices from unauthorized use. Laptops should have password protection. Many handheld devices can be configured with password protection, and these protections should be enabled when available. If password protection is not provided, additional steps must be taken to protect electronic health information on the handheld, including extra precautions over the physical control of the device.
- Laptop computers and handheld devices are often used to transmit and receive data wirelessly. These wireless communications must be protected from eavesdropping and interception. Cybersecurity experts recommend not transmitting electronic health information across public networks without encryption.

Transporting data with mobile devices is inherently risky. There must be an overriding justification for this practice that rises above mere convenience. The U.S. Department of Health and Human Services (HHS) has developed guidance on the risks and possible mitigation strategies for remote use of and access to electronic health information.

Health Technology Sourcebook, Third Edition

Where it is absolutely necessary to commit electronic health information to a mobile device, cybersecurity experts recommend that the data be encrypted. Mobile devices that cannot support encryption should not be used. Encrypted devices are readily obtainable at a modest cost—much less than the cost of mitigating a data breach.

If it is absolutely necessary to take a laptop containing electronic health information out of a secure area, you should protect the information on the laptop's hard drive through encryption.

Policies specifying the circumstances under which devices may be removed from the facility are very important, and all due care must be taken in developing and enforcing these policies. The primary goal is to protect the patient's information, so considerations of convenience or custom (e.g., working from home) must be considered in that light.

In today's increasingly mobile world, it is certainly tempting to use mobile technology to break away from the office and perform work from the comfort of home. Those who have responsibility for protecting patient information must recognize that this responsibility does not end at the office door. Good privacy and security practices must always be followed.

MAINTAIN GOOD COMPUTER HABITS

The medical practitioner is familiar with the importance of healthy habits to maintain good health and reduce the risk of infection and disease. The same is true for IT systems, including EHR systems—they must be properly maintained so that they will continue to function properly and reliably in a manner that respects the importance and the sensitive nature of the information stored within them. As with any health regimen, simple measures go a long way.

Configuration Management

New computers and software packages are delivered with a dizzying array of options and little guidance on how to configure them so that the system is secure. In the face of this complexity, it can

Tips for Cybersecurity in Health Care

be difficult to know what options to permit and which to turn off. While a publication of this length cannot go into detail on this topic, there are some rules of thumb:

- Uninstall any software application that is not essential to running the practice (e.g., games, instant messaging platforms, photo-sharing tools). If the purpose of a software application is not obvious, look at the software company's website to learn more about the application's purposes and uses. Also, check with the EHR developer to see if the software is critical to the EHR's function.
- Do not simply accept defaults or "standard" configurations when installing software. Step through each option, understand the choices, and obtain technical assistance where necessary.
- Find out whether the EHR vendor maintains an open connection to the installed software (a "back door") in order to provide updates and support. If so, ensure a secure connection at the firewall and request that this access be disabled when not in use.
- Disable remote file sharing and remote printing within the operating system configuration. Allowing these could result in the accidental sharing or printing of files to locations where unauthorized individuals could access them.

Software Maintenance

Most software requires periodic updating to keep it secure and to add features. Vendors may send out updates in various ways, including automated downloads and customer-requested downloads.

Keeping software up-to-date is critical to maintaining a secure system since many of these updates address newly found vulnerabilities in the product. In larger enterprises, this "patching" can be a daily task, where multiple vendors may issue frequent updates. In the small practice, there may not be the resources to continually monitor for new updates and apply them in good time. Small practices may instead wish to automate updates to occur weekly (e.g., use Microsoft Windows Automatic Update). However, practices

Health Technology Sourcebook, Third Edition

should monitor for critical and urgent patches and updates that require immediate attention. Messages from vendors regarding these patches and updates should be monitored and acted upon as soon as possible.

Operating System Maintenance

Over time, an operational system tends to accumulate outdated information and settings unless regular maintenance is performed. Just as medical supplies have to be monitored for their expiration dates, material that is out-of-date on a computer system must be dealt with. Things to check include:

- User accounts of former employees are appropriately and timely disabled. If an employee is to be involuntarily terminated, disable access to the account before the notice of termination is served.
- Computers and any other devices, such as copy machines, that have had data stored on them are "sanitized" before disposal. Even if all the data on a hard drive has been deleted, it can still be recovered with commonly available tools. To avoid the possibility of an unintended data breach, follow the guidelines for disposal found in the National Institute of Standards and Technology (NIST) Special Publication 800-88 "Guidelines for Media Sanitation."
- Old data files are archived for storage if needed or cleaned off the system if not needed, subject to applicable data retention requirements.
- Software that is no longer needed is fully uninstalled (including "trial" software and old versions of current software).

How Do You Know If Staff Members Have Downloaded Programs They Are Not Supposed To?

There are several commercial applications and services (e.g., anti-malware and antivirus programs) that can be set up to report or even stop the download of rogue/unapproved software. They can conduct vulnerability and configuration scans, and some

Tips for Cybersecurity in Health Care

applications/services can conduct general security audits as well (e.g., other technical, administrative, and physical safeguards). Work with your IT team or other resources to perform malware, vulnerability, configuration, and other security audits on a regular basis.

USE A FIREWALL

Unless a small practice uses an EHR system that is totally disconnected from the Internet, it should have a firewall to protect against intrusions and threats from outside sources. While antivirus software will help find and destroy malicious software that has already entered, a firewall's job is to prevent intruders from entering in the first place. In short, the antivirus can be thought of as infection control, while the firewall has the role of disease prevention.

A firewall can take the form of a software product or a hardware device. In either case, its job is to inspect all messages coming into the system from the outside (either from the Internet or from a local network) and decide, according to predetermined criteria, whether the message should be allowed in.

Configuring a firewall can be technically complicated, and hardware firewalls should be configured by trained technical personnel. Software firewalls, on the other hand, are often preconfigured with common settings that tend to be useful in many situations. Software firewalls are included with some popular operating systems, providing protection at the installation stage. Alternatively, separate firewall software is widely available from computer security vendors, including most of the suppliers of antivirus software. Both types of firewall software normally provide technical support and configuration guidance to enable successful configuration by users without technical expertise.

When Should a Hardware Firewall Be Used?

Large practices that use a local area network (LAN) should consider a hardware firewall. A hardware firewall sits between the LAN and the Internet, providing centralized management of firewall settings. This increases the security of the LAN since it ensures that the firewall settings are uniform for all users.

Health Technology Sourcebook, Third Edition

If a hardware firewall is used, it should be configured, monitored, and maintained by a specialist in this subject.

INSTALL AND MAINTAIN ANTIVIRUS SOFTWARE

The primary way that attackers compromise computers in the small office is through viruses and similar code that exploits vulnerabilities on the machine. These vulnerabilities are ubiquitous due to the nature of the computing environment. Even a computer that has all of the latest security updates to its operating system and applications may still be at risk because of previously undetected flaws. In addition, computers can become infected by seemingly innocent outside sources, such as CDs, e-mail, flash drives, and web downloads. Therefore, it is important to use a product that provides continuously updated protection. Antivirus software is widely available and well-tested to be reliable and costs relatively little.

After the implementation of EHRs, it is important to keep antivirus software up-to-date. Antivirus products require regular updates from the vendor in order to protect against the newest computer viruses and malware. Most antivirus software automatically generates reminders about these updates, and many are configurable to allow for automated updating.

Without antivirus software, data may be stolen, destroyed, or defaced, and attackers could take control of the machine.

How Can Users Recognize a Computer Virus Infection?

Some typical symptoms of an infected computer include:
- System will not start normally (e.g., "blue screen of death").
- System repeatedly crashes for no obvious reason.
- Internet browser goes to unwanted webpages.
- Antivirus software does not appear to be working.
- Many unwanted advertisements pop up on the screen.
- The user cannot control the mouse/pointer.

Tips for Cybersecurity in Health Care

PLAN FOR THE UNEXPECTED

Sooner or later, the unexpected will happen. Fire, flood, hurricane, earthquake, and other natural or human-made disasters can strike at any time. Important health-care records and other vital assets must be protected against loss from these events. There are two key parts to this practice: creating backups and having a sound recovery plan.

In the world of business, creating a backup is routine. In the small practice, however, it may be that the staff members are only familiar with a home computing environment, where backups are rarely considered until a crash happens, by which time it is too late. From the first day, a new EHR is functioning in practice; the information must be backed up regularly and reliably. A reliable backup is one that can be counted on in an emergency, so it is important not only that all the data be correctly captured but also that it can quickly and accurately be restored. Backup media must be tested regularly for their ability to restore properly.

Whatever medium is used to hold the backup (e.g., magnetic tape, CD, DVD, removable hard drive), it must be stored safely so that it cannot be wiped out by the same disaster that befalls the main system. Depending on the local geography or type of risk, this could mean that backups should be stored many miles away. One emerging option for backup storage is cloud computing, which may be a viable option for many since it involves no hardware investment and little technical expertise. However, cloud backup must be selected with care. The backed-up data must be as secure as the original.

Critical files can be manually copied onto backup media although this can be tedious and potentially error-prone. If possible, an automated backup method should be used.

Some types of backup media are reusable, such as magnetic tape and removable hard drives. These media can wear out over time and after multiple backup cycles. It is especially important to test them for reliable restore operations as they age. Storage of backup media must be protected with the same type of access controls.

Recovery planning must be done so that when an emergency occurs, there is a clear procedure in place. In a disaster, it is possible that health-care practices will be called upon to supply medical records and information rapidly. The practice must be prepared to access their backups and restore functionality, which requires knowledge about what data was backed up, when the backups were done (time frame and frequency), where the backups are stored, and what types of equipment are needed to restore them. If possible, this information must be placed for safekeeping at a remote location where someone has responsibility for producing it in the event of an emergency.

Is It OK to Store Your Backup Media at Home?

A fireproof, permanently installed home safe, which only the health-care provider knows the combination for, may be the most feasible choice for many practices to store backup media. This would not place the backup out of the danger zone of a widespread disaster (earthquake, hurricane, nuclear), but it would provide some safety against local emergencies such as fire and flood. Fireproof portable boxes or safes where nonstaff have the combination are inadequate.

CONTROL ACCESS TO PROTECTED HEALTH INFORMATION

To minimize the risk to electronic health information when effectively setting up EHR systems, it is important to set up passwords. The password, however, is only half of what makes up a computer user's credentials. The other half is the user's identity or username. In most computer systems, these credentials (username and password) are used as part of an access control system in which users are assigned certain rights to access the data within. This access control system might be part of an operating system (e.g., Windows) or built into a particular application (e.g., an e-prescribing module); often, both are true. In any case, configure your EHR implementation to grant electronic health information access only to people with a "need to know."

For many situations in small practices, setting file access permissions may be done manually using an access control list. This can only be done by someone with authorized rights to the system. Prior to setting these permissions, it is important to identify which files should be accessible to which staff members.

Tips for Cybersecurity in Health Care

Additional access controls that may be configured include role-based access control, in which a staff member's role within the practice (e.g., physician, nurse, billing specialist) determines what information may be accessed. In this case, care must be taken to assign staff to the correct roles and then to set the access permissions for each role correctly with respect to the need to know. The combination of regulations and the varieties of access control possibilities make this one of the more complex processes involved in setting up an EHR system in a small practice.

What If Electronic Health Information Is Accessed without Permission?

Under certain circumstances, such an incident is considered a breach that has to be reported to the HHS (and/or a state agency if there is such a requirement in the state's law). Having good access controls and knowledge of who has viewed or used information (i.e., access logs) can help prevent or detect these data breaches.

USE STRONG PASSWORDS AND CHANGE THEM REGULARLY

Passwords are the first line of defense in preventing unauthorized access to any computer. Regardless of the type or operating system, a password should be required to log in. Although a strong password will not prevent attackers from trying to gain access, it can slow them down and discourage them. In addition, strong passwords, combined with effective access controls, help prevent casual misuse (e.g., staff members pursuing their personal curiosity about a case even though they have no legitimate need for the information).

Strong passwords are ones that are not easily guessed. Since attackers may use automated methods to try to guess a password, it is important to choose a password that does not have characteristics that could make it vulnerable.

Strong passwords should not include the following:
- Words found in the dictionary, even if they are slightly altered (e.g., replacing a letter with a number).
- Personal information such as birth date; names of self, family members, or pets; Social Security number; or

Health Technology Sourcebook, Third Edition

anything else that could easily be learned by others. Remember: If a piece of information is on a social networking site, it should never be used in a password.

Below are some examples of strong password characteristics:
- At least eight characters in length (the longer, the better)
- A combination of uppercase and lowercase letters, one number, and at least one special character, such as a punctuation mark

Finally, systems should be configured so that passwords must be changed on a regular basis. While this may be inconvenient for users, it also reduces some of the risks that a system will be easily broken into with a stolen password.

Passwords and Strong Authentication

Strong, or multifactor, authentication combines multiple different authentication methods, resulting in stronger security. In addition to a username and password, another authentication method is used (e.g., a smartcard, key fob, or fingerprint or iris scan).

Under federal regulations permitting the e-prescribing of controlled substances, multifactor authentication must be used.

What about Forgotten Passwords?

Anyone can forget a password, especially if the password is long. To discourage people from writing down their passwords and leaving them in unsecured locations, plan for password resetting. This could involve (1) allowing two different staff members to be authorized to reset passwords or (2) selecting a product that has built-in password reset capabilities.

LIMIT NETWORK ACCESS

Ease of use and flexibility make contemporary networking tools very appealing. Web 2.0 technologies, such as peer-to-peer file

Tips for Cybersecurity in Health Care

sharing and instant messaging, are popular and widely used. Wireless routing is a quick and easy way to set up broadband capability within a home or office. However, because of the sensitivity of health-care information and the fact that it is protected by law, tools that might allow outsiders to gain access to a health-care practice's network must be used with extreme caution.

Wireless routers that allow a single incoming Internet line to be used by multiple computers are readily available for less than $100. For the small practice that intends to rely on wireless networking, special precautions are in order. Unless the wireless router is secured, its signal can be picked up from some distance away, including, for example, the building's parking lot, other offices in the same building, or even nearby homes. Since electronic health information flowing over the wireless network must be protected by law, it is crucial to secure the wireless signal so that only those who are permitted to access the information can pick up the signal. Wireless routers must be set up to operate only in encrypted mode.

Devices brought into the practice by visitors should not be permitted access to the network since it is unlikely that such devices can be fully vetted for security on short notice. Setting up a network to safely permit guest access is expensive and time-consuming, so the best defense is to prohibit casual access. When a wireless network is configured, each legitimate device must be identified to the router, and only then can the device be permitted access.

Peer-to-peer applications, such as file sharing and instant messaging, can expose the connected devices to security threats and vulnerabilities, including permitting unauthorized access to the devices on which they are installed. Check to make sure peer-to-peer applications have not been installed without explicit review and approval. It is not sufficient to just turn these programs off or uninstall them. A machine containing peer-to-peer applications may have exploitable bits of code that are not removed even when the programs are removed.

A good policy is to prohibit staff from installing software without prior approval.

Health Technology Sourcebook, Third Edition

CONTROL PHYSICAL ACCESS

Not only must assets, such as files and information, be secured, but the devices themselves that make up an EHR system must also be safe from unauthorized access. The single most common way that electronic health information is compromised is through the loss of devices, whether this happens accidentally or through theft. Incidents reported to the Office for Civil Rights (OCR) show that more than half of all these data loss cases consist of missing devices, including portable storage media (e.g., thumb or flash drives, CDs, or DVDs), laptops, handhelds, desktop computers, and even hard drives ripped out of machines, lost and stolen backup tapes, and entire network servers.

Should a data storage device disappear—no matter how well an office has taken care of its passwords, access control, and file permissions—it is still possible that a determined individual could access the information on it. Therefore, it is important to limit the chances that a device may be tampered with, lost, or stolen.

Securing devices and information physically should include policies limiting physical access, for example, securing machines in locked rooms, managing physical keys, and restricting the ability to remove devices from a secure area.

Where Should You Place Your Server That Stores Electronic Health Information?

When considering where to locate a server containing electronic health information (such as within an EHR), two main factors should be considered: physical and environmental protection. Physical protection should be focused on preventing unauthorized individuals from accessing the server (e.g., storing the server in a locked room accessible only to staff). Environmental protections should focus on protecting the server from fire, water, and other elements (e.g., never store a server in a restroom; instead, store the server off the floor, away from water and windows, and in a temperature-regulated room).

Part 10 | Additional Help and Information

Chapter 50 | **Glossary of Terms Related to Health Technology**

accuracy: The degree to which a measurement (e.g., the mean estimate of a treatment effect) is true or correct. An estimate can be accurate, yet not be precise, if it is based on an unbiased method that provides observations having great variation or random error (i.e., not close in magnitude to each other).

adherence: A measure of the extent to which patients undergo, continue to follow, or persist with a treatment or regimen as prescribed, for example, taking drugs, undergoing a medical or surgical procedure, doing an exercise regimen, or abstaining from smoking.

benchmarking: A quality assurance process in which an organization sets goals and measures its performance in comparison to those of the products, services, and practices of other organizations that are recognized as leaders.

beta (β): The probability of a type II (false-negative) error. In hypothesis testing, β is the probability of concluding incorrectly that an intervention is not effective when it has a true effect. (1 – β) is the power to detect an effect of an intervention if one truly exists.

bias: In general, a systematic (i.e., not due to random error) deviation in an observation from the true nature of an event. In clinical trials, bias may arise from any factor other than the intervention of interest that systematically distorts the magnitude of an observed treatment effect from the true effect. Bias diminishes the accuracy (though not necessarily the precision) of an observation. Biases may arise from inadequacies in the design, conduct,

This glossary contains terms excerpted from documents produced by several sources deemed reliable.

Health Technology Sourcebook, Third Edition

analysis, or reporting of a study. Among the main forms of bias are selection bias, performance bias, detection bias, attrition bias, reporting bias, and publication bias. Confounding of treatment effects can arise from various sources of bias.

biocompatibility: A measure of how a biomaterial interacts in the body with the surrounding cells, tissues, and other factors.

bioengineering: The application of concepts and methods of engineering, biology, medicine, physiology, physics, materials science, chemistry, mathematics, and computer sciences to develop methods and technologies to solve health problems in humans.

bioinformatics: The branch of biology that is concerned with the acquisition, storage, display, and analysis of biological information.

biomarker: An objectively measured variable or trait that is used as an indicator of a normal biological process, a disease state, or the effect of a treatment. It may be a physiological measurement (height, weight, blood pressure, etc.), blood component or other biochemical assays (red blood cell (RBC) count, viral load, hemoglobin A1c (HbA1c) level, etc.), genetic data (presence of a specific genetic mutation), or measurement from an image (coronary artery stenosis, cancer metastases, etc.).

biomaterial: Any matter, surface, or construct that interacts with biological systems. Biomaterials can be derived from nature or synthesized in the laboratory using metallic components, polymers, ceramics, or composite materials. Medical devices made of biomaterials are often used to replace or augment a natural function.

biomedical imaging: The science and the branch of medicine concerned with the development and use of imaging devices and techniques, to obtain internal anatomic images and to provide biochemical and physiological analysis of tissues and organs.

biosensors: A device that uses biological material, such as deoxyribonucleic acid (DNA), enzymes, and antibodies, to detect specific biological, chemical, or physical processes and then transmits or reports this data.

blood-brain barrier (BBB): A highly selective, semi-impermeable boundary that divides the brain from the rest of the body. It allows the passage of vital molecules through specialized transport proteins and diffusion mechanisms.

brain–computer interface (BCI): A system that uses the brain's electrical signals to allow individuals with limited mobility to learn to use their

Glossary of Terms Related to Health Technology

thoughts to move a computer cursor or other devices such as a robotic arm or a wheelchair.

cardiovascular disease (CVD): Also called "heart disease" it is a class of diseases that involve the heart, the blood vessels (arteries, capillaries, and veins), or both.

clinical decision support (CDS): An interactive software-based system designed to assist physicians and other health professionals as well as patients with diagnostic and treatment decisions and reminders.

computational modeling: The use of mathematics, statistics, physics, and computer science to study the mechanism and behavior of complex systems by computer simulation.

computed tomography (CT): A computerized x-ray imaging procedure in which a narrow beam of x-rays is aimed at a patient and quickly rotated around the body, producing signals that are processed by the machine's computer, to generate cross-sectional images—or "slices"—of the body.

computerized provider order entry (CPOE): A computer application that allows a physician's orders for diagnostic and treatment services (such as medications, laboratory, and other tests) to be entered electronically instead of being recorded on order sheets or prescription pads. The computer compares the order against standards for dosing, checks for allergies or interactions with other medications, and warns the physician about potential problems.

contrast agent: A substance used to enhance the imaged appearance of structures, processes, or fluids within the body in biomedical imaging.

control group: The group of participants in a trial that receives a standard treatment or a placebo. The control group may also be made up of healthy volunteers. Researchers compare results from the control group with results from the experimental group to find and learn from any differences.

controlled clinical trial: A prospective experiment in which investigators compare outcomes of a group of patients receiving an intervention to a group of similar patients not receiving the intervention. Not all clinical trials are randomized controlled trials (RCTs) though all RCTs are clinical trials.

cost-benefit analysis: A comparison of alternative interventions in which costs and outcomes are quantified in common monetary units.

deep brain stimulation: A neurosurgical treatment utilizing a neurostimulator placed in the brain to deliver electrical signals to specific parts of the

Health Technology Sourcebook, Third Edition

brain to help control unwanted movements, such as in Parkinson disease (PD), or regulate the firing of neurons in the brain to help control the symptoms of disorders such as epilepsy or depression.

disease management: A systematic process of managing the care of patients with specific diseases or conditions (particularly chronic conditions) across the spectrum of outpatient, inpatient, and ancillary services. The purposes of disease management may include: reducing acute episodes, reducing hospitalizations, reducing variations in care, improving health outcomes, and reducing costs. Disease management may involve continuous quality improvement or other management paradigms. It may involve a cyclical process of following practice protocols, measuring the resulting outcomes, feeding those results back to clinicians, and revising protocols as appropriate.

drug delivery systems: Engineered technologies for the targeted delivery and/or controlled release of therapeutic agents.

effectiveness: The benefit (e.g., for health outcomes) of using a technology for a particular problem under general or routine conditions, for example, by a physician in a community hospital or by a patient at home.

efficacy: The benefit of using a technology for a particular problem under ideal conditions, for example, in a laboratory setting, within the protocol of a carefully managed randomized controlled trial (RCT), or at a "center of excellence."

elastography: A medical imaging technique that measures the elasticity or stiffness of a tissue. The technique captures snapshots of shear waves, a special type of sound wave, as they move through the tissue.

electronic health record (EHR): A real-time patient health record with access to evidence-based decision support tools that can be used to aid clinicians in decision-making. The EHR can automate and streamline a clinician's workflow, ensuring that all clinical information is communicated.

electronic medical record (EMR): An electronic record of health-related information on an individual that can be created, gathered, managed, and consulted by authorized clinicians and staff within one health-care organization.

electronic prescribing (e-prescribing): A technology where health-care providers can enter prescription information into a computer device—such as a tablet, laptop, or desktop computer—and securely transmit the prescription to pharmacies using a special software program and connectivity to a

Glossary of Terms Related to Health Technology

transmission network. When a pharmacy receives a request, it can begin filling the medication right away.

endoscope: A thin illuminated flexible or rigid tube-like optical system used to examine the interior of a hollow organ or body cavity by direct insertion.

endpoint: A measure or indicator chosen for determining an effect of an intervention.

evidence-based medicine: The use of current best evidence from scientific and medical research to make decisions about the care of individual patients. It involves formulating questions relevant to the care of particular patients, searching the scientific and medical literature, identifying and evaluating relevant research results, and applying the findings to patients.

extracellular matrix (ECM): The ECM is a collection of extracellular molecules secreted by support cells that provides structural and biochemical support to the surrounding cells.

fluorescence: The emission of light by a substance that has absorbed light or other electromagnetic radiation. The absorbed and emitted light are usually different wavelengths and therefore produce different colors.

follow-up: The ability of investigators to observe and collect data on all patients who were enrolled in a trial for its full duration. To the extent that data on patient events relevant to the trial are lost, for example, among patients who move away or otherwise withdraw from the trial, the results may be affected, especially if there are systematic reasons why certain types of patients withdraw. Investigators should report on the number and type of patients who could not be evaluated so that the possibility of bias may be considered.

functional magnetic resonance imaging (fMRI): An MRI-based technique for measuring brain activity. It works by detecting the changes in blood oxygenation and flow that occur in response to neural activity—when a brain area is more active, it consumes more oxygen, and to meet this increased demand, blood flow increases to the active area. fMRI can be used to produce activation maps showing which parts of the brain are involved in a particular mental process.

gamma ray: Electromagnetic radiation of the shortest wavelength and the highest energy.

genomics: The branch of molecular genetics that studies the genome, that is, the complete set of deoxyribonucleic acid (DNA) in the chromosomes of

Health Technology Sourcebook, Third Edition

an organism. This may involve the application of DNA sequencing, recombinant DNA, and related bioinformatics to sequence, assemble, and analyze the structure, function, and evolution of genomes. Whereas genetics is the study of the function and composition of individual genes, genomics addresses all genes and their interrelationships in order to understand their combined influence on the organism.

health information exchange (HIE): The electronic movement of health-related information across organizations within a region, community, or hospital system and according to nationally recognized standards.

health information technology (health IT): The application of information processing involving both computer hardware and software that deals with the storage, retrieval, sharing, and use of health-care information, data, and knowledge for communication and decision-making.

health technology assessment (HTA): The systematic evaluation of properties, effects, and/or impacts of health-care technology. It may address the direct, intended consequences of technologies as well as their indirect, unintended consequences. Its main purpose is to inform technology-related policy-making in health care. HTA is conducted by interdisciplinary groups using explicit analytical frameworks drawn from a variety of methods.

image-guided robotic interventions: Medical procedures, primarily minimally invasive surgery, performed through a small incision or natural orifice using robotic tools operated remotely by a surgeon with visualization by devices such as cameras small enough to fit into a minimal incision.

in vitro: A laboratory experiment or process performed in a test tube, culture dish, or elsewhere outside a living animal.

incidence: The rate of occurrence of new cases of a disease or condition in a population at risk during a given period of time, usually one year.

indication: A clinical symptom or circumstance indicating that the use of a particular intervention would be appropriate.

induced pluripotent stem cell (iPSC): A stem cell that is formed by the introduction of stem-cell-inducing factors into a differentiated cell of the body, typically a skin cell.

interoperability: It refers to the ability of health information systems to work together within and across organizational boundaries in order to advance the effective delivery of health care for individuals and communities.

Glossary of Terms Related to Health Technology

ionizing radiation: A type of electromagnetic radiation that can strip electrons from an atom or molecule—a process called "ionization." Ionizing radiation has a relatively short wavelength on the electromagnetic spectrum (EMS). Examples of ionizing radiation include gamma rays and x-rays. Lower energy ultraviolet, visible light, infrared, microwaves, and radio waves are considered nonionizing radiation.

magnetic resonance elastography (MRE): A special MRI technique to capture snapshots of shear waves that move through the tissue and create "elastograms" or images that show tissue stiffness. MRE is used to noninvasively detect hardening of the liver caused by chronic liver disease (CLD). MRE also has the potential to diagnose diseases in other parts of the body.

magnetic resonance imaging (MRI): A noninvasive imaging technology used to investigate the anatomy and function of the body without the use of damaging ionizing radiation. It is often used for disease detection, diagnosis, and treatment monitoring. It is based on sophisticated technology that excites and detects changes in protons found in the water that makes up living tissues.

microfluidics: A multidisciplinary field including engineering, physics, chemistry, and biotechnology involving the design of systems for the precise control and manipulation of fluids on a small, submillimeter scale. Typically, fluids are moved, mixed, separated, or processed in various ways.

microscopy: Using microscopes to view samples and objects that cannot be seen with the unaided eye.

minimally invasive surgery: A surgical procedure typically utilizing one or more small incisions through which laparoscopic surgical tools are inserted and manipulated by a surgeon. Minimally invasive surgery can reduce damage to surrounding healthy tissue, decrease the need for pain medication, and reduce patient recovery time.

mobile health (mHealth): An abbreviation for mobile health, which is the practice of medicine and public health supported with mobile devices such as mobile phones for health services and information.

molecular imaging: A discipline that involves the visualization of molecular processes and cellular functions in living organisms. With the inclusion of a biomarker, which interacts chemically with tissues and structures of interest, many imaging techniques can be used for molecular imaging, including ultrasound, x-rays, magnetic resonance imaging (MRI), optical imaging,

Health Technology Sourcebook, Third Edition

positron emission tomography (PET), and single photon emission computed tomography (SPECT).

nanoparticle: Ultrafine particles between 1 and 100 nanometers in size. The size is similar to that of most biological molecules and structures. Nanoparticles can be engineered for a wide variety of biomedical uses, including diagnostic devices, contrast agents, physical therapy applications, and drug delivery vehicles. A nanoparticle is approximately 1/10,000 the width of a human hair. Nanoparticles are generally 1,000 times smaller than microparticles.

nanotechnology: It is science, engineering, and technology conducted at the nanoscale, which is about 1–100 nanometers. Nanoscience and nanotechnology are the study and application of extremely small things and can be used across all the other science fields, such as chemistry, biology, physics, materials science, and engineering.

negative predictive value: An operating characteristic of a diagnostic test; negative predictive value is the proportion of persons with a negative test who truly do not have the disease, determined as follows: (true negatives, (true negatives + false negatives)). It varies with the prevalence of the disease in the population of interest.

neuroimaging: It includes the use of a number of techniques to image the structure and function of the brain, spinal cord, and associated structures.

nuclear medicine: A medical specialty that uses radioactive tracers (radiopharmaceuticals) to assess bodily functions and to diagnose and treat disease. Diagnostic nuclear medicine relies heavily on imaging techniques that measure cellular function and physiology.

optical imaging: A technique for noninvasively looking inside the body, as is done with x-rays. Unlike x-rays, which use ionizing radiation, optical imaging uses visible light and the special properties of photons to obtain detailed images of organs and tissues as well as smaller structures, including cells and molecules.

patient-reported outcomes: Results that are self-reported by patients or obtained from patients (or reported on their behalf by their caregivers or surrogates) by an interviewer without interpretation or modification of the patient's response by other people, including clinicians.

personal health record (PHR): An electronic application through which individuals can maintain and manage their health information (and that of

Glossary of Terms Related to Health Technology

others for whom they are authorized) in a private, secure, and confidential environment.

personalized medicine: The tailoring of health care (including prevention, diagnosis, therapy) to the particular traits (or circumstances or other characteristics) of a patient that influence response to a health-care intervention. These may include genomic, epigenomic, microbiomic, sociodemographic, clinical, behavioral, environmental, and other personal traits, as well as personal preferences. Personalized medicine generally does not refer to the creation of interventions that are unique to a patient but the ability to classify patients into subpopulations that differ in their responses to particular interventions. (It is also known as "personalized health care.")

photon: A particle of light or electromagnetic radiation. The energies of photons range from high-energy gamma rays and x-rays to low-energy radio waves.

placebo: An inactive substance or treatment given to satisfy a patient's expectation for treatment. In some controlled trials (particularly of drug treatments), placebos that are made to be indistinguishable by patients (and providers when possible) from the true intervention are given to the control group to be used as a comparative basis for determining the effect of the investigational treatment.

point of care (POC): Testing and treating of patients at sites close to where they live. Rapid diagnostic tests are used to obtain immediate, on-site results.

polymer: A large molecule composed of many repeating subunits. Polymers range from familiar synthetic plastics such as polystyrene to natural biopolymers such as deoxyribonucleic acid (DNA). Polymers have unique physical properties, including strength, flexibility, and elasticity.

positron emission tomography (PET): These scans use radiopharmaceuticals to create three-dimensional (3D) images. The decay of the radiotracers used with PET scans produces small particles called "positrons." When positrons react with electrons in the body, they annihilate each other. This annihilation produces two photons that shoot off in opposite directions. The detectors in the PET scanner measure these photons and use this information to create images of internal organs.

precision medicine: The tailoring of health care (particularly diagnosis and treatment using drugs and biologics) to the particular traits of a patient that influence response to a health-care intervention. Though it is sometimes

Health Technology Sourcebook, Third Edition

used synonymously with personalized medicine, precision medicine tends to emphasize the use of patient molecular traits to tailor therapy.

prevalence: The number of people in a population with a specific disease or condition at a given time, usually expressed as a ratio of the number of affected people to the total population.

progenitor cells: They are cells that are similar to stem cells, but instead of the ability to become any type of cell, they are already predisposed to develop into a particular type of cell.

prosthetics: The design, fabrication, and fitting of artificial body parts.

quality assurance: Activities intended to ensure that the best available knowledge concerning the use of health care to improve health outcomes is properly implemented. This involves the implementation of health-care standards, including quality assessment and activities to correct, reduce variations in, or otherwise improve health-care practices relative to these standards.

radiation: The emission of energy as electromagnetic waves or as moving subatomic particles, especially high-energy particles that cause ionization.

regenerative medicine: A broad field that includes tissue engineering but also incorporates research on self-healing—where the body uses its own systems, sometimes with the help of foreign biological material, to rebuild tissues and organs.

rehabilitation engineering: The use of engineering science and principles to develop technological solutions and devices to assist individuals with disabilities and aid the recovery of physical and cognitive functions lost because of disease or injury.

reliability: The extent to which an observation that is repeated in the same, stable population yields the same result (i.e., testa–retest reliability) and also the ability of a single observation to distinguish consistently among individuals in a population.

robotic surgery: Surgery performed through very small incisions or natural orifices using thin finger-like robotic tools controlled remotely by the surgeon through a telemanipulator or computer interface.

safety: A judgment of the acceptability of risk (a measure of the probability of an adverse outcome and its severity) associated with using a technology in a given situation, for example, for a patient with a particular health problem, by a clinician with certain training, or in a specified treatment setting.

Glossary of Terms Related to Health Technology

scaffold: A structure of artificial or natural materials on which tissue is grown to mimic a biological process outside the body or to replace a disease or damaged tissue inside the body.

sensitivity: An operating characteristic of a diagnostic test that measures the ability of a test to detect a disease (or condition) when it is truly present. Sensitivity is the proportion of all diseased patients for whom there is a positive test, determined as follows: (true positives, (true positives + false negatives)).

sensors: In medicine and biotechnology, sensors are tools that detect specific biological, chemical, or physical processes and then transmit or report this data. Some sensors work outside the body, while others are designed to be implanted within the body. Sensors help health-care providers and patients monitor health conditions. Sensors are also used to monitor the safety of medicines, foods, and other environmental substances that may be encountered.

stem cell: An undifferentiated cell of a multicellular organism that is capable of giving rise to more of the same cell type indefinitely and has the ability to differentiate into many other types of cells that form the structures of the body.

technology: The application of scientific or other organized knowledge— including any tool, technique, product, process, method, organization, or system—to practical tasks. In health care, technology includes drugs; diagnostics, indicators, and reagents; devices, equipment, and supplies; medical and surgical procedures; support systems; and organizational and managerial systems used in prevention, screening, diagnosis, treatment, and rehabilitation.

telehealth: The use of communication technologies to provide and support health care at a distance.

tissue engineering: An interdisciplinary and multidisciplinary field that aims at the development of biological substitutes that restore, maintain, or improve tissue function.

ultrasound: A form of acoustic energy, or sound, that has a frequency that is higher than the level of human hearing. As a medical diagnostic technique, high-frequency sound waves are used to provide real-time medical imaging image inside the body without exposure to ionizing radiation. As a therapeutic technique, high-frequency sound waves interact with tissues to destroy diseased tissue such as tumors or to modify tissues or target drugs to specific locations in the body.

Health Technology Sourcebook, Third Edition

utility: The relative desirability or preference (usually from the perspective of a patient) for a specific health outcome or level of health status.

validity: The extent to which a measure or variable accurately reflects the concept that it is intended to measure.

x-ray: A form of high-energy electromagnetic radiation (EMR) that can pass through most objects, including the body. X-rays travel through the body and strike an x-ray detector (such as a radiographic film or a digital x-ray detector) on the other side of the patient, forming an image that represents the "shadows" of objects inside the body.

Chapter 51 | **Directory of Agencies That Provide Information about Health Technology**

GOVERNMENT AGENCIES

Agency for Healthcare Research and Quality (AHRQ)
5600 Fishers Ln.
Rockville, MD 20857
Phone: 301-427-1364
Website: www.ahrq.gov

Centers for Disease Control and Prevention (CDC)
1600 Clifton Rd.
Atlanta, GA 30329-4027
Toll-Free: 800-CDC-INFO
(800-232-4636)
Toll-Free TTY: 888-232-6348
Website: www.cdc.gov
E-mail: cdcinfo@cdc.gov

***Eunice Kennedy Shriver* National Institute on Child Health and Human Development (NICHD)**
P.O. Box 3006
Rockville, MD 20847
Toll-Free: 800-370-2943
Toll-Free Fax: 866-760-5947
Website: www.nichd.nih.gov
E-mail: NICHDInformation
ResourceCenter@mail.nih.gov

Federal Trade Commission (FTC)
600 Pennsylvania Ave., N.W.
Washington, DC 20580
Phone: 202-326-2222
Website: www.ftc.gov

Resources in this chapter were compiled from several sources deemed reliable; all contact information was verified and updated in November 2022.

Health Technology Sourcebook, Third Edition

Health Resources and Services Administration (HRSA)
5600 Fishers Ln.
Rockville, MD 20857
Phone: 301-443-3376
Toll-Free: 800-221-9393
Toll-Free TTY: 877-897-9910
Website: www.hrsa.gov

National Cancer Institute (NCI)
9609 Medical Center Dr.
Bethesda, MD 20892
Phone: 240-276-6600
Toll-Free: 800-4-CANCER
(800-422-6237)
Website: www.cancer.gov
E-mail: NCIinfo@nih.gov

National Human Genome Research Institute (NHGRI)
31 Center Dr., MSC 2152, 9000 Rockville Pike
Bldg. 31, Rm. 4B09
Bethesda, MD 20892-2152
Phone: 301-402-0911
Fax: 301-402-2218
Website: www.genome.gov

National Institute of Arthritis and Musculoskeletal and Skin Diseases (NIAMS)
1 AMS Cir.
Bethesda, MD 20892-3675
Phone: 301-495-4484
Toll-Free: 877-22-NIAMS
(877-226-4267)
TTY: 301-565-2966
Fax: 301-718-6366
Website: www.niams.nih.gov
E-mail: NIAMSinfo@mail.nih.gov

National Institute of Biomedical Imaging and Bioengineering (NIBIB)
6707 Democracy Blvd.
Ste. 202
Bethesda, MD 20892-5469
Phone: 301-496-8859
Website: www.nibib.nih.gov
E-mail: info@nibib.nih.gov

National Institute of Diabetes, Digestive and Kidney Diseases (NIDDK)
31 Center Dr., MSC 2560
Bldg. 31, Rm. 9A06
Bethesda, MD 20892-2560
Phone: 301-496-3583
Toll-Free: 800–472–0424
Website: www.niddk.nih.gov
E-mail: healthinfo@niddk.nih.gov

National Institute of Standards and Technology (NIST)
100 Bureau Dr.
Gaithersburg, MD 20899
Phone: 301-975-2000
Website: www.nist.gov

National Institute on Deafness and Other Communication Disorders (NIDCD)
1 Communication Ave.
Bethesda, MD 20892-3456
Toll-Free: 800-241-1044
TTY: 800-241-1055
Website: www.nidcd.nih.gov
E-mail: nidcdinfo@nidcd.nih.gov

Directory of Agencies That Provide Information about Health Technology

National Institute on Mental Health (NIMH)
6001 Executive Blvd., MSC 9663
Rm. 6200
Bethesda, MD 20892-9663
Toll-Free: 866-615-6464
Website: www.nimh.nih.gov
E-mail: nimhinfo@nih.gov

National Institutes of Health (NIH)
9000 Rockville Pike
Bethesda, MD 20892
Phone: 301-496-4000
TTY: 301-402-9612
Website: www.nih.gov

Substance Abuse and Mental Health Services Administration (SAMHSA)
5600 Fishers Ln.
Rockville, MD 20857
Toll-Free: 877-SAMHSA-7
(877-726-4727)
Toll-Free TTY: 800-487-4889
Website: www.samhsa.gov
E-mail: samhsainfo@samhsa.hhs.
gov

U.S. Congressional Budget Office (CBO)
Ford House Office Bldg.
4th Fl. Second and D St., S.W.
Washington, DC 20515-6925
Phone: 202-226-2602
Website: www.cbo.gov
E-mail: communications@cbo.gov

U.S. Department of Energy (DOE)
1000 Independence Ave., S.W.
Washington, DC 20585
Phone: 202-586-5000
Fax: 202-586-4403
Website: www.energy.gov
E-mail: the.secretary@hq.doe.gov

U.S. Department of Health and Human Services (HHS)
200 Independent Ave., S.W.
Washington, DC 20201
Toll-Free: 877-696-6775
Website: www.hhs.gov

U.S. Department of Justice (DOJ)
950 Pennsylvania Ave., N.W.
Washington, DC 20530-0001
Phone: 202-514-2000
TTY: 800-877-8339
Website: www.justice.gov

U.S. Department of Labor (DOL)
200 Constitution Ave., N.W.
Washington, DC 20210
Toll-Free: 866-4-USA-DOL
(866-487-2365)
Website: www.dol.gov

U.S. Food and Drug Administration (FDA)
10903 New Hampshire Ave.
Silver Spring, MD 20993-0002
Toll-Free: 888-INFO-FDA
(888-463-6332)
Website: www.fda.gov

Health Technology Sourcebook, Third Edition

U.S. Library of Congress (LOC)
101 Independence Ave., S.E.
Washington, DC 20540
Phone: 202-707-5000
Website: www.loc.gov

U.S. National Library of Medicine (NLM)
8600 Rockville Pike
Bethesda, MD 20894
Phone: 301-594-5983
Toll-Free: 888-FIND-NLM
(888-346-3656)
Website: www.nlm.nih.gov
E-mail: nlmcommunications@nih.gov

PRIVATE AGENCIES

AdvaMed
1301 Pennsylvania Ave., N.W.
Ste. 400
Washington, DC 20004
Phone: 202-783-8700
Fax: 202-783-8750
Website: www.advamed.org

American Academy of Family Physicians (AAFP)
11400 Tomahawk Creek Pkwy.
Leawood, KS 66211-2680
Phone: 913-906-6000
Toll-Free: 800-274-2237
Fax: 913-906-6075
Website: www.aafp.org
E-mail: aafp@aafp.org

American Academy of Pediatrics (AAP)
345 Park Blvd.
Itasca, IL 60143
Toll-Free: 800-433-9016
Fax: 847-434-8000
Website: www.aap.org

American Association for the Advancement of Science (AAAS)
1200 New York Ave., N.W.
Washington, DC 20005
Phone: 202-326-6400
Website: www.aaas.org

American Federation for Medical Research (AFMR)
500 Cummings Center
Ste. 4400
Beverly, MA 01915
Phone: 978-927-8330
Fax: 978-524-0498
Website: afmr.org

American Heart Association (AHA)
7272 Greenville Ave.
Dallas, TX 75231
Phone: 214-570-5943
Toll-Free: 800-AHA-USA-1
(800-242-8721)
Website: www.heart.org

Directory of Agencies That Provide Information about Health Technology

American Medical Association (AMA)
AMA Plaza, 330 N. Wabash Ave.
Ste. 39300
Chicago, IL 60611-5885
Phone: 312-464-4782
Toll-Free: 800-262-3211
Website: www.ama-assn.org

American Optometric Association (AOA)
243 N. Lindbergh Blvd.
St. Louis, MO 63141-7881
Phone: 314-991-4100
Fax: 314-991-4101
Website: www.aoa.org

American Society of Health-System Pharmacists (ASHP)
4500 East-West Hwy.
Ste. 900
Bethesda, MD 20814
Toll-Free: 866-279-0681
Fax: 301-657-1251
Website: www.ashp.org
E-mail: CustServ@ashp.org

American Society of Ophthalmic Plastic and Reconstructive Surgery (ASOPRS)
1041 Grand Ave.
Ste. 132
St. Paul, MN 55105
Phone: 612-601-3168
Website: www.asoprs.org
E-mail: info@asoprs.org

Americans for Medical Progress (AMP)
444 N. Capitol St., N.W.
Ste. 417
Washington, DC 20001
Phone: 202-624-8810
Website: www.amprogress.org

Biotechnology Innovation Organization (BIO)
1201 New York Ave., N.W.
Ste. 1300
Washington, DC 20005
Phone: 202-962-9200
Website: www.bio.org/contact-bio
E-mail: info@bio.org

Cincinnati Children's Hospital Medical Center
3333 Burnet Ave.
Cincinnati, OH 45229-3026
Phone: 513-636-4200
Toll-Free: 800-344-2462
Website: www.cincinnatichildrens.org

Cleveland Clinic
9500 Euclid Ave.
Cleveland, OH 44195
Phone: 216-444-2200
Toll-Free: 800-223-2273
Website: www.my.clevelandclinic.org

Health Technology Sourcebook, Third Edition

Drug, Chemical & Associated Technologies Association (DCAT)
One Washington Blvd.
Ste. 6
Robbinsville, NJ 08691
Phone: 609-208-1888
Toll-Free: 800-640-DCAT
(800-640-3228)
Fax: 609-208-0599
Website: www.dcat.org
E-mail: info@dcat.org

Health Volunteers Overseas (HVO)
1900 L St., N.W.
Ste. 310
Washington, DC 20036
Phone: 202-296-0928
Fax: 202-296-8018
Website: www.hvousa.org/
contact-us
E-mail: info@hvousa.org

Healthcare Information and Management Systems Society (HIMSS)
350 N. Orleans St.
Ste. S10000
Chicago, IL 60654
Phone: (312-664-HIMSS)
312-664-4467
Fax: 312-664-6143
Website: www.himss.org

Immunize.org
2136 Ford Pkwy.
Ste. 5011
St. Paul, MN 55116
Phone: 651-647-9009
Fax: 651-647-9131
Website: www.immunize.org
E-mail: admin@immunize.org

Materials Research Society (MRS)
506 Keystone Dr.
Warrendale, PA 15086-7537
Phone: 724-779-3003
Fax: 724-779-8313
Website: www.mrs.org
E-mail: info@mrs.org

Mental Health America (MHA)
500 Montgomery St.
Ste. 820
Alexandria, VA 22314
Phone: 703-684-7722
Toll-Free: 800-969-6642
Fax: 703-684-5968
Website: www.
mentalhealthamerica.net

National Alliance on Mental Illness (NAMI)
4301 Wilson Blvd.
Ste. 300
Arlington, VA 22203
Phone: 703-524-7600
Toll-Free: 800-950-6264
Website: www.nami.org

Directory of Agencies That Provide Information about Health Technology

National Safety Council (NSC)
1121 Spring Lake Dr.
Itasca, IL 60143-3201
Phone: 630-285-1121
Toll-Free: 800-621-7615
Fax: 630-285-1434
Website: www.nsc.org
E-mail: customerservice@nsc.org

National Scoliosis Foundation (NSF)
5 Cabot Pl.
Stoughton, MA 02072
Toll-Free: 800-NSF-MYBACK
(800-673-6922)
Fax: 781-341-8333
Website: www.scoliosis.org
E-mail: nsf@scoliosis.org

Palo Alto Medical Foundation (PAMF)
795 El Camino Real
Palo Alto, CA 94301
Phone: 650-321-4121
Toll-Free: 888-398-5677
Website: www.pamf.org

Pan American Health Organization (PAHO)
525 23rd St., N.W.
Washington, DC 20037
Phone: 202-974-3000
Fax: 202-974-3663
Website: www.paho.org/hq

Radiological Society of North America (RSNA)
820 Jorie Blvd.
Ste. 200
Oak Brook, IL 60523-2251
Phone: 630-571-2670
Toll-Free: 800-381-6660
Fax: 630-571-7837
Website: www.rsna.org/ContactUs.aspx
E-mail: customerservice@rsna.org

INDEX

INDEX

Page numbers followed by 'n' indicate a footnote. Page numbers in *italics* indicate a table or illustration.

A

AAC *see* augmentative and alternative communication
abdominal aortic aneurysm (AAA), machine learning (ML) 234
ablation techniques, image-guided robotic interventions 390
ACA *see* Affordable Care Act
accuracy
    artificial intelligence (AI) 288
    continuous glucose monitoring (CGM) 200
    light therapy and brain function 416
    medical chatbots 33
    precision medicine 378
    stem cells 516
    wearable devices 177
acute respiratory distress syndrome (ARDS), messenger RNA (mRNA) 262
AD *see* Alzheimer disease
ADA.gov
    publication
        mobility aids 483n
adenine, genomics 239
AdvaMed, contact information 594

Advanced Molecular Detection (AMD), overview 225–231
adverse drug reactions (ADRs), data privacy 218
Affordable Care Act (ACA), described 546
Agency for Healthcare Research and Quality (AHRQ)
    contact information 591
    publications
        artificial intelligence (AI) 286n
        health information technology 143n
        medical scribes 160n
age-related macular degeneration (AMD)
    low vision 435
    stem cells 516
AI *see* artificial intelligence
ALDs *see* assistive listening devices
ALS *see* amyotrophic lateral sclerosis
alternative site testing (AST), continuous glucose monitoring (CGM) 202
Alzheimer disease (AD)
    artificial intelligence (AI) in health care 15
    neurotechnology 273
    rehabilitation engineering 430
ambulance, wireless medical devices 181

601

Health Technology Sourcebook, Third Edition

AMD *see* age-related macular degeneration

American Academy of Family Physicians (AAFP), contact information 594

American Academy of Pediatrics (AAP), contact information 594

American Association for the Advancement of Science (AAAS), contact information 594

American Federation for Medical Research (AFMR), contact information 594

American Heart Association (AHA), contact information 594

American Medical Association (AMA), contact information 595

American Optometric Association (AOA), contact information 595

American sign language (ASL), assistive devices 480

American Society of Health-System Pharmacists (ASHP), contact information 595

American Society of Ophthalmic Plastic and Reconstructive Surgery (ASOPRS), contact information 595

Americans for Medical Progress (AMP), contact information 595

amyotrophic lateral sclerosis (ALS), assistive devices 481

anesthesia
  advanced therapies 418
  cochlear implants 453
  medical technology 5
  virtual colonoscopy 293

angioplasty, smart operating rooms 536

ANN *see* artificial neural network

anonymity
  infectious diseases 221

medical chatbots 32

mental health apps 328

antibacterial ointment, drug delivery systems 528

antibiotic drug, surface plasmon resonance imaging (SPRI) 310

antibiotic resistance, infectious disease 220

antibiotic-resistant microbes (AMRs), Advanced Molecular Detection (AMD) 227

anti-inflammatory drugs, virtual colonoscopy 295

antimicrobial-resistant pathogens, Advanced Molecular Detection (AMD) 230

antiretroviral therapy (ART), described 108

antivirus software, firewall 569

anxiety
  assistive devices 475
  COVID-19 105
  health technology assessment (HTA) 39
  mental health apps 329

APDS *see* artificial pancreas device system

API *see* application programming interface

application programming interface (API), HIPAA 550

applied research, medical technology 6

Argonne National Laboratory (ANL) publication
  light therapy 413n

arrhythmia, radiofrequency thermal ablation (RFA) 417

arthritis
  cartilage engineering 412
  digital innovations 195
  prosthetic engineering 461
  virtual colonoscopy 295

602

Index

artificial cloning *see* cloning
artificial hands, rehabilitation
   engineering 430
artificial intelligence (AI)
   advanced therapies 410
   augment patient care 319
   cardiovascular disease (CVD) 292
   colon cancer 231
   diagnostic imaging 286
   digital health 7
   oncology 523
   overview 13–30
   stem cells 515
artificial legs, rehabilitation
   engineering 429
artificial neural network, machine
   learning (ML) 18
artificial pancreas device system
   (APDS), overview 335–339
artificial retina, overview 446–449
asexual reproduction, cloning 264
ASL *see* American sign language
assistive devices
   neurotechnology 274
   overview 471–495
   rehabilitation engineering 428
assistive listening devices (ALDs),
   cochlear implant 476
assistive technology (AT)
   overview 471–476
   rehabilitation engineering 430
   telehealth visits 68
AST *see* alternative site testing
AT *see* assistive technology
atomic force microscope (AFM),
   nanotechnology 510
attention deficit hyperactivity disorder
   (ADHD), genetic disease 242
augment patient care, overview 319–326
augmentative and alternative
   communication (AAC), assistive
   device 476

B

BAN *see* body area network
Barrett's esophagus, image-guided
   robotic interventions 391
BBB *see* blood–brain barrier
BCI *see* brain–computer
   interface
BGD *see* blood glucose device
big data, overview 211–222
billing codes, mobile medical
   applications 191
biocompatibility
   cancer treatment 352
   tissue engineering and regenerative
    medicine 404
biodegradable stent, smart operating
   rooms 536
biofilms, surface plasmon resonance
   imaging (SPRI) 310
bioinformatics, Advanced
   Molecular Detection (AMD)
   technologies 225
biomarkers
   cancer treatment 356, 370
   cardiovascular disease
    (CVD) 292
   deep learning (DL) 519
   live cell imaging 305
biomaterial
   nonlinear optical imaging 307
   smart operating rooms 533
   tissue engineering and regenerative
    medicine 403
Biomedical Data to Knowledge
   (BD2K), genomics 216
biomedical imaging
   deep learning (DL) 520
   wearable sensors 16
biomolecules
   nanotechnology 350
   tissue engineering and regenerative
    medicine 409

603

Health Technology Sourcebook, Third Edition

biopsy
  augment patient care 324
  cancer screening and diagnosis 523
  cancer treatment 358
  fiber optic enabled sensitive
    surgery tools 398
  genomics 214
  liver elastography 298
  radiofrequency thermal ablation
    (RFA) 422
biosensors
  cancer treatment 359
  preventive medicine 173
  surface plasmon resonance imaging
    (SPRI) 310
  tissue engineering and regenerative
    medicine 403
biotechnology
  advanced therapies 410
  drug delivery systems 530
  Human Genome Project 383
Biotechnology Innovation
  Organization (BIO), contact
  information 595
birth defects
  telehealth 113
  vision problems 435
black box
  deep learning (DL) 520
  machine learning (ML) 19
blockchain, overview 503–505
blood glucose device (BGD)
  artificial pancreas device system
    (APDS) 336
  diabetes 96
blood pressure
  cardiovascular disease (CVD) 291
  machine learning (ML) 235
  mental health treatment 329
  mobile medical applications 195
  nanotechnology 352
  obesity 97

rehabilitation engineering 430
remote patient monitoring
  (RPM) 75
telecritical care 538
telehealth 46, 116
wearable technology 179
wireless patient monitoring 207
blood–brain barrier (BBB), cancer
  treatment 351
blood sugar
  artificial pancreas device system
    (APDS) 339
  continuous glucose monitoring
    (CGM) 198
  diabetes 95
  health information exchange (HIE)
    146
  telehealth 46
Blue Button, overview 157–160
Bluetooth
  Internet of Things (IoT) 500
  remote patient monitoring (RPM)
    79
  wireless medical devices 180
body area network (BAN),
  overview 173–176
body mass index (BMI),
  cardiovascular disease (CVD) 291
Braille, assistive device technology 442
brain tumor
  nanotechnology 357
  oncology 524
  radio frequency thermal
    ablation 422
brain–computer interface (BCI)
  assistive technology (AT) 481
  overview 465–468
  rehabilitation engineering 429
BRCA1, DNA microarray
  technology 249
BRCA2, DNA microarray
  technology 249

604

Index

breathing patterns, self-management apps 329
Bridge2AI, genomics 245

C

cancer
  biomarker testing 370
  emerging artificial intelligence (AI) applications 523
  genetics 247, 253
  GI Genius 231
  image scanning system 16
  medical technology 7
  nanotechnology 350
  NIH-supported technologies 535
  proton beams 347
  radiofrequency thermal ablation (RFA) 417
  telehealth technology 87
  telerehabilitation 90
  virtual colonoscopy 294
cardiovascular disease (CVD)
  pancreas 335
  telehealth chronic conditions 97
cartilage engineering, overview 412–413
catheters, medical technology 5
CBT see cognitive behavioral therapy
CDS see clinical decision support
CEHRT see Certified Electronic Health Record Technology
Center for Limb Loss and Mobility (CLiMB)
  publication
    prosthetic engineering 459n
Centers for Disease Control and Prevention (CDC)
  contact information 591
  publications
    Advanced Molecular Detection (AMD) 225n

big data in the age of genomics 214n
  COVID-19 vaccines 258n
  genetic testing 245n
  SARS-CoV-2 rapid testing 311n
Centers for Medicare & Medicaid Services (CMS)
  publications
    Blue Button® 2.0 157n
    e-prescribing 148n
    medicare benefits 53n
    telehealth 53n
central nervous system (CNS), nanotechnology 368
cerebral palsy (CP), assistive devices 475
Certified Electronic Health Record Technology (CEHRT), HIPAA privacy 550
CEs see Covered Entities
CGM see continuous glucose monitoring
chemotherapy
  biomarker test 373
  nanotechnology 363
  proton therapy 348
  radiofrequency thermal ablation (RFA) 423
  telehealth and cancer care 88
Cherenkov radiation, radiotherapy 367
chromosomes
  cloning 269
  defined 240
chronic diseases
  chronic conditions 94
  clinical artificial intelligence (AI) tools 326
  communication technology 136
  mobile apps 195
  telehealth 59
  wireless medical devices 184

605

Cincinnati Children's Hospital Medical Center, contact information 595

circulating tumor cells (CTCs), nanotechnology 356

cirrhosis, elastography 298

Clear Guide ONE, biopsy guidance 534

Cleveland Clinic, contact information 595

Clinical Center (CC) publication
  radiofrequency thermal ablation 416n

clinical decision support (CDS)
  artificial intelligence (AI) 30
  health information technology 144
  overview 277–279
  scribes 162

clinical exome, genomic testing 247

clinical trials
  biomarker testing 376
  low vision and blindness rehabilitation 445
  machine learning (ML) in drug development 19
  nanotechnology 368
  National Institute of Biomedical Imaging and Bioengineering (NIBIB) 405
  patient-derived xenografts (PDXs) 344

cloning, overview 264–271

cloud computing
  cybersecurity 571
  Internet of Things (IoT) 500

clustered regularly interspaced short palindromic repeats (CRISPR), overview 251–257

CNS see central nervous system

cochlear implant
  assistive devices for communication 476
  overview 449–457

cognitive aids, assistive technologies 472

cognitive behavioral therapy (CBT), smartphone 332

cognitive disabilities, assistive devices 475

colonography, virtual colonoscopy 293

colonoscopy, overview 291–297

comirnaty, messenger RNA (mRNA) 259

community mental health centers (CMHCs), telehealth 55

computed tomography (CT)
  cardiovascular disease (CVD) 292
  image-guided robotic interventions 390
  medical technology 7
  radiofrequency thermal ablation (RFA) 416

computer-assisted surgical system, robot-assisted surgery (RAS) 392

computerized provider order entry (CPOE), health information technology 144

contact tracing, monitoring patients 325

continuous, noninvasive blood pressure (cNIBP), wireless patient monitoring 207

continuous glucose monitoring (CGM)
  artificial pancreas device system (APDS) 336
  overview 198–206

conventional therapies, rehabilitation engineering 429

coronavirus
  clustered regularly interspaced short palindromic repeats (CRISPR) 254
  messenger RNA (mRNA) 258
  point-of-care testing 313

Index

coronavirus disease 2019 *see* COVID-19
Covered Entities (CEs)
  HIPAA privacy rule 547
  mobility aids 484
COVID-19
  Advanced Molecular Detection (AMD) program 230
  augment patient care 322
  chronic health conditions 96
  drug delivery systems 528
  follow-up care 129
  HIPAA compliance 555
  medical chatbots 33
  messenger RNA (mRNA) 258
  point-of-care testing 312
  remote patient monitoring (RPM) 78
  telehealth 52, 103
CP *see* cerebral palsy
CRISPR-Cas9, genome editing 251
Crohn's disease, drug delivery systems 529
cross-modal plasticity, vision and hearing loss 440
CT *see* computed tomography
CTCs *see* circulating tumor cells
cultural humility training, telehealth for HIV care 110
Cures Act, Office of the National Coordinator for Health Information Technology (ONC) 543
CVD *see* cardiovascular disease
cybersecurity
  digital health 9
  overview 563–576
  phishing attack 155
cystic fibrosis (CF)
  assistive devices 475
  clustered regularly interspaced short palindromic repeat (CRISPR) 252
  genetic disease 241
cytosine, genomics 239

D

data analysis
  cancer treatment 346
  genomics 215
  oncology 525
data brokers, wearable devices 558
data intelligence, big data 214
data portability, HIPAA 548
data security, laws and regulations 560
DEAL *see* DNA-encoded antibody libraries
deep brain stimulation
  light therapy 414
  neurotechnology 273
deep learning (DL), cancer screening and diagnosis 523
deep neural networks
  enhanced image analysis 16
  stem cells and artificial intelligence (AI) 516
deep vein thrombosis (DVT), sensors 172
deoxyribonucleic acid (DNA)
  contributions to medical technology 7
  genetic testing 245
  Human Genome Project 382
  laboratory technologies 226
depression
  COVID-19 105
  distress screening tool 88
  implications of vision loss 437
  light therapy 414
  neurotechnology 274
  passive symptom tracking 330
  population health 50
  postpartum telehealth services 118
diabetes
  assistive devices 475
  continuous glucose monitor (CGM) 204
  described 124

Health Technology Sourcebook, Third Edition

diabetes, *continued*
  diabetic retinopathy 285
  glucose 198
  health information exchange
    (HIE) 146
  pancreas 335
  remote patient monitoring
    (RPM) 75
  robotic pill 529
  telehealth 46
  video appointments 100
diabetic retinopathy
  described 285
  low vision 435
diagnostic tests
  Advanced Molecular Detection
    (AMD) 225
  DNA microarray 250
  medical technology 5
  Patients over Paperwork 59
  point-of-care (POC) testing 311
  provider-to-provider telehealth 100
diets
  genetic sensor 173
  glucose 198
digital fingerprint, hash 503
digital health
  health IT 549
  mental health intervention 333
  overview 153–165
disabilities
  genetic tests 247
  health equity 60
  rehabilitation engineering 427
  rehabilitative and assistive
    technology (AT) 471
distributed denial of service (DDoS),
  Internet of Things (IoT) 505
DNA *see* deoxyribonucleic acid
DNA-encoded antibody libraries
  (DEAL), sensing in vitro 360
Down syndrome, genetic diseases 242

Drug, Chemical & Associated
  Technologies Association (DCAT),
  contact information 596
drug delivery systems, overview 527–531
drug resistance
  gene therapy 367
  surface plasmon resonance imaging
    (SPRI) 309
drugs
  applications of cloned animals 268
  chemotherapeutics 369
  cochlear implants 453
  described 35
  drug delivery systems 527
  drug development 20
  medical technology 7
  mobile apps 194
  neurotechnology 274
  passive tumor accumulation 351
  patch 178
  regenerative medicine 405
  virtual colonoscopy 295

E

e-consults, virtual health-care
  services 127
e-prescription, overview 148–150
Ebola, big data for disease
  surveillance 221
ECM *see* extracellular matrix
ecosystem
  big data and healthcare 211
  biomanufacturing initiative 411
  HIPAA and privacy rules 548
EGFR gene, biomarker testing 371
EHIE *see* electronic health information
  exchange
EHRs *see* electronic health records
elastography
  described 297
  see also liver elastography

608

Index

electrical surgery, cochlear
implants 455
electrocardiogram (ECG)
health related wearable
technology 179
medical technology 5
wireless patient monitoring 208
electroconvulsive therapy, cochlear
implants 455
electromagnetic compatibility (EMC),
wireless medical devices 185
electromagnetic interference (EMI)
cybersecurity 565
wireless medical devices 181
electromagnetic radiation,
nanotechnology 366
electronic clinical quality measure
(eCQMs), clinical decision support
(CDS) 279
electronic health information
exchange (EHIE)
overview 145–148
HIPAA 541
HITECH 545
electronic health records (EHRs)
artificial intelligence (AI) tools 325
big data and healthcare services 213
big data for disease surveillance 218
blockchain technology 504
Blue Button 159
cybersecurity 564
electronic medical records
(EMRs) 153
health information
technology 138, 144
health information technology
legislation and regulations 545
medical scribes 160
telehealth for maternal health
services 113
electronic medical records (EMRs)
e-prescription 148
overview 153–157

electrophysiology, rehabilitation
engineering 429
electrosurgical unit (ESU), robot-
assisted surgery (RAS) 393
electrotherapeutic equipment, medical
technology 5
embryonic stem cells, cloning 264
emergency medical services (EMS),
wireless patient monitoring 206
emergency room (ER)
artificial intelligence (AI) tools 321
blood glucose monitoring
devices 200
health information exchange (HIE)
technology 147
remote patient monitoring
(RPM) 78
telehealth for chronic
conditions 98
telehealth in emergency
departments 128
wireless patient monitoring 207
EMI *see* electromagnetic interference
encryption
electronic medical and health
records 154
security and privacy risks of
wearable devices 559
endoscope
colon cancer detection 231
robot-assisted surgery
(RAS) 393
smart operating rooms 535
Enhanced Permeability and Retention
(EPR) effect, nanotechnology for
cancer 351
epidemic simulation data management
system, big data for infectious
disease surveillance 222
epidemiologic foundation, big data in
the age of genomics 215
epidemiologic study, big data 215

Health Technology Sourcebook, Third Edition

epidemiology, Advanced Molecular Detection (AMD) 225

ER *see* emergency room

Escherichia coli, human genome 381

Eunice Kennedy Shriver National Institute on Child Health and Human Development (NICHD)
contact information 591
publications
assistive devices 476n
rehabilitative and assistive technology 471n

evidence-based medicine, big data in the age of genomics 216

extracellular matrix (ECM)
nanotechnology 353
surface plasmon resonance imaging (SPRI) 309
tissue engineering and regenerative medicine 403

F

family-centered care, telehealth for children 119

fatigue
chronic health conditions 96
COVID-19 104
Edmonton Symptom Assessment System (ESAS-r) 88
elastography 299
messenger RNA (mRNA) 260
minimally invasive surgery 390
prosthetic engineering 460

fcMRI *see* functional connectivity magnetic resonance imaging

federal privacy law, HIPAA 541

Federal Trade Commission (FTC), contact information 591

FHW *see* frontline health worker

fibrosis
tissue healing and regeneration 409

liver elastography 298
radiofrequency thermal ablation (RFA) 419

firewall, cybersecurity in health care 569

fitness care manager, telerehabilitation 92

fitness trackers
categorization of wearables 177
Internet of Things (IoT) 499
security and privacy risks of wearable devices 558

flexible endoscope, fluorescent capabilities 535

flu
age of genomics 215
medical chatbots 33

fluorescence
induced pluripotent stem cell (iPSC) 305
light therapy and brain function 415
medical images 520
microarray technology 249

fMRI *see* functional magnetic resonance imaging

Fogarty International Center (FIC)
publication
big data for infectious disease surveillance 217n

follow-up appointments
chronic health conditions 95
health information exchange (HIE) 145
telehealth 46

fragile X syndrome (FXS), genetic testing 246

frontline health worker (FHW), artificial intelligence (AI) 28

functional connectivity magnetic resonance imaging (fcMRI), neuroimaging technique 290

610

Index

functional magnetic resonance imaging (fMRI)
  artificial intelligence (AI) 16
  neurotechnology 273

G

gamma rays, augmenting radiotherapy 366
gene cloning, overview 264–271
gene editing
  artificial intelligence (AI) 244
  overview 251–257
gene therapy
  blindness rehabilitation 439
  cancer therapies 367
  CRISPR's 255
genetic testing
  biomarker testing 371
  health technology assessment (HTA) 38
  overview 245–248
genomic medicine
  knowledge integration (KI) 216
  pharmacogenomics 243
giant magnetoresistive (GMR) biosensors, nanotechnology for cancer 360
glucagon
  artificial pancreas device system (APDS) 335
  continuous glucose monitor (CGM) 206
glucose
  artificial pancreas device system (APDS) 335
  chronic health conditions 96
  diabetes care 124
  Internet of Things (IoT) 501
  maternal telehealth 116
  next-generation sequencing (NGS) 378
  overview 198–206

glucose meter
  artificial pancreas device system (APDS) 335
  continuous glucose monitor (CGM) 206
  mobile medical apps 186
  remote patient monitoring (RPM) 76
gluten-free food, mobile medical applications 190
GMPs *see* good manufacturing practices
good manufacturing practices (GMPs), artificial retina 447
guanine, genomes 239

H

HCMI *see* Human Cancer Models Initiative
health equity
  described 60
  health information technology 135
  maternal health care 111
health information exchange (HIE)
  HIPAA 541
  overview 145–148
  see also electronic health information exchange
health information technology
  Cures Act 543
  digital health 7
  overview 135–140
Health Information Technology for Economic and Clinical Health (HITECH) Act
  legislation and regulations 545
  medical scribes 162
Health Insurance Portability and Accountability Act (HIPAA)
  big data 213
  COVID-19 555

Health Technology Sourcebook, Third Edition

Health Insurance Portability and
Accountability Act (HIPAA),
continued
digital health 155
health information privacy law and
policy 541
mobile medical applications 191
overview 547–551
health IT toolkit, technology and
health care 144
Health Professional Shortage Areas
(HSPA), telehealth 55
Health Resources and Services
Administration (HRSA), contact
information 592
health technology assessment (HTA),
overview 35–39
Health Volunteers Overseas (HVO),
contact information 596
Healthcare Information and
Management Systems Society
(HIMSS), contact information 596
health-care-associated infections
(HAIs), Advanced Molecular
Detection (AMD) program 227
HealthIT.gov
publications
artificial intelligence for health
and health care 285n
Blue Button 157n
clinical decision support 277n
cybersecurity in health
care 563n
health information exchange
(HIE) 145n
health information privacy law
and policy 541n
health IT 138n, 143n, 543n
HIPAA and health information
portability 547n
hearing aids
cochlear implants 450

medical technology 5
overview 482–483
rehabilitative and assistive
technology (AT) 472
wearable devices 179
hearing loop system, assistive listening
devices (ALDs) 477
heart attack
artificial intelligence (AI) and
machine learning (ML)
technologies 13
sensors 171
heart rate
artificial intelligence (AI) 16
mobile medical
applications 194, 329
remote monitoring 80
sensors 171
TeleCritical Care 538
hematocrit, blood glucose
monitoring 199
hemophilia, genome editing 252
HIE *see* health information exchange
HIFU *see* high-intensity focused
ultrasound
high-intensity focused ultrasound
(HIFU), cancer 355
HIPAA *see* Health Insurance
Portability and Accountability Act
HIV *see* human immunodeficiency
virus
HTA *see* health technology assessment
Human Cancer Models Initiative
(HCMI), cancer 345
Human Genome Project
medical technology 7
overview 381–385
human immunodeficiency virus (HIV)
assistive devices 475
genome editing 252
screening and detection
technologies 227

612

Index

human immunodeficiency virus (HIV), *continued*
 telehealth 106
 virtual health-care services 97
Huntington disease, nanomedicine 511
hyperglycemia, artificial pancreas device system (APDS) 336
hypodermic needles, medical technology 5

I

ICU *see* intensive care unit
identical twins, cloning 264
image-guided robotic interventions, overview 389–392
immune system
 drug delivery systems 528
 gene therapy 255
 nano-enabled immunotherapy 364
 regenerative medicine 404
Immunize.org, contact information 596
immunotherapy
 CRISPR 256
 nano-enabled immunotherapy 364
 small business technology 346
implantable cardioverter defibrillators (ICDs), radio frequency identification (RFID) 183
implanted devices, body area networks (BANs) 175
in vitro
 medical technology 5
 nanotechnology 359, 407
 technology assessment (TA) 38
infectious diseases
 drug delivery systems 527
 genome sequencing 215
 magnetic resonance imaging (MRI) 7

inflammatory bowel disease (IBD), colon and rectal cancer 294
influenza
 big data 215
 personal health record (PHR) systems 195
 wastewater surveillance 230
Influenzanet, big data for infectious disease surveillance 219
information technology (IT)
 cybersecurity in health care 563
 electronic health record (EHR) 138
infrared system, assistive listening devices (ALDs) 477
infusion pump
 glucose monitoring system 335
 magnetic resonance elastography (MRE) 300
Innovative Molecular Analysis Technologies (IMAT), activities to promote technology research collaborations (APTRC) 345
insomnia, intervention apps 331
insulin
 alternative site testing (AST) 202
 digestive enzymes 335
 mobile apps 186
 telehealth 95, 124
insurance
 Affordable Care Act (ACA) 546
 Blue Button 158
 chronic conditions 102
 continuous glucose monitor (CGM) 205
 electronic health records (EHRs) 139
 genomic biomarker testing 372
 health equity 60
 Medicare 78
 proton therapy 347
 smart contracts 504
 spatial big data 221
 virtual colonoscopy 294

intellectual property, health technology assessment 39
intensive care unit (ICU)
　predicting health trajectories 321
　telecritical care 537
interprofessional consults, e-consults 127
International Trade Administration (ITA)
　publication
　　medical technologies 5n
Internet of Medical Things (IoMT), remote patient monitoring (RPM) 505
Internet of Things (IoT), overview 499–501
inventory control, radio frequency identification (RFID) 182
investigators
　medical insurance 219
　nanomedicine 511
　patient-derived xenografts (PDXs) 344
　primitive version of the tissue 406
ionic radiation therapy, cochlear implant 455
IoT *see* Internet of Things
IT *see* information technology

J

joint pain
　cartilage engineering 412
　messenger ribonucleic acid (mRNA) 260

K

kidney failure
　artificial pancreas device system (APDS) 335
　radio frequency thermal ablation 421

knowledge integration (KI), age of genomics 216

L

lab-on-a-chip, photonic integrated circuits (PICs) 399
laser capture microdissection, Barrett's esophagus 392
leber congenital amaurosis, CRISPR 256
light spectrum, nanoscience and nanotechnology 510
light therapy, overview 413–416
liposomal doxorubicin (Doxil), passive tumor accumulation 352
liposomes, drug delivery vehicles 530
liquid biopsy
　machine learning (ML) techniques 244
　nanotechnology 361
literacy guide, health information technology 144
lithography, nanotechnology 359
live cell imaging, overview 305–306
liver elastography, overview 297–301
LMICs *see* low- and middle-income countries
long-term care (LTC), point-of-care diagnostic testing 314
low- and middle-income countries (LMICs), artificial intelligence (AI) 24

M

machine learning (ML)
　artificial intelligence (AI) tools 322
　autism spectrum disorder (ASD) 290
　brain–computer interface (BCI) 465

Index

machine learning (ML), *continued*
colon cancer 231
deep learning (DL) approach 520
digital health 8
drug development 20
genomics 244
MACRA *see* Medicare Access and CHIP Reauthorization Act
magnetic nanoparticles (MMPs), liquid biopsy 362
magnetic resonance elastography (MRE), liver elastography 298
magnetic resonance imaging (MRI)
artificial intelligence (AI) 287
cancer 357
cochlear implants 455
image-guided robotic interventions 389
medical technology 5
radiofrequency thermal ablation (RFA) 416
surgical care 324
magnetic resonance (MR) scanners *see* magnetic resonance imaging (MRI)
malaria, big data for infectious disease surveillance 221
malicious software, wearable health-care devices 561
Materials Research Society (MRS), contact information 596
MD *see* muscular dystrophy
MDDS *see* medical device data system
medical apps policy
digital health 7
smartphones 186
medical device data system
digital health 9
mobile medical apps 197
medical history
electronic medical records (EMRs) 153
medical chatbots 32
wearable devices 180

medical imaging, artificial intelligence (AI) 286
Medical Implant Communications Service (MICS), body area networks 175
medical scribes, digital health records 160
medical technology
artificial intelligence (AI) 28
overview 5–7
remote patient monitoring (RPM) 76
smart operating rooms of the future 534
Medicare
biomarker testing 376
colon and rectal cancer 294
continuous glucose monitor (CGM) 205
e-prescription 150
health information technology legislation and regulations 544
remote patient monitoring (RPM) 101
telehealth services 53, 73
Medicare Access and CHIP Reauthorization Act (MACRA), health information technology legislation and regulations 544
Medicare Fee-For-Service (FFS) Program, big data 213
medication errors, electronic health information exchange (eHIE) 146
MedlinePlus
publications
elastography 297n
genome editing and CRISPR-Cas9 251n
NIH-supported technologies of the future 533n
surgery of the future 533n

615

Health Technology Sourcebook, Third Edition

mental health
autism spectrum disorder
(ASD) 290
health information technology
legislation and regulations 543
human immunodeficiency virus
(HIV) 108
low vision and blindness
rehabilitation 437
medical chatbots 33
obesity 97
rehabilitative and assistive
technology (AT) 475
technology and the future 327
telehealth 45, 68
Mental Health America (MHA),
contact information 596
merit-based incentive payment
system (MIPS), Medicare Access
and CHIP Reauthorization Act
(MACRA) 544
MERS *see* Middle East Respiratory
Syndrome
messenger RNA (mRNA),
overview 258–263
meter malfunctions, continuous
glucose monitoring (CGM) 202
mHealth *see* mobile health
microarray technology,
overview 249–251
microfluidics, tissue engineering and
regenerative medicine 407
microneedle patch, drug delivery
systems 528
microscopes
genomics 239
machine learning (ML) 19
nanotechnology 509
microscopic needles, drug delivery
systems 529
Middle East Respiratory Syndrome
(MERS), Internet reports 221

minimally invasive surgery
health technology assessment
(HTA) 35
image-guided robotic
interventions 389
radiofrequency thermal ablation
(RFA) 416
MIPS *see* merit-based incentive
payment system
mitigation
cybersecurity in health care 565
electronic health records
(EHRs) 156
mobile medical applications 189
ML *see* machine learning
MMAs *see* mobile medical applications
MMPs *see* magnetic nanoparticles
mobile apps
device software functions 188
digital health 9
remote patient monitoring
(RPM) 79
smart operating rooms 533
visual disabilities 489
wearable health-care devices 561
mobile devices
cybersecurity in health care 565
mental health treatment 327
visual disabilities 489
wearable health-care devices 559
mobile health (mHealth)
Blue Button 159
digital health 7
health information technology 137
wearable health-care device 557
mobile medical applications,
overview 186–197
mobility aids
assistive technologies 472
overview 483–489
molecular imaging, deep learning (DL)
for better medical images 519

Index

morphology, live cell imaging 305
motion analysis, rehabilitative
 technologies 473
MRI *see* magnetic resonance
 imaging
MS *see* multiple sclerosis
multimodal imaging
 nanotechnology for cancer 357
 visual impairment 442
multiple sclerosis (MS)
 Alzheimer disease (AD) 16
 rehabilitative technology 475
muscle pain, COVID-19 105, 260
muscular dystrophy (MD),
 rehabilitative technology 475
mutations
 biomarker testing 371
 genetic disease 241
 new cancer technologies 345
 oncology 524
 therapeutic cloning 270
 whole-genome sequencing
  (WGS) 229

N

nano-enabled immunotherapy, cancer
 treatment technology 364
nanomedicine
 overview 510–513
 passive tumor accumulation 352
nanoparticles
 artificial retina 447
 augmenting radiotherapy 365
 drug delivery systems 528
 in vitro diagnostic devices 358
 light therapy 414
 passive tumor accumulation 351
nanoscience, overview 509–510
nanoscintillator, light therapy 414
nanotechnology,
 overview 509–513

National Aeronautics and Space
 Administration (NASA)
 publication
  fiber-optic nerves enable
   sensitive surgery tools 395n
National Alliance on Mental Illness
 (NAMI), contact information 596
National Cancer Institute (NCI)
 contact information 592
 publications
  AI applications in
   oncology 523n
  biomarker testing 370n
  cancer research and
   treatment 251n
  nanotechnology 350n
  new enabling cancer
   technologies 343n
  proton therapy 347n
  telerehabilitation 90n
National Eye Institute (NEI)
 publications
  artificial retina 446n
  low vision and blindness
   rehabilitation 435n
National Human Genome Research
 Institute (NHGRI)
 contact information 592
 publications
  artificial intelligence, machine
   learning, and genomics 239n
  cloning 264n
  DNA microarray
   technology 249n
  genomics 239n
  Human Genome Project 381n
  messenger RNA (mRNA) 258n
  microarray technology 249n
  pharmacogenomics 239n
National Institute of Arthritis and
 Musculoskeletal and Skin Diseases
 (NIAMS), contact information 592

Health Technology Sourcebook, Third Edition

National Institute of Biomedical
Imaging and Bioengineering
(NIBIB)
contact information 592
publications
artificial intelligence (AI) 13n
deep learning 519n
drug delivery systems 527n
image-guided robotic
interventions 389n
NIBIB tissue engineering
and regenerative
medicine 403n
rehabilitation engineering 427n
sensors 171n
National Institute of Dental and
Craniofacial Research (NIDCR)
publications
tissue engineering and
regenerative medicine 403n
National Institute of Diabetes,
Digestive and Kidney Diseases
(NIDDK)
contact information 592
publications
continuous glucose
monitoring 198n
virtual colonoscopy 293n
National Institute of Mental Health
(NIMH)
contact information 593
publication
mental health treatment 327n
National Institute of Standards and
Technology (NIST)
contact information 592
publications
big data 211n
body area networks 173n
broadband coherent anti-
stokes raman scattering
microscopy 306n

NIST and the national
biotechnology and
biomanufacturing
initiative 410n
stem cells 515n
surface plasmon resonance
imaging 309n
National Institute on Aging (NIA)
publication
anti-inflammatory drug 412n
National Institute on Deafness and
Other Communication Disorders
(NIDCD), contact information 592
National Institutes of Health (NIH)
contact information 593
publications
artificial intelligence 291n
brain–computer interface 465n
machine learning 234n
multi-photon microscopy
system 306n
nanomedicine 510n
neuroimaging 290n
National Nanotechnology Initiative
(NNI)
publication
nanotechnology 509n
National Safety Council (NSC),
contact information 597
National Science Foundation (NSF)
publication
disability and rehabilitation
engineering (DARE) 427n
National Scoliosis Foundation (NSF),
contact information 597
National Wastewater Surveillance
System (NWSS)
needle-electrode, radiofrequency
thermal ablation (RFA) 419
neuroengineering, disability and
rehabilitation engineering
(DARE) 432

Index

neuroimaging
  Alzheimer disease (AD) 16
  functional connectivity
    magnetic resonance imaging
      (fcMRI) 290
neurological disorders
  Alzheimer disease (AD) 16
  brain–computer interface
    (BCI) 465
neuromodulation
  light therapy 414
  neurotechnology 273
neurons
  brain–computer interface
    (BCI) 466
  light therapy 413
  vision and hearing loss 446
neurostimulation
  cochlear implants 455
  rehabilitation engineering 430
neurotechnology,
  overview 273–274
next-generation genomic sequencing
  (NGS), Advanced Molecular
  Detection (AMD) 226
N95, point-of-care diagnostic
  testing 314
nonlinear optical imaging,
  described 306–307
norovirus, wastewater
  surveillance 230
nuclear magnetic resonance
  (NMR), in vitro diagnostic
  devices 360
nuclear medicine, radioisotopes 7
nucleic acids
  active tumor targeting 353
  artificial intelligence (AI) 525
  gene therapy 367
NY-ESO-1, clustered regularly
  interspaced short palindromic
  repeats (CRISPR) 256

O

Office of Disease Prevention and
  Health Promotion (ODPHP)
  publication
    health communication
    and health information
    technology 135n
Office of Technology Transfer (OTT)
  publication
    multi-photon microscopy
    system 306n
OI see osteogenesis imperfecta
Omicron, whole-genome sequencing
  (WGS) 229
Omnigraphics
  publications
    medical chatbots 31n
    neurotechnology 273n
oncology
  artificial intelligence (AI) 523
  radiofrequency thermal ablation
    (RFA) 416
  telehealth cancer care 87
operating systems
  software firewalls 569
  wearable health-care
    devices 559
operational field assessment
  (OFA), continuous surveillance
  monitoring 208
ophthalmologist
  diabetic retinopathy 285
  low vision 435
optical imaging
  biomarkers 519
  silica-hybrid nanoparticles 358
organoids, advanced next-generation
  human cancer models 345
orthopedics
  artificial intelligence (AI) 234
  image-guided robotic
    interventions 390

Health Technology Sourcebook, Third Edition

orthotic devices, assistive technology (AT) 472

osteoarthritis, cartilage engineering 412

OsteoDetect software, wrist fracture analysis 233

osteogenesis imperfecta (OI), complex rehabilitative technology 475

osteoporosis, artificial-intelligence-based analysis 292

P

pacemakers
  health-care professionals 183
  medical technology 5

pain management
  health information technology 35
  telerehabilitation 93

Palo Alto Medical Foundation (PAMF), contact information 597

Pan American Health Organization (PAHO), contact information 597

pandemic
  artificial intelligence (AI) 322
  COVID-19 104
  medical chatbots 33
  telehealth 57

paralysis
  assistive devices 476
  neurotechnology 274
  rehabilitation engineering 430

paramedics, wireless patient monitoring 206

Parkinson disease (PD)
  genetic variants 242
  neurotechnology 273
  radiofrequency thermal ablation (RFA) 422
  remote patient monitoring (RPM) 76

PAT *see* photoacoustic tomography

pathogens, Advanced Molecular Detection (AMD) 225

pathologist, rehabilitative technology 474

patient management, mobile apps 188

patient-derived xenografts (PDXs), described 343–344

patient-specific treatment, artificial intelligence (AI) 319

PD *see* Parkinson disease

PDT *see* photodynamic therapy

PDXs *see* patient-derived xenografts

pedometer, telerehabilitation program 92

PEG *see* polyethylene glycol

personal health record (PHR)
  defined 586
  health information technology 550
  mobile apps 193

personal protective equipment (PPE)
  point-of-care testing (POC) 314
  telehealth technology 125

personalized medicine *see* precision medicine

personnel tracking, radio frequency identification (RFID) 182

PET *see* positron emission tomography

pharmacogenomics, described 243

phishing attack, described 154

photoacoustic imaging, nanotechnology 358

photoacoustic tomography (PAT), cancer treatment 357

photodynamic therapy (PDT), nanotechnology for cancer 352

photon
  defined 587
  nonlinear optical imaging 308
  radiotherapy 366

PHR *see* personal health record (PHR)

Index

physical activity
  continuous glucose monitoring
    (CGM) 202
  diabetes care appointments 124
pneumonia, comirnaty (COVID-19
  vaccine mRNA) 262
point of care (POC)
  defined 587
  e-prescription 148
  health information exchange
    (HIE) 146
polyethylene glycol (PEG),
  nanotechnology for cancer 352
polymer
  coherent anti-stokes raman
    scattering (CARS) 308
  nanotechnology for cancer 352
polyps
  GI Genius 231
  virtual colonoscopy 293
portable document format (PDF),
  accessing documents for
  telehealth 83
positron emission tomography (PET)
  defined 587
  nanotechnology for cancer 357
  new cancer technologies 343
posttraumatic stress disorder (PTSD)
  assistive devices 475
  mental health apps 331
PPE *see* personal protective equipment
precision medicine
  artificial intelligence (AI) 319
  big data in genomics 215
  biomarker testing 371
  defined 587
  genomics 243
  medical technology 7
  overview 377–379
prescription medications
  accessing telehealth services 82
  Blue Button 160

privacy law, overview 541–542
progenitor cells
  defined 588
  tissue engineering and regenerative
    medicine 407
proliferation
  artificial intelligence (AI) in
    diagnostic imaging 286
  health technology assessment
    (HTA) 35
  Internet of Things (IoT) 499
  nanotechnology for cancer 355
  tissue engineering and regenerative
    medicine 408
prostate hyperplasia,
  radiofrequency thermal
  ablation (RFA) 421
prostatectomy, image-guided robotic
  interventions 390
prostate-specific membrane
  antigen (PSMA), new cancer
  technologies 346
prosthetic engineering,
  overview 459–463
prosthetics
  defined 588
  low vision and blindness
    rehabilitation 443
  rehabilitation engineering 429
  robotics and biomechanics 460
protected health information
  cybersecurity in health care 572
  HIPAA Flexibility after the
    COVID-19 555
proton beam radiation therapy, cancer
  treatment 347
PSMA *see* prostate-specific membrane
  antigen
psychosis, passive symptom
  tracking 330
PTSD *see* posttraumatic stress
  disorder

621

Health Technology Sourcebook, Third Edition

public health emergency (PHE)
  point-of-care (POC) diagnostic
    testing 312
  remote patient monitoring
    (RPM) 76
  telehealth 57
  telehealth for COVID-19 102
  telehealth privacy and legal
    considerations 553
pulmonary embolism (PE),
  sensors 172
pulse oximeter
  remote patient monitoring
    (RPM) 76
  sensors 171
  telehealth for chronic conditions 95

Q

QOL *see* quality of life
QPP *see* quality payment program
quality of care
  artificial intelligence (AI) 30
  big data 213
  information technology (IT) 145
  patient care 320
  telehealth services 125
quality of life (QOL)
  assistive technology (AT) 471
  Internet of Things (IoT) 501
  proton therapy 349
  rehabilitation engineering 431
  telehealth 49
  wearables 180
quality payment program (QPP),
  reauthorization act 544

R

radiation
  cancer therapy 347
  chemotherapy 364

  diagnostic imaging 287
  medical applications 186
  tumor therapy 416
Radiation Emergency Medical
  Management (REMM), medical
  applications 186
radiation injuries, medical
  applications 186
radio frequency (RF)
  body area networks (BAN) 173
  robotic interventions 391
  tissue barriers 355
radio frequency identification (RFID),
  medical devices 180
radiofrequency thermal ablation
  (RFA), overview 416–423
radiographs, fracture analysis 234
Radiological Society of North
  America (RSNA), contact
  information 597
radiologist
  decision support 30
  diagnostic imaging 286
  tumors 524
radiotherapy, cancer 358
Raman spectroscopic imaging,
  cancer 357
ransomware, medical records 154
RBCs *see* red blood cells
red blood cells (RBCs)
  continuous glucose monitoring
    (CGM) 199
  nanotechnology 350
regenerative medicine
  overview 403–409
  stem cells 515
rehabilitation engineering,
  overview 427–432
rehabilitation robotics, rehabilitation
  engineering 428
rehabilitative technologies, assistive
  technology (AT) 473

622

Index

REMM *see* Radiation Emergency Medical Management
remote communication, telehealth 555
remote desktop protocol (RDP), medical records 156
remote patient monitoring (RPM)
  COVID-19 105
  overview 75–80
  telehealth 88
remote physiologic monitoring (RPM), patient monitoring 78
remote therapeutic monitoring (RTM), patient monitoring 80
reproductive cloning, artificial cloning 264
retinal implants, low vision 445
retinal prosthesis, vision restoration 445
RFA *see* radiofrequency thermal ablation
ribonucleic acid (RNA)
  microarray technology 249
  molecular detection 227
RNA *see* ribonucleic acid (RNA)
robotic prostatectomy, robotic interventions 390
robotic surgery
  patient care 324
  surgical systems 392
robotics
  biomechanics 460
  operating rooms 533
  rehabilitation engineering 432
  robotic interventions 389
  surgical care 324
RPM *see* remote patient monitoring

S

safer technologies program (STeP), described 562

sanger sequencing, Advanced Molecular Detection (AMD) program 228
scaffold
  defined 589
  tissue engineering 403
scanning tunneling microscope (STM), nanotechnology 509
schizophrenia
  artificial intelligence (AI) 16
  mobile technology 334
SCI *see* spinal cord injury
screen readers
  assistive technology (AT) 472
  telehealth 62
self-stitching surgical robot, defined 535
sensors
  artificial intelligence (AI) 325
  defined 589
  digital health 8
  Internet of Things (IoT) 500
  overview 171–173
  prosthetic engineering 460
  regenerative medicine 403
service animals, visual impairment 489
sexually transmitted diseases (STDs), Advanced Molecular Detection (AMD) program 227
sickle cell disease (SCD)
  genetic variants 241
  nanotechnology 511
silhouette inductor, assistive listening devices (ALDs) 478
simulation
  body area network (BAN) 174
  medical images 520
  predictive analytics 222
  rehabilitative technologies 473
single-nucleotide polymorphisms (SNPs), microarray technology 249

Health Technology Sourcebook, Third Edition

skilled nursing facilities (SNFs),
    telehealth care 55
sleep problems
    COVID-19 96
    self-management apps 329
smart operating room,
    overview 533–536
smartphones
    digital health technologies 8
    HIPAA privacy rule's right 550
    implementation of telehealth 51
    Internet of Things (IoT) 499
    low vision and blindness
        rehabilitation 436
    machine learning (ML) in artificial
        intelligence (AI) 17
    mobile medical applications 186
    mobile mental health treatment 327
    wearable health-care devices 560
smartwatches
    sensors 171
    wearable devices 558
social phobia, mobile mental health
    treatment 332
soft tissue
    augment patient care 324
    radiofrequency thermal ablation
        (RFA) 417
    smart operating rooms 535
software as a medical device (SAMD),
    digital health technologies 9
somatic cell
    cloning 265
    genome editing and CRISPR 252
spatial cognition, low vision and
    blindness rehabilitation 440
spina bifida, rehabilitative and assistive
    technologies 475
spinal cord
    brain–computer interface
        (BCI) 465
    neurotechnology 273

rehabilitation engineering 430
rehabilitative and assistive
    technologies 475
spinal cord injury (SCI)
    rehabilitation engineering 430
    rehabilitative and assistive
        technologies 475
stem cell
    cloning 264
    defined 589
    health technology assessment
        (HTA) 38
    live cell imaging 305
    low vision and blindness
        rehabilitation 439
    stem cells and artificial
        intelligence (AI) 515
    tissue engineering and regenerative
        medicine 405
stent
    medical technology 5
    smart operating rooms 536
stress
    augment patient care 320
    cartilage engineering 412
    continuous glucose monitoring
        (CGM) 202
    health communication and health
        information technology 136
    injury prevention research 462
    mental health apps 329
    mobile medical applications 191
    rehabilitative and assistive
        technologies 475
    telehealth 48, 70, 106, 118
stroke
    artificial-intelligence-based
        analysis 291
    augment patient care 322
    brain–computer interface
        (BCI) 465
    e-consults 127

624

Index

stroke, *continued*
  low vision and blindness
    rehabilitation 445
  medicare telehealth-care
    benefits 55
  neurotechnology 273
  rehabilitation engineering 428
  rehabilitative and assistive
    technologies 473
  sensors 171
substance abuse
  health information technology
    legislation and regulations 543
  maternal telehealth care 115
Substance Abuse and Mental
  Health Services Administration
  (SAMHSA)
  contact information 593
  publications
    telehealth 47n, 51n, 60n
surface plasmon resonance imaging
  (SPRI), overview 309–310
surgical implant, cochlear
  implants 453
surgical robots
  artificial intelligence (AI) 323
  fiber-optic enabled sensitive
    surgery tools 398

T

targeted drug delivery *see* drug
  delivery systems
TBI *see* traumatic brain injury
T-cell therapies, genome editing 256
tDCS *see* transcranial direct current
  stimulation
technology assessment (TA)
  machine learning (ML) 23
  overview 35–39
telebehavioral care, advanced
  cancer 100

tele-emergency care, described 126
telehealth
  chronic health conditions 94
  digital health 7
  human immunodeficiency virus
    (HIV) care 109
  intensive care unit (ICU) 537
  Internet services 82
  legal considerations 553
  overview 45–65
  primary care appointments 122
telemedicine
  chatbots 34
  COVID-19 104
  digital health 7
  human immunodeficiency virus
    (HIV) 110
  medicare benefits 57
telementoring, human
  immunodeficiency virus
  (HIV) 109
tele-oncology, cancer care 87
tele-palliative care, cancer care 89
TelePrEP, human immunodeficiency
  virus (HIV) 110
telerehabilitation
  overview 90–94
  rehabilitation engineering 429
telomeres
  cloning 269
  Human Genome Project 384
therapeutic cloning, described 269
3-D microdevice, new cancer
  technologies 343
3D near-infrared imaging,
  image-guided robotic
  interventions 390
thymine, genomics 239
tissue engineering, overview 403–409
TME *see* tumor microenvironment
TMS *see* transcranial magnetic
  stimulation

625

Health Technology Sourcebook, Third Edition

transcranial direct current stimulation (tDCS), rehabilitative and assistive technology (AT) 473

transcranial magnetic stimulation (TMS)
  neurotechnology 273
  rehabilitative technologies 473

transfer learning, medical images 520

traumatic brain injury (TBI), assistive devices 475

treatment strategies
  cloning 268
  gene therapy 367

tremor-reducing instrument, future technologies 536

tumor
  chemotherapy 363
  genomics 214
  image-guided robotic interventions 390
  nanotechnology for cancer 351
  neurotechnology 274
  oncology 524
  patient-derived xenografts (PDXs) 343
  precision medicine 377
  radiofrequency thermal ablation (RFA) 417
  smart operating rooms of the future 535

tumor microenvironment (TME), nanotechnology for cancer 354

tumor mutational burden, biomarker testing 374

21st Century Cures Act, health information technology legislation and regulations 543

Tylenol, blood glucose monitoring devices 199

type 2 diabetes
  blood glucose monitoring devices 204

chronic health conditions 95

pancreas 335

U

ulcerative colitis, virtual colonoscopy 294

ultrasound
  biopsy guidance 534
  image-guided robotic interventions 390
  maternal telehealth 117
  medical technology 5
  nanotechnology for cancer 355
  radiofrequency thermal ablation (RFA) 418

ultrasound elastography, image testing 298

uric acid, blood glucose monitoring devices 199

U.S. Agency for International Development (USAID)
  publication
    artificial intelligence in global health 24n

U.S. Congressional Budget Office (CBO), contact information 593

U.S. Consumer Product Safety Commission (CPSC)
  publication
    wearable technology 176n

U.S. Department of Energy (DOE)
  contact information 593
  publication
    medical imaging, diagnostics, and treatment 5n

U.S. Department of Health and Human Services (HHS)
  contact information 593
  publications
    blockchain for healthcare 503n

626

Index

U.S. Department of Health and Human Services (HHS) publications, *continued*
  electronic medical records in healthcare 153n
  health equity in telehealth 60n
  physical therapy and remote patient monitoring 75n
  school-based telehealth 122n
  telehealth 45n, 81n, 125n
  telehealth and cancer care 87n
  telehealth and COVID-19 102n
  telehealth and remote patient monitoring 75n
  telehealth for chronic conditions 94n
  telehealth for families of children with special health care needs 118n
  telehealth for HIV care 106n
  telehealth for maternal health services 111n
  telehealth privacy for patients 553n
  virtual visit 67n
  wearable device security 176n
U.S. Department of Homeland Security (DHS) publications
  consumer mobile healthcare devices 557n
  wireless patient monitoring 206n
U.S. Department of Labor (DOL), contact information 593
U.S. Department of Veterans Affairs (VA) publication
  telecritical care 537n

U.S. Food and Drug Administration (FDA)
  contact information 593
  publications
    artificial intelligence and colon cancer 231n
    artificial intelligence and machine learning 13n
    artificial intelligence for detecting wrist fractures 233n
    artificial pancreas device system 335n
    blood glucose monitoring devices 198n
    cochlear implant 449n
    computer-assisted surgical systems 392n
    COVID-19 vaccine 258n
    digital health 7n
    hearing aids 482n
    mobile medical applications 186n
    precision medicine 377n
    wireless medical devices 180n
U.S. Government Accountability Office (GAO)
  publications
    artificial intelligence in health care 13n, 319n
    machine learning in drug development 19n
    Internet of Things (IOT) 499n
U.S. Library of Congress (LOC)
  contact information 594
  publication
    GPS and wayfinding apps 489n
U.S. National Library of Medicine (NLM)
  contact information 594
  publication
    health technology assessment 35n

V

vaccination
detection program 229
follow-up care 129
health equity 71
health records 158
routes of delivery 528
vaccine
COVID-19 103
current medical practice 528
data privacy 218
immunotherapy 365
infertility in women 262
technology assessment 35
vacuum suspension system, injury
prevention research 461
Verigene®, detection and
diagnosis 356
virtual colonoscopy,
overview 293–297
virtual exercises, life for
individuals 429
virtual reality
life for individuals 429
rehabilitative
technologies 473
virtual rehabilitation, life for
individuals 429
visual disorders, blindness
rehabilitation 436
visual impairment
blindness rehabilitation 435
mobile apps 489
visual prostheses, blindness
rehabilitation 442
voice recognition
artificial intelligence (AI)
innovation 17
assistive devices 472
rehabilitation engineering 428
VR *see* virtual reality

W

wearable devices
mobile medical apps 7
overview 176–180
telehealth 7, 15
wheelchairs
brain-controlled assistive
devices 274
described 484
Internet of Things (IoT) 501
mobility aids 472
rehabilitation methods 428
surgical appliances 5
tongue drive system
(TDS) 430
white canes, mobile apps for visual
impairment 489
whole-exome sequencing, biomarker
tests 374
whole-genome sequencing (WGS)
biomarker tests 374
defined 227
Wilson disease, genetic
variants 241
Wireless Medical Telemetry
Service (WMTS), radio
frequency 180
wireless patient monitoring,
emergency medical services
(EMS) 206
wireless technology
emergency medical services
(EMS) 207
medical devices 180

X

X chromosome, cloned animals 267
x-ray
brain disorders 413
computed tomography (CT) 581

Index

x-ray, *continued*
    computer-aided detection 233
    ionizing radiation 585
    medical technology 5
    radiation therapy 366
    telehealth 45, 101
    virtual colonoscopy 293

Z

Zika
    artificial intelligence (AI) predictive
      analytics 27
    influenza-like illnesses 219
zinc deficiency, fetal growth
    retardation 173